THIRD EDITION

FOUNDATIONS OF EMS SYSTEMS

BRUCE J. WALZ, PHD

JASON J. ZIGMONT, PHD, CHSE-A

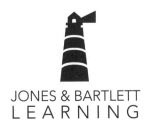

JONES & BARTLETT
LEARNING

World Headquarters
Jones & Bartlett Learning
5 Wall Street
Burlington, MA 01803
978-443-5000
info@jblearning.com
www.jblearning.com

Jones & Bartlett Learning books and products are available through most bookstores and online booksellers. To contact Jones & Bartlett Learning directly, call 800-832-0034, fax 978-443-8000, or visit our website, www.jblearning.com.

Production Credits

General Manager, Safety and Trades: Doug Kaplan
General Manager and Executive Publisher: Kimberly Brophy
VP, Product Development and Executive Editor: Christine Emerton
Director, PSG Editorial Development: Carol B. Guerrero
Senior Development Editor: Janet Morris
VP, Sales, Public Safety Group: Matthew Maniscalco
Director of Sales, Public Safety Group: Patricia Einstein
Vendor Manager: Nora Menzi
Director of Ecommerce and Digital Marketing: Eric Steeves

Director of Marketing Operations: Brian Rooney
VP, Manufacturing and Inventory Control: Therese Connell
Composition and Project Management: Integra Software Services Pvt. Ltd.
Cover Design: Kristin E. Parker
Rights & Media Specialist: Robert Boder
Media Development Editor: Shannon Sheehan
Cover Image: © Annette Shaff/Shutterstock.
Printing and Binding: Edwards Brothers Malloy
Cover Printing: Edwards Brothers Malloy

Library of Congress Cataloging-in-Publication Data
Names: Walz, Bruce J., author. | Zigmont, Jason J., author.
 Title: Foundations of EMS systems / Bruce J. Walz, Jason J. Zigmont.
 Other titles: Foundations of emergency medical services systems
 Description: Third edition. | Burlington, Massachusetts : Jones & Bartlett
 Learning, [2017] | Includes index.
 Identifiers: LCCN 2016034000 | ISBN 9781284041781
 Subjects: | MESH: Emergency Medical Services | Emergency Treatment--methods |
 Emergency Responders
 Classification: LCC RA645.5 | NLM WX 215 | DDC 362.18--dc23 LC record available at https://lccn.loc.gov/2016034000

6048

Printed in the United States of America
20 19 18 17 16   10 9 8 7 6 5 4 3 2 1

In memory of my father.
—Bruce J. Walz

To my loving wife whose support and encouragement drives me to always help others.
—Jason J. Zigmont

Contents

Foreword

Following is the foreword from the first edition of this book. The foreword was written by Daniel L. Storer, MD, who at the time was adjunct professor with the Department of Emergency Medicine at the University of Cincinnati College of Medicine. Dr. Storer passed away on September 21, 2004. His service and many contributions to EMS education, air medical services, and EMS in general are greatly missed. It was a privilege to have known Dr. Storer. May his life and dedication be an inspiration to all who seek a future role in EMS.

Bruce J. Walz, PhD

It is an honor and a pleasure to contribute to this textbook. This book is an excellent example of a growing testimony that EMS providers are professionals and not just technicians. The intended use for this text is as an introductory textbook for use in a survey course on EMS systems at the college level. However, this text can serve as an excellent introduction for anyone interested in a better understanding of EMS systems. This text will be useful to EMS administrators, EMS medical directors, EMS educators, and anyone searching for a reference to explain EMS and how its systems are structured. The text is clearly stated and organized in an easy-to-use manner. Currently there are no other texts written specifically for this purpose. In addition to being unique in its intended use, the text's content follows the vision and recommendations of the EMS Agenda for the Future, which is a consensus document published in 1996 to reflect the current vision for the future of EMS in this country. The Agenda addresses 14 attributes of EMS, including EMS education. The author, Bruce J. Walz, PhD, NREMT-P, is a professor and chair of the Department of Emergency Health Services at the University of Maryland, Baltimore County (UMBC). Dr. Walz has long been a recognized EMS education leader, dedicated to excellence in education and the promotion of EMS providers as professionals. He is a charter member of the National Association of EMS Educators and served as the organization's president in 1998. During a visit to UMBC, I observed a class of Emergency Health Services students learning how to evaluate articles from the medical literature for significance. Research is emphasized both in Dr. Walz's EMS educational program and his textbook. Research is important to every academic program. This textbook and the achievements of the author are examples of how EMS education is being elevated to new educational and professional heights. I recommend this textbook to anyone searching for a better understanding of EMS and its systems, whether they are new to EMS or seasoned EMS administrators, educators, and providers.

Daniel L. Storer, MD
Adjunct Professor, Department of Emergency Medicine
University of Cincinnati College of Medicine

Preface

Welcome to *Foundations of EMS Systems*. This book is the third edition of *Introduction to EMS Systems*, which was published in 2002 as an overview text for students, administrators, government officials, and others who needed to know about the emergency medical services (EMS) system. This new edition continues to serve those same users as well as being an introductory text in the Fire and Emergency Services Higher Education (FESHE) EMS series.

Historically, the focus of EMS has been the delivery of prehospital clinical care. And although this should remain the focus, recent trends have placed a greater emphasis on operational and economic aspects of EMS delivery. The Affordable Care Act is driving change in how EMS will be funded as well as fostering the development of innovative approaches to healthcare delivery, such as the community paramedic concept. This changing environment makes it even more important for students and practitioners of EMS to have a broad understanding of the foundations and basic concepts of a modern EMS system.

Development of this Book

As an EMS educator for over 30 years, I have taught all aspects of EMS including clinical as well as management and operational courses. In the 1990s, I was teaching an introductory EMS course in the Department of Emergency Health Services (EHS) at the University of Maryland, Baltimore County (UMBC). Semester after semester I struggled with trying to find an appropriate textbook for the course. Many books were clinically focused, and no one book covered all the management topics. Books written for medical directors came close but were either too expensive or written to a higher level. So it seemed like the only alternative was to write my own book. The approach used in the first edition, *Introduction to EMS Systems*, was to use the 14 attributes of an EMS system as presented in the EMS Agenda for the Future: A Systems Approach as the basis for each chapter. Chapters began with a case study and whenever possible presented the topic in a historical perspective. This approach was similar to the way I was presenting my lectures in my introductory EMS course.

Over time, I made changes to my course and began combining chapters and attributes. For instance, the chapters on information systems, research, and evaluation are best taught together as a unit. The same is true for public access and communications. I also ended up handing the course off to a new faculty member who arranged the course material differently.

I am a member of the advisory committee on the National EMS Management Curriculum at the National Fire Academy (NFA) that developed the FESHE EMS curriculum. As part of my work on the FESHE introductory course, Foundations of EMS Systems, the committee identified specific topic areas in the course. Again, these topic areas were a consolidation of the 14 attributes.

As I began to plan for revising the first edition, it became apparent that writing 14 separate chapters correlated to the attributes was not the best way to go. The revision was also to serve as the first in a series of FESHE EMS texts. Drawing on my experience teaching from the text, as well as the deliberations of the FESHE curriculum committee, is what led to the current arrangement of topics into chapters in the second edition text.

Given the breadth and depth of EMS and the many changes that have taken place in the field since I wrote the first edition, I concluded that in addition to changes in the text, a broader perspective was needed to give proper coverage to the text material. This led to my decision to invite two colleagues to be coauthors. Kurt Krumperman brings a private EMS service perspective as well as experience with federal EMS legislation and agencies and expertise in disaster response. Jason Zigmont is an EMS educator and writer for EMS trade publications and has a doctorate in adult learning. Their contributions have strengthened many of the topics and chapters covered in the second edition.

This current edition retains the format of the previous edition; however, all chapters have been reviewed and updated to reflect current practices and trends at the time of publication. Because this edition is more of a revision than a rewrite, the main coauthors, Walz and Zigmont, completed this edition of the text.

Organization of this Book

As stated earlier, the text is designed to follow the FESHE Foundations of EMS course. It also integrates my many years of teaching an introductory course as well as the input and guidance of the coauthors. Each chapter is focused on offering guidance to EMS managers on topics essential to the delivery of quality EMS care.

- **In the Beginning**: The text begins with an introductory chapter that is essentially a large case study designed to not only introduce, in chapter 1, the 14 attributes of an EMS system but also to show how these are integrated to provide an effective and efficient EMS response. Chapter 2 presents the history of EMS from the beginning of recorded history to present day. The reader should keep in mind that covering the entire history of EMS is beyond the scope of this introductory text.

- **Human Resources**: The next two chapters (3 and 4) deal with the human resources that make up the heart of EMS. The various providers and personnel who are the human face of EMS are presented and discussed. Because training is required for all levels of EMS provider as well as personnel who support the system, chapter 4 discusses the education and training requirements of EMS personnel.

- **Transportation**: When one thinks of EMS, the vision of an ambulance running along with lights and siren comes to mind. Chapter 5 is dedicated to the most common aspect of EMS, transportation of the patient to a receiving facility. The chapter also provides an overview of the various approaches used to deliver EMS services.

- **Practicing Medicine in the Field**: Because EMS involves the practice of medicine, chapters 6 and 8 address the medical aspects of EMS as well as the all-important role of the physician in EMS. Medical oversight by a physician is necessary not only as a means for providers to practice medicine in the field but also to provide overall quality assurance to all aspects of EMS.

- **EMS Role in the Community**: A community could have the best EMS system in the world, but if local residents do not know how to contact it for service or understand its organization and capabilities, the system is essentially worthless. Chapters 7 and 11 address attributes of an EMS system that work together to connect the system with the public it is designed to serve. Chapter 11 introduces the concept of prevention and the role of EMS as an entity well suited to assist in improving community public health.

- **Legal and Financial Considerations**: Chapter 10 provides background on the legislative and legal foundation of EMS and the role played by federal, state, and local entities in the support and development of EMS services. The delivery of high-quality EMS is not without cost. How these costs are covered is the focus of chapter 9, which addresses system finance.

- **Disaster Response**: One needs to only recall the tragic events of September 11, 2001, to appreciate the importance of EMS as a critical part of disaster response. The basic concepts of disaster mitigation as well as the role of EMS in a disaster situation are covered in chapter 12.

- **Research and Evaluation**: As EMS systems evolve and become more complex, it is important to ask if such evolution is achieving the basic goal of EMS, which is to transport the right patient, to the right resources, under the care of the right provider, while providing the right treatment efficiently and economically. To answer this question, it is necessary for EMS systems and others to engage in system evaluation and research, which, however, cannot be carried out if the necessary data and information are not available. Chapters 13 and 14 address information systems, evaluation, and research.

Features of this Book

Because this book is written to provide an introduction to EMS, the text is presented in such a manner to allow either the casual reader or the student enrolled in a course to better understand the material.

- **FESHE Correlation**: The content in this book meets the criteria described in the FESHE course for Foundations of EMS Systems. For this reason, a correlation to the FESHE course is included in this book to illustrate how this content meets national guidelines for EMS education.

- **National EMS Educational Standards**: Information on the latest practices in the field is based on the National EMS Educational Standards, which explain the educational requirements and corresponding provider levels that are the standards set forth for the EMS community.

- **14 Attributes of an EMS System**: Built on the premise of the 14 attributes of the EMS system that was presented in the EMS Agenda for the Future, this book offers students a national and modern perspective on the EMS field.

- **EMS as an Evolving Field**: The book presents a historical review of the development of EMS, explains the current state of the field, and looks to the future to help students fully understand the EMS profession.

- **Current photos, graphics, and tables**: New and updated photos, graphics, and tables are included in this edition to illustrate key points and help students remain current with the latest information from the field.

New to this Edition

Because EMS is both an evolving system and a technical field, change is constantly occurring both in the clinical aspects of patient care and in the delivery of EMS services. This change has been especially evident in EMS over the past few years due to the significant changes in the scope of practice and education of EMS providers. Even the titles of prehospital providers have changed to better reflect their role and function in EMS. To address these changes, this text has been updated from the original *Introduction to EMS Systems* written in 2002. Material and approaches new to this edition include:

- An updated *History of EMS* chapter to cover events and significant developments in EMS of the last decade.

- Current information in the *System Finances* chapter on reimbursement for EMS services as the result of the Affordable Care Act.

- Updated federal legislation and federal agency activity related to EMS.

- An updated *EMS and Disaster Response* chapter reflecting changes in disaster response and mitigation as the result of recent natural and terrorist events, with a special emphasis on NIMS integration.

- Information on the expanding role of prehospital providers as an integrated part of the health care system including the role of the community paramedic.

About the Authors

Bruce J. Walz, PhD, is a professor in the Department of Emergency Health Services and Special Assistant to the Provost for Strategic Initiatives, at the University of Maryland, Baltimore County (UMBC). As a professor, he teaches management and clinical courses as well as serving on graduate thesis committees. He has been in the University System of Maryland since 1979, having served with the Maryland Fire and Rescue Institute until 1987 when he joined the faculty of UMBC. He served as department chair from 1994 to 2016.

Bruce Walz has been involved in many aspects of EMS education and development. Most notably, he served as a group leader for the development of the 1998 National Standard Paramedic Curriculum and the 1999 National Standard Intermediate Curriculum. He headed the educational infrastructure workgroup for the development of the National EMS Education Standards. He is a charter member of the National Association of EMS Educators and served as president in 1998. He is a past president of Advocates for EMS. Additionally, he served as a site visitor for the Committee on Accreditation of Educational Programs for the EMS Professions (CoAEMSP) and is on the editorial board of Prehospital Emergency Care. He wrote the chapter on education in the National Association of EMS Physician's medical director's handbook, *Prehospital Systems and Medical Oversight*. He has presented at numerous international, national, and regional EMS conferences.

In addition to his professional experience, Bruce Walz has been active in the volunteer fire service since 1970. He has served in many administrative and line positions, including president and chief officer. In 1975, he was certified as one of the first 50 Cardiac Rescue Technicians in the state of Maryland. In 1990, he became a nationally registered paramedic. He is an approved Maryland paramedic instructor. He is a nationally certified Fire Officer IV and Fire Instructor IV.

Jason J. Zigmont, PhD, Paramedic, is a learning innovator and founder of Learning in Healthcare. He has previously worked as the System Director of Learning Innovation for OhioHealth. In this role he provides leadership for an integrated clinical learning infrastructure that includes Simulation, Learning Consulting, Learning Management System, and Continuing Medical Education (CME) and Nursing Continuing Education (CE). Jason served on the Society for Simulation in Healthcare's education committee and headed the subcommittee on preparation for the Certified Healthcare Simulation Educator.

He holds a PhD in Adult Learning specifically focused on Experiential Learning. He is a paramedic and EMS instructor who has served in both paid and volunteer EMS and fire departments for over 15 years. He founded VolunteerFD.org and was a regular columnist for JEMS. Jason's mission in life is to improve health care through learning. His research focuses on creating learning initiatives that have demonstrated outcomes in clinical quality, customer service, work life, and finance.

Acknowledgments

The publisher and authors would like to thank the following individuals who participated in the development of this book.

We gratefully acknowledge the contributors of the first edition who provided the solid foundation upon which to build this new edition:

- William Hathaway, MS
- Brian Maguire, DrPH
- Jeffrey Mitchell, PhD
- Roger Stone, MD
- Kevin Seaman, MD
- Mathew J. Levy, DO
- Jennifer Lee Jenkins, MD
- Mic Gunderson

For the support of faculty, staff, and students of the Department of Emergency Health Services, UMBC, we offer our appreciation.

Kurt Krumperman, Ph.D., for his assistance in revising the first edition and serving as a co-author of Foundations of EMS Systems.

Diane Flint, MS, NRP, clinical assistant professor in the Department of Emergency Health Services, UMBC, for her great assistance in reviewing and revising the chapters on system finance and human resources to reflect current trends in the industry and profession.

To those who reviewed previous versions of this manuscript, our sincere thanks.

From the Authors

Bruce J. Walz, PhD
Professor, Department of Emergency Health Services
Special Assistant to the Provost for Strategic Initiatives
University of Maryland, Baltimore County
Baltimore, Maryland

Jason J. Zigmont, PhD, Paramedic
Learning Innovator and Founder
Learning in Healthcare
West Haven, CT

Introduction

A mother takes her five-year-old daughter outside to play on the family swing set. The little girl is the youngest of four children, and the swing has been in the backyard for some time. The mother absent-mindedly pushes the little girl, who keeps asking to "go higher, go higher." Suddenly, a rope breaks, stressed by many years of use and exposure to the weather. The little girl is propelled forward and flies through the air. She lands in a tumble on the hard ground and remains motionless. The panic-stricken mother cries out, "My baby, my baby!" The next-door neighbor, who is working in his garden, looks up and sees the crumpled little girl lying on the lawn. He immediately runs over to help. The sobbing mother kneels by her daughter and turns her onto her back. The little girl has abrasions on her face and arms, her right leg is angulated outward, and she is listless. The neighbor arrives and remarks that she seems to be breathing. He takes out his cellular phone and calls 9-1-1.

At the local fire station, approximately one mile from the accident location, the crew is finishing their morning checkouts. Three miles away at the intersection of two major cross streets, a paramedic unit of the local ambulance company is staged according to a systems status management plan.

The local 9-1-1 center receives the neighbor's call for help. The center has an enhanced wireless 9-1-1 computer system that displays the caller's location via GPS input from the cellular phone. The call taker confirms the incident location, asks the neighbor to remain on the line, and transfers the call to the ambulance company dispatcher and the fire board. Simultaneously, the local engine company and the staged ambulance begin their response to the little girl's home. The 9-1-1 dispatcher begins to interrogate the neighbor to determine the child's condition. After accomplishing this, she gives him prearrival first aid instructions, which the neighbor relays to the frantic mother.

The engine crew, consisting of four personnel, two of whom are trained as emergency medical technicians (EMTs) and the other two as emergency medical responders (EMRs), arrive on the scene. The EMTs stabilize the little girl's head and neck, check for an open airway, and assess her pulse. Oxygen is applied and the child's right leg is stabilized. One of the firefighters comforts the mother and obtains information about the incident and the little girl.

The ambulance arrives, and the paramedic assesses the child. She determines that the girl has a closed head injury as well as a fractured right femur. She contacts her dispatch center and requests a helicopter for evacuation to a pediatric trauma center located 57 miles away. While waiting for the helicopter, the paramedic intubates the child and establishes an intraosseous infusion in the uninjured leg. The child is fully immobilized on a pediatric spine board and loaded into the ambulance. The engine company responds to the local high school athletic field to establish a landing zone for the helicopter. The ambulance arrives and awaits the approaching helicopter. The paramedic is patched through by radio to the pediatric trauma center and updates the attending physician on the child's status; she remains stable.

The helicopter, staffed by a critical care flight nurse and a critical care flight paramedic, arrives, and the little girl and her mother are placed on board. The ambulance paramedic transfers her findings to the flight crew. The helicopter lifts off and is on its way to the trauma center. The flight paramedic relays information to the medical staff via medical communications radio. Upon landing, a pediatric traumatologist resident and a nurse anesthetist meet the helicopter on the landing pad. The team rapidly moves the patient to the resuscitation area. A social worker greets the overwhelmed mother and escorts her to a quiet area.

The little girl is quickly surrounded by a team of healthcare providers, all working in controlled chaos under the direction of a pediatric traumatologist. The child is assessed, blood is drawn for analysis, and the little patient is sent for a CAT scan. The traumatologist receives the lab results, CAT scan report, and x-rays. He determines that the child has a small epidural hematoma, a transverse fracture of the right femur, and two fractured right ribs. The senior resident advises that the little girl is starting to come around and resist the endotracheal tube. The attending physician advises the resident to sedate her so as not to increase intracranial pressure. She is moved to the ICU, and an orthopedic specialist is called to manage her fractured femur. The traumatologist visits with the mother and father, who has recently arrived, and informs them that their daughter should be all right. She will be kept sedated for a few days. The bleeding in her head has stopped and surgery is not indicated. The leg will be cast and the ribs will not need any special treatment. After visiting with the parents, the traumatologist returns to his office and dictates a report of the incident, which will be reviewed by the hospital quality management team with a copy forwarded to the staff epidemiologist. The first-year resident writes up the case for presentation at resident rounds the following week.

After transferring the little girl to the helicopter, the ambulance returns to service. The paramedic completes her report and makes a note that this would be a good case to present during bimonthly case reviews. She also makes a mental note to call the pediatric trauma center to find out how the girl is doing.

Two days after the incident, a graduate student from a nearby university interviews the child's parents. The student informs the parents that he is doing research on pediatric trauma and asks if they would mind answering a few questions. The parents agree, and the student adds another case to his research database.

The little girl progresses well and is taken off sedation three days postincident. Her mental functions are good and there is no indication of permanent damage. A social worker continues to assist and support the family. She arranges for the parents to receive instruction on how to manage their daughter's recovery and interaction with her siblings.

One week postincident, the child returns home with her leg cast. She is surrounded by her siblings and relatives. Life in the family returns to near normal. The mother returns with the little girl to the trauma center on a regular basis for follow-up care and evaluation. The cast is eventually removed, and the little girl is sent for physical therapy. Six months later, the social worker contacts the parents for a follow-up evaluation. The case of the little girl is finally closed, and she again leads a normal life.

1

Introduction to Emergency Medical Systems

Objectives

Upon completion of this chapter, the reader should be able to:

- State the three main parts of a system.

- List the 15 components of an EMS system as defined by the EMSS Act of 1973.

- List the additional components necessary for a well-functioning EMS system.

- List the 14 attributes of an EMS system as presented in the *EMS Agenda for the Future*.

- List the seven critical patient groups.

- State the impact on EMS of passage of the Patient Protection and Affordable Care Act.

The Emergency Medical Services System

The scenario in the *Introduction* describes a typical incident handled by a well-coordinated emergency medical services (EMS) system (**Figure 1-1**). The little girl was able to return to normal life because a diverse group of components came together in an orderly fashion to assist her. This coordinated effort is known as an EMS system.

In order to understand an EMS system, you must first understand what makes up the system. As shown in **Figure 1-2**, a system has three major components—input, process, and output. Input is what enters the system. The input is processed or changed in some way by the system or is affected by it with the resulting product being the output. The transformation process is sometimes referred to as a "black box," a term derived from the many complicated electronic components of early missile systems. Field soldiers may not have understood what each component of a weapons system did within the box—just that it worked in some particular way to produce a particular outcome.

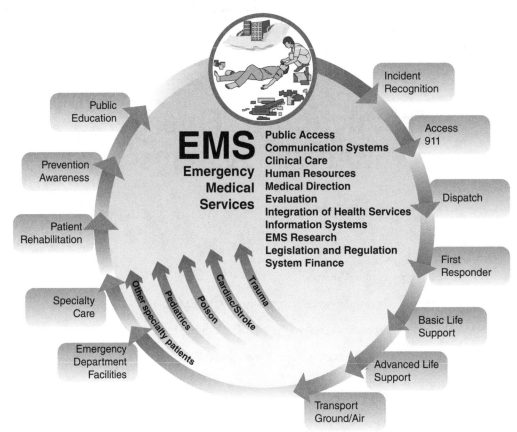

Reproduced from National Highway Traffic Safety Administration. www.ems.gov

FIGURE 1-1 The EMS system.

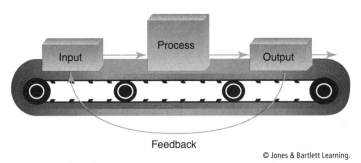

© Jones & Bartlett Learning.

FIGURE 1-2 All systems have three basic components.

There are many different types of systems. Some are open, meaning that they interact with the environment, while others are closed. Systems can also be described as manmade or natural; concrete, such as the circulatory system; or abstract, such as the social system. Systems can also be simple or complex. Complex systems are made up of a series of subsystems.

The first case study illustrates the concept of a system. The input was the injured child. The process was the response, her treatment, and rehabilitation. The output was a healthy child able to live a normal and productive life. This system, known as an EMS system, is not a simple one; it is very complex and consists of a number of components and subsystems.

Components of an EMS System

The components of an EMS system were originally specified in the **Emergency Medical Services Systems (EMSS) Act of 1973**, which was passed as Public Law No. 93-154 by the U.S. Congress. This law defined an EMS system and provided funding for systems that met these requirements. The components, as specified in this legislation, are outlined in **Figure 1-3**.

The law defined an EMS system as follows:

The term "emergency medical services system," which provides for the arrangement of personnel, facilities, and equipment for the effective and coordinated delivery in an appropriate geographical area of health care services under emergency conditions (occurring either as the result of the patient's condition or of a natural disaster or similar situations) and which is administered by a public or nonprofit private entity that has the authority and the resources to provide effective administration of the system.

The 15 components were delineated as a means to assist local planners and administrators in establishing EMS systems and as benchmarks for evaluating existing programs.

Communications
Manpower
Training of Personnel
Use of Public Safety Agencies
Transportation
Mutual Aid Agreements
Facilities
Accessibility of Care
Critical Care Units
Transfer of Patients
Standard Medical Record Keeping
Independent Review and Evaluation
Consumer Information and Education
Consumer Participation
Disaster Linkage

FIGURE 1-3 15 Components of an EMS system.

Revision of the 15 Components

Since 1973, the 15 components have remained a vital part of any EMS system. However, other necessary components have been identified that must be considered in the functioning of contemporary EMS systems. These components include medical direction, system financing, regulation and policy, and trauma systems.

Medical Direction

EMS involves the practice of medicine, but there is no mention of physician involvement in the 15 components of the development or delivery of EMS. Thus, many EMS systems were developed without direct physician involvement or oversight. As EMS matured, the need for direct physician involvement and oversight became apparent, leading to the recognition and establishment of medical direction as an integral part of EMS. Most states now require medical direction as a requirement for licensure both of the system and of individual EMS providers.

System Finance

Federal funds were available for the initial development of EMS systems. However, the need to plan for and integrate long-term funding resources for EMS systems was not delineated. Consequently, as federal funds for EMS dried up, many systems were left without a dedicated means of support. Likewise, changes to insurance and Medicare reimbursement schedules have strained the ability of systems to properly finance EMS operations.

Regulation and Policy

The EMSS Act of 1973 contained specific requirements for the development of an EMS system using federal funds. The act encouraged the development of an EMS lead agency and the necessary authority for the EMS system to function. However, with the demise of federal funding, many states did not have regulations or legislation in place to effectively administer an EMS system. As EMS systems developed and became more complex, laws and regulations to control and regulate the systems became more of a necessity. This was especially true as new players, such as commercial providers and public trusts, entered the field of EMS.

Trauma Systems

Although trauma resulting from auto crashes was one of the major forces behind the development of EMS, the initial 15 components did not specifically address the concept of a regional or statewide trauma care system. Facilities and critical-care units addressed part of the trauma system, but there was no total, coordinated approach. Problems in trauma care came to the forefront with the passage of the Trauma Care Systems Planning and Development Act of 1990. An example of a trauma center is shown in **Figure 1-4**.

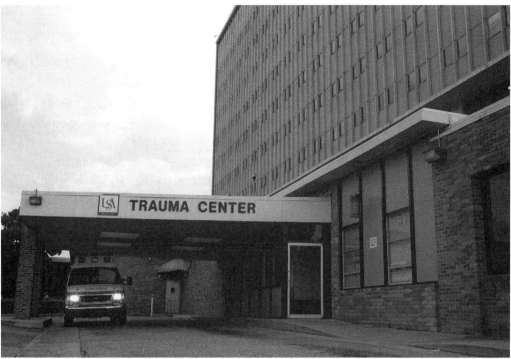

© Michelle Rolls-Thomas/AP Photo.

FIGURE 1-4 Trauma centers have become an integral part of the EMS system.

EMS Agenda for the Future

The traditional 15 components have served EMS well for 30 years. However, as the nature of healthcare delivery has changed, especially in areas related to technology and cost containment, the components of an EMS system need to be redefined. This redefinition is presented in the *EMS Agenda for the Future*, a consensus document that outlines a future approach for EMS. Supported by the National Highway Traffic Safety Administration and the Health Resources and Services Administration, Maternal and Child Health Bureau, the agenda puts forth a vision for out-of-facility EMS:

> *EMS of the future will be community-based health management that is fully integrated with the overall health care system. It will have the ability to identify and modify illness and injury risks, provide acute illness and injury care and follow-up, and contribute to treatment of chronic conditions and community health monitoring. EMS will be integrated with other health care providers and public health and public safety agencies. It will improve community health and result in more appropriate use of acute health care resources. EMS will remain the public's emergency medical safety net.*

The 14 Attributes of an EMS System

Similar to the 15 components, the **emergency medical services attributes** presented in the agenda define a modern EMS system. The 14 attributes are listed in **Figure 1-5**.

Integration of Health Services

Historically, EMS has been viewed as a public safety function. However, the focus of EMS has changed to that of a provider of emergency out-of-facility medical care. EMS is recognized as a legitimate component of the overall healthcare system and is integral to the **public health** of a community.

With passage of the Patient Protection and Affordable Care Act (ACA) in 2010, the role of EMS as a provider of patient care changed. Now EMS is seen as a provider of patient care services and not just as a means to transport patients to the hospital. Community paramedic programs provide preventive care to patients in an out-of-facility environment. Advanced practice paramedics, functioning as part of an integrated healthcare system and utilizing telemedicine, provide diagnostic and treatment services directly to patients in a variety of home and healthcare settings. Such programs help to reduce cost and improve health system efficiency by reducing unnecessary and costly transport to an emergency department.

EMS Research

Early EMS practice was based on conjecture and "best guesses." The goal of research in EMS is to provide a scientific basis for how EMS is delivered and practiced. Like all of medicine, EMS is striving to establish **evidence-based best practices**. Research also provides a basis for continued improvement of the system.

Integration of Health Services
EMS Research
Legislation and Regulation
System Finance
Human Resources
Medical Direction
Education Systems
Public Education
Prevention
Public Access
Communication Systems
Clinical Care
Information Systems
Evaluation

FIGURE 1-5 14 Attributes of an EMS system.

Legislation and Regulation

To be effective and receive the necessary resources to function, 9-1-1 transport EMS must be recognized as an official and regulated activity of government. Although overlooked in the 15 components, legislation and regulation continue to provide the legal basis for patient care and EMS system operation.

System Finance

Many EMS systems were established through the EMSS Act of 1973 and supported by federal funding. When federal funding was phased out, systems had to rely on other funding sources to survive. Insurance and Medicare funding continue to struggle to meet the needs of EMS systems. New funding models bought about by the ACA are not only changing the funding of EMS but also influencing the role of EMS as an integral part of the healthcare system. However, regardless of the sources, secure funding is necessary for the continued development of EMS systems.

Human Resources

This attribute is a modernization of the original components of manpower, training, and public safety involvement (**Figure 1-6**). Passage of the ACA provides the potential for greatly expanding the role of EMS providers in the healthcare system.

Medical Direction

EMS involves the practice of medicine, but early EMS systems were developed without a requirement for physician input or oversight. The addition of this attribute recognizes the role of the physician in patient care and in the medical oversight of EMS operations.

With the introduction of specialized advanced practice EMS providers using telemedicine, the role of medical direction in a modern EMS system is even more important.

Education Systems

This attribute expands on the original training component. Education is recognized as an ongoing need of EMS providers as well as a necessity for the professional growth of EMS providers.

Public Education

The original components of consumer information and education addressed the need to not only make the public aware of EMS, but also to have input from citizens regarding system development and operation. This attribute focuses on the need to educate the public about health concerns and the operation and value of EMS systems.

Prevention

The original concept of EMS was as a reactive service to support injured and sick people. Now, the trend is changing to become proactive and to provide opportunities to reduce injury, illness, and death through prevention. This role of EMS has been greatly expanded through passage of the ACA.

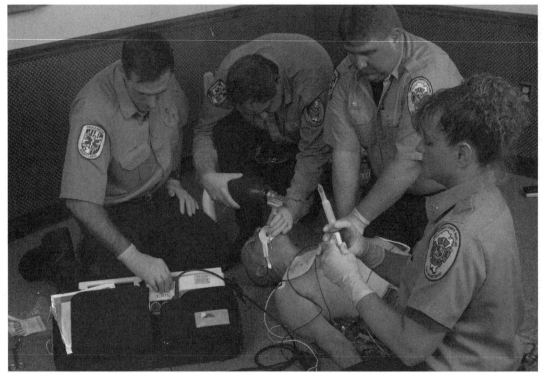

© Jones & Bartlett Learning.

FIGURE 1-6 EMS responders on scene.

Public Access

The idea of universal access to all people who need EMS has been a foundation of EMS system development. This attribute is a carryover of the original component specified in 1973 of public access.

Communication Systems

Communication remains the foundation of all EMS systems. With new technology, communication has the potential to play an even bigger part in access to and delivery and coordination of EMS.

Clinical Care

This attribute recognizes the need for effective, efficient, and efficacious care by trained professionals during all aspects of patient care, both on scene and at the appropriate medical facility. This attribute differs from the components of facilities and critical care units that focus only on hospital-based care. Development of advanced practice paramedics is one example of a contemporary change in clinical care.

Information Systems

In 1973, when the first EMS systems were being formed, the importance and necessity of information and its management could not have been foreseen. Now, all aspects of life are intimately connected with data and information management. This attribute addresses the importance of data collection, management, and analysis in EMS.

Evaluation

No system or service can continue to function without some means of measuring its effectiveness. One of the original components of this attribute was review and evaluation. This component focuses on the overall evaluation of an EMS system. The evaluation attribute addresses not only system-outcome measures but all aspects of EMS system operation, both structural and clinical. This component will become even more important as new reimbursement models for EMS based on system efficiency replace traditional transport-based schemes.

Comparison of Components and Attributes

It should be noted that although these attributes define a modern EMS system, many of the attributes are similar to the original 15 components. This is because an EMS system needs certain basic components to function as a system. Two examples of these components are human resources, which replaces the manpower component; and communication systems, which provides a broader view of the basic role of communications.

The attributes also recognize the changes in healthcare management that have occurred over the past years. The first attribute, integration of health services, is designed to ensure that EMS is part of the total healthcare delivery system. It also acknowledges the linkages to other community health resources. The next section of this chapter addresses EMS subsystems. These are combined into the attribute of clinical care.

Critical Patient Areas

The EMSS Act not only outlined the 15 components of a comprehensive regional EMS system but also identified seven **critical patient areas**. Each of these special patient populations has specific needs or care that is best met through an established subsystem of the total community EMS system. One such resource is a burn unit. The seven critical patient groups are the following:

1. Major accidental trauma;
2. Burn injuries;
3. Spinal cord injuries;
4. Acute coronary care/heart attacks;
5. Poisonings;
6. High-risk infants and mothers; and
7. Behavioral and psychiatric emergencies.

These patient groups provide unique challenges for system planners and administrators. Each group has special needs and can be viewed as a separate system within the larger scheme of the local EMS system. For instance, much attention in EMS system development has been focused on the trauma patient. Central to the survival of a trauma victim is the need for rapid evacuation to a medical facility capable of providing intensive resuscitative and surgical care. To meet this need, many EMS systems have established specialized trauma centers and transport components as well as communication systems to ensure that the trauma victim receives the right care, at the right time, and in the right facility. However, such systems cannot be divorced from the total community EMS system. Just as a helicopter can be used to transport a trauma victim from the scene of an accident, it can also be used as part of a community-wide coronary care system to provide interfacility transport of cardiac patients to specialty centers. The hallmark of a well-coordinated EMS system is the total integration of all components as well as the flexibility to provide for the special needs of diverse patient populations.

WRAP UP

Summary

EMS systems are a complex assemblage of components designed to serve the needs of diverse patient populations. Input into the system in the form of patients in need of emergency or emergent care is processed through a coordinated response and treatment process and emerges as either treated and recovering patients or patients stabilized for transfer to other parts of the much larger health care system.

Regardless of the nature of the system, a system will not work if it lacks coordination, integration, support, and constant feedback and review. By developing an understanding of EMS systems, the student of EMS will be better prepared to function optimally as a viable component of an EMS system. It is important for the student of EMS to have a working knowledge of the components of a modern EMS system.

It is also important for the student to recognize that EMS, like all fields of medicine, is constantly evolving. As research, medicine, delivery systems, and social and political systems change, so too does EMS to meet the demand to provide the right treatment, for the right patient, at the right time, with the right outcome. One such example of the changing nature of EMS is the recognition in the ACA that EMS is not just a public safety service, but also an integral part of a community's public health.

Key Terms

black box

components processes

critical patient areas

emergency medical services (EMS) system

emergency medical services attributes

Emergency Medical Services Systems (EMSS) Act of 1973

EMS Agenda for the Future

evidence-based best practices

input

output

process

public health

public safety agencies

subsystems

system

trauma care system

Review Questions

1. Draw a diagram of a system and label the three main components.
2. List the 15 original components defined by the EMSS Act of 1973.
3. Compare the 15 components to the 14 attributes of an EMS system.
4. State the importance of the *EMS Agenda for the Future*.
5. List the seven patient groups that need special attention in an EMS system.

2

History of Emergency Medical Systems

Objectives

Upon completion of this chapter, the reader should be able to:

- Identify significant events and people that have shaped the development of EMS.

- Summarize the history of EMS in the United States.

History of Emergency Medical Systems

A student once commented that "the problem with history is there is so much of it." Volumes have been written concerning both our history and the history of health care in the United States, so writing a single chapter requires a good deal of condensing. This chapter attempts to put the development of emergency medical services (EMS) systems within the context of the United States' growth as a nation, noting the significant events and developments that have led to its current EMS system.

The basic tenet of EMS is that the patient will be treated by the right people, in the right place, at the right time. In order to accomplish this, three key elements must be in place. First, we must have personnel with the medical knowledge, technology, and facilities necessary to effectively intervene. Second, we must have the communications and transportation equipment and technology in place to ensure that the patient can be treated in a timely manner. Third, we need society's support—conceptually, politically, and financially—in order to mold the first two elements into a system.

Preindustrial Era (1600–1850)

The importance of this era to EMS development is almost negligible, but it is useful to consider, if only to see where we started and to realize how far we have come. During the first 250 years of its history, the United States evolved from a scattering of settlements in the "new world" to a nation poised to fight a bloody civil war. From a few early colonists huddled along the East Coast, the United States had grown to a country of more than 23 million people, with states and territories extending from the Atlantic to the Pacific. During the colonial period and the early years of the republic, 95% of the population was involved in agriculture, and except for the large plantations of the South, these farms were relatively small family endeavors in remote and isolated areas. Several cities developed during this time as mercantile centers engaged in trade with Europe. The Industrial Revolution that had swept through England during this era, however, was only beginning to reach the United States. Transportation and communication were constrained to travel by foot, horse, or watercraft until well into the 1800s. The first practical steam-powered locomotive was not developed until 1825, and Samuel Morse's telegraph was not patented until 1837 (Brunner, 1999).

Early death due to illness and injury was a common occurrence that affected virtually every family. The major cause of death by far was infectious diseases. Malaria and respiratory illnesses such as influenza, pneumonia, and tuberculosis routinely afflicted much of the population. With little understanding of public health, the developing towns and cities often lacked a pure water supply and proper sewage treatment, which led to dysentery, diarrhea, and typhoid. In addition to these endemic or community-based diseases, there were periodic epidemics such as yellow fever, smallpox, and cholera (Rothstein, 1987). Fatalities from the scourges of modern society—heart attack, cancer, and accidents—were minor by comparison.

For treatment and care, the individual primarily depended on family members and a wide range of home remedies. If outside assistance was desired and available it might include physicians, but it might also include Native American doctors, botanical healers, and nostrum dealers whose patent medicines promised to cure a wide range of illnesses.

In England, clear distinctions existed among physicians, surgeons, and pharmacists; in the colonies these distinctions were often blurred, depending on need and training. If a physician was treating an illness he would focus on the outward signs and prescribe interventions. For centuries these interventions were based on the "humoral theory," which explained illness in terms of imbalances in the four humors: blood, phlegm, black bile, and yellow bile. Complementary theories focused on the tone of the blood vessels and nerves as well as on the balance of acids and bases (King, 1997).

In order to adjust these tones and balances, two treatment therapies developed. The first, evacuation, sought to rid the body of fluids that disrupted balance and tone. This was accomplished by various methods: drugs to increase urination, sweating, vomiting, and bowel movements; plasters to create blisters; and bleeding blood vessels by cutting, cupping, or leeches. Drugs such as opium were used to calm hyperactivity, and an appropriate diet was prescribed. The adage "feed a cold and starve a fever" is clearly traceable to this therapy. There is strong evidence to suggest that George Washington's death was considerably hastened by an overzealous application of bleeding, which was then termed "heroic medicine" (Starr, 1982). If the patient survived the illness and treatment, the second therapy, restorative, was begun. This regimen consisted of an array of tonics, drugs, and food, as well as cold water and even electrical stimulation. All were applied with the intent of building up and further strengthening the body (King, 1997).

Surgical procedures were equally primitive. Armed with only a basic, and frequently incorrect, notion of how the human body functioned, surgeons had no effective means of controlling pain,

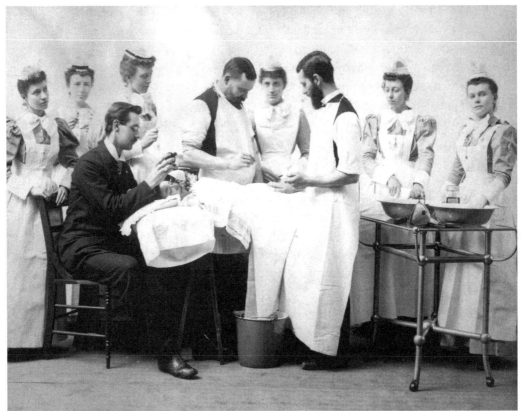

© Everett Historical/Shutterstock.

Figure 2-1 Early surgical procedure.

visualizing internal injuries, replenishing blood loss, or dealing with infections, which they neither understood nor had the medicines to effectively treat.

A well-trained surgeon would be called upon to lance boils, remove superficial tumors, externally manipulate intestines to reduce hernias, pull teeth, and treat burns. A surgeon could splint fractures and remove bullets, arrows, and splinters, although infection frequently followed. Severe injuries to the head and torso were virtually untreatable, although some surgeons would remove a portion of the skull in a process called **trepanning** to reduce pressure on the brain (Boyd, Edlich, & Micik, 1983).

Severe injuries to the extremities were usually addressed by amputations, which were gruesome, but often successful if the dressings were properly tended. With only opium or alcohol available as an anesthetic, the patient was held steady by strong assistants—speed was essential. A skilled surgeon could remove a leg in less than two minutes, but doing so was not without risk. A well-known British surgeon of the time, who prided himself on his speed, is reported to have amputated his patient's leg and his scrotum as well, inadvertently slashed his assistant, who subsequently died of infection, and caused the death by heart attack of an observer who thought he had also been slashed (Boyd et al., 1983).

Pharmacists fulfilled a major role in health care during this period, providing the drugs prescribed by physicians and surgeons as well as prescribing medicines of their own. By the 1800s, more than 200 remedies were a regular part of a pharmacist's inventory, providing the means to balance and strengthen the body's systems. Although most of the remedies were of marginal benefit, several are still in use or were found to contain effective ingredients. A favored drug, cinchona, or Peruvian bark, was prescribed as early as the 1600s as a cure for fevers, including malaria. In fact, the drug contained quinine, which is still used to treat malaria, although it would have been ineffective against other fevers. Ipecac, a drug that was used to induce vomiting and to remove "foul humors," is still used to remove poisons from the stomach. Opium was used in several forms and was effective as a sedative and antidiarrheal agent.

A seriously ill or injured patient during this time did not have a general hospital to go to for care. Most care was provided in the home with supportive care provided by family members. As towns and cities developed, however, there was a growing need for facilities to care for those who did not have families to rely on. These facilities, called **alms houses**, provided care to a broad class of the needy, including orphans and poor, mentally ill, or sick and injured people who did not have family support or could not afford to purchase care. As time went on, this diverse, needy population was segmented and sent to more specialized facilities. Many of these alms houses would later become **general hospitals**, as in Maryland where the Baltimore County Alms House became the Baltimore City Hospital (Starr, 1982). Another facility that developed during this time was the **city dispensary** (**Figure 2-2**). Several were

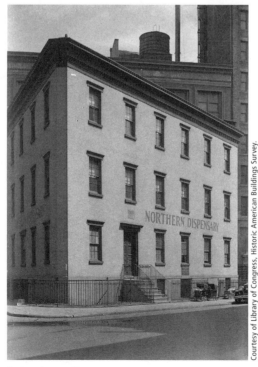

Courtesy of Library of Congress, Historic American Buildings Survey.

Figure 2-2 Dispensary or "alms house."

founded in the late 1700s in major commercial centers such as Philadelphia (1786), New York (1791), Boston (1796), and Baltimore (1800) (Stan, 1982).

Dispensaries were similar to alms houses in that they ministered to the poor, but unlike alms houses they focused on medical care. Because dispensaries brought together a large group of patients requiring medical care, they became excellent training facilities for medical schools. Over time, many of these dispensaries were incorporated as **outpatient departments** in medical-school teaching hospitals.

The medical training of physicians during this era was haphazard and, in fact, formal training was not even required in order to open a practice. A few physicians studied at the universities of Europe, but the majority received their training through apprenticeships or were self-taught. As time went on, medical schools were established at American colleges and universities, and by 1850 there were 42 medical colleges. The majority of these programs were in rural Western areas and were generally poor quality with a small, nonsalaried faculty presenting lectures. To obtain a degree, a student was expected to first attend and then repeat lectures, which might include dissection labs, during two four-month sessions over two years (Starr, 1982). Many programs required students to bring their own **cadavers**, which led to a justifiable distrust of medical institutions by the public, particularly by people who had just lost a family member. Several contemporary medical schools, which had their beginnings in this time period, have interesting histories of townspeople storming the grounds in search of deceased loved ones.

With the proliferation of training programs and the growing numbers of people holding themselves out as physicians, several state medical societies were temporarily successful in having state licensure laws established in the 1830s, but the concept was unpopular and all such laws were subsequently repealed in the same era (Starr, 1982).

One could easily write off the entire era from an EMS perspective, except for three events: the early efforts to provide **resuscitation** to victims of sudden death, which led to the establishment of humane societies in the United States; the discovery and use of general anesthesia in surgical operations; and the development and use of ambulances in the healthcare field.

Resuscitation

Although there are early records in texts and works of art from different cultures depicting what appear to be attempts at resuscitating victims, for most of Western history, death was believed to be irreversible except through divine intervention. Galen, an ancient Greek physician (120–210 C.E.) whose writings were regarded as inviolate for centuries, believed that the "furnace of life" was turned on at birth and turned off at death and could not be restarted (Eisenberg, 1957). Not until the Renaissance (14th–16th centuries) did people began to question Galen's teachings of human anatomy, and not until the Enlightenment period (18th century) did physicians and scientists of the day begin to actively intervene in cases of sudden death. Still acting on an incomplete understanding of the physiology of the body, a variety of methods were tried to restore breathing, including warming, tickling, suspending the body upside down, compressing the chest in a variety of ways, applying electricity, and blowing air and smoke into the lungs and rectum.

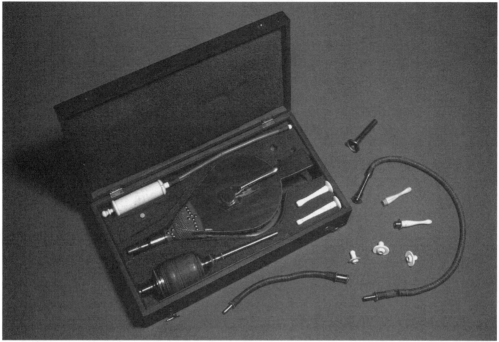

© Science & Society Picture Library/Getty.

Figure 2-3 Bellows for resuscitation.

Interestingly, in 1732, a Scottish physician named William Tassach used **mouth-to-mouth ventilation** to revive a miner overcome by smoke and fumes. The fact that his experience was recorded and the information was circulated has led to the recognition of him as the first physician to use mouth-to-mouth ventilation. Unfortunately, the technique enjoyed only a short period of support; it was later rejected in favor of the bellows and rediscovered some 240 years later (Eisenberg, 1957). Based on several reported successes at resuscitation, in 1767 a group in Amsterdam, responding to the large number of deaths due to drowning, established the Amsterdam Rescue Society. Following their success, similar societies were established in Italy, France, Russia, and England. American physicians who had trained in Europe formed similar rescue societies in Philadelphia (1780), New York (1784), and Boston (1786) (Eisenberg, 1957). Although modern healthcare providers would certainly disagree with some of the medical techniques advocated, the ideas of **preplanning** an emergency response, education, and keeping sound statistics are remarkably similar to the EMS systems of today. There was also a strong current of volunteerism in these efforts, in that rescuers normally refused compensation for their efforts.

Anesthesia

The use of **general anesthetics** in surgery began in 1842 with Dr. Crawford Long, who removed a tumor from a patient who was inhaling ether (Brunner, 1999). After a demonstration by Dr. William Morton at the Massachusetts General Hospital in 1846, the use of general anesthesia was quickly adopted and was in general use by both sides during the American Civil War. The advantage was obvious for both the patient and the surgeon, and the use of general anesthesia was the first step toward the development of modern surgical procedures.

Transportation

Baron Dominique-Jean Larrey, chief physician in Napoleon's army, is credited with developing the first **prehospital** transport system in 1792 (Eisenberg, 1957). Using a fast two-wheeled horse-drawn cart, casualties were **triaged** and treated in the field and then evacuated to aid stations if required. In the United States the concept was known, but it was only after several large Civil War engagements that an organized system of evacuation of the wounded was developed (**Figure 2-4**).

As the preindustrial era ended, none of the elements necessary to establish an effective EMS system existed or could even be conceived. Medical knowledge and facilities were just beginning to move away from their ancient forms and institutions. Transportation and communication were slow and based on the same means that had been used for centuries. Health care remained primarily a concern for the individual and his or her family and focused primarily on alleviating the ravages of infectious diseases.

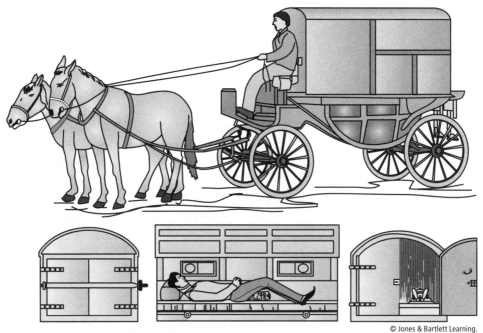

© Jones & Bartlett Learning.

Figure 2-4 Illustration of Larrey's ambulance.

Industrial Era (1850–1970)

During this 120-year period, the U.S. population grew from 23 million to 203 million as a result of natural growth and as succeeding waves of immigrants arrived to seek new lives. Industrialization and innovation brought new products and inventions that fundamentally changed Americans' lives and expectations.

Railroads, automobiles, and then aircraft reduced to a few hours the travel time between distant locations and to a few minutes the travel time between neighboring locations. Communication went from the useful but cumbersome telegraph to telephones, radio, and television, making information and the knowledge of events almost instantaneous.

Large cities developed as American culture moved from an agricultural base to an industrial base. Accompanying this change, municipal, state, and federal governments assumed greater responsibility for the health and welfare of the citizenry.

During this era, Americans were called on to fight a succession of major wars and to endure cyclical economic hardships, from recessions to depressions. Though painful, each contained lessons that brought about changes in the role of government and health care. As a result of a rising standard of living, and improved health care and public health programs, **mortality rates** dropped significantly. In 1850, life expectancy was 38 years; by 1900, it was 48 years; and by 1970, it had nearly doubled to 71 years.

Medical interventions gained credibility during this period, and reliance on physicians and hospitals became routine. Medical science was revolutionized through the development of new technologies and understandings. Following the invention of the stethoscope in 1816, new tools were developed to assist physicians in evaluating their patients and understanding and treating their illnesses and injuries.

With the use of anesthesia, surgical procedures proliferated. No longer constrained by time because of patients' pain, physicians tried and perfected new procedures. **Antiseptic techniques**, which were finally accepted near the end of the 1800s, coupled with the discovery of blood types, which allowed the safe transfusion of blood, helped to make many surgical operations routinely successful. The gruesome amputations in the field hospitals of the Civil War were in stark contrast to 1960s operating rooms, where kidneys, livers, and hearts were changing owners in operations that made front-page news.

This era also witnessed the successful organization of American medicine through the creation of the American Medical Association (AMA), which was established in 1846. Though it struggled initially, the AMA became powerful by the turn of the 20th century and was able to establish standards for physicians, medical schools, and hospitals. Hospitals, which had at the beginning of the era functioned chiefly as institutions of last resort for the poor, became integral to the practice of medicine and the training of physicians and nurses. In addition to the overall improvements in medicine, several developments during this time period had a direct bearing on the development of EMS systems.

Causes of Death

One of the more significant events that occurred during this era was the change in the leading causes of death. In 1900, most deaths were caused by pneumonia, influenza, tuberculosis, and diarrhea (Brunner, 1999). As a result of public health measures and medical care that could prevent as well as treat many infectious diseases, by 1970 the leading causes of death were heart disease, cancer, and cerebrovascular disease. In addition, accidents became the leading cause of death for individuals between the ages of 1 and 37 (Brunner, 1999).

First Aid Training

As industrial development continued and society became more mobile, there was an increasing need for a standardized approach to the delivery of immediate life-saving care to the sick and injured. This standardization came in the form of **Basic and Advanced Red Cross First Aid**. These courses, offered by the American Red Cross, remained the standard for prehospital care well into the 1970s.

Although most people associate first aid care and emergencies with the American Red Cross (ARC), the original mission of the ARC was to provide assistance to victims of war (Picken, 1923). The American Red Cross was incorporated in 1881 under the leadership of Clara Barton, a nurse who

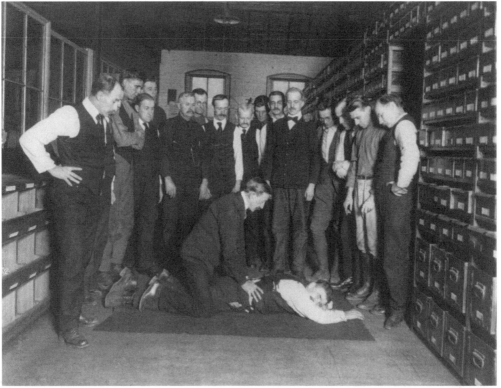

Courtesy of Library of Congress.

Figure 2-5 Teaching first aid methods.

treated soldiers during the Civil War and developed the concept of "treat them where they lie," but did not begin offering first aid training until 1909.

The concept of first aid training, now called **first responder** training, developed in the mining towns of Pennsylvania. Because of the hazards associated with coal mining, miners formed first aid clubs to teach each other first aid skills. The early teams received training from members of the St. John's Ambulance Association in England. As more and more teams were formed, first aid contests developed between the teams. Hearing about these **first aid clubs**, members of the American Red Cross Executive Committee observed a first aid club contest in 1908. In 1909, the ARC Central Committee organized the Red Cross First Aid Bureau. The bureau was managed by Colonel Charles Lynch, who was detailed to the ARC from the U.S. Army Medical Corps. In 1910, Colonel Lynch authored the first ARC first aid textbook, *Red Cross First Aid*, which remained the standard for ambulance personnel training until the widespread acceptance of emergency medical technician (EMT) training in the late 1970s. (See chapter 7 for additional information on training EMS personnel.)

Resuscitator Calls

The 1930s and 1940s saw the development of portable oxygen-powered devices to help revive patients in **respiratory arrest** (not breathing). These large, heavy, mechanical devices were also used to administer supplemental oxygen to a breathing patient. Familiar brands of these devices

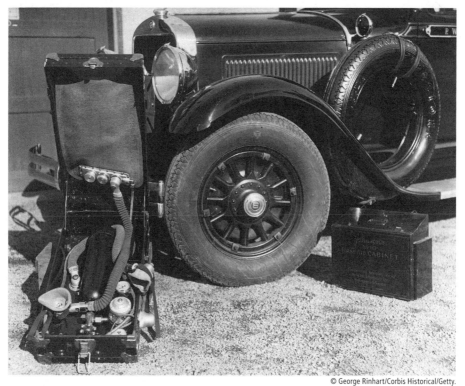

© George Rinhart/Corbis Historical/Getty.

Figure 2-6 Inhalator car.

were the E&J resuscitator-inhalator-aspirator, MSA pneolator, and Emerson resuscitator (Ohio Trade and Industrial Education Service, 1959).

Firefighters during this time period did not have modern self-contained breathing apparatus, and canister masks were just coming into use. As a result of this lack of respiratory protection, firefighters were routinely overcome by smoke and the products of combustion. To revive these firefighters, fire departments organized **resuscitation squads** and special vehicles to respond with an oxygen-powered resuscitator on what were called resuscitator runs. These early responses were, for many fire departments, the beginning of their involvement in the provision of EMS.

Motor Vehicle Injuries

America's love affair with the automobile resulted in increased road traffic, and inevitably the number of auto accidents—or auto crashes—began to climb. It was the concern over death and injury from auto crashes that brought the federal government into EMS. In the 1920s, the first uniform nationwide traffic codes were established. The Federal-Aid Highway Act of 1956 provided funding for the development of interstate highways and standards for road design and safety. The Kennedy administration was the first to express concern over the increasing number of Americans killed in traffic crashes. In 1965, a presidential commission published *Health, Medical Care, and Transportation of the Injured*, which addressed the treatment and survival of auto crash victims. Perhaps the most significant federal response to highway deaths came in 1966 with passage of the Highway Safety Act of 1966. This act created the **National Highway Traffic Safety Administration (NHTSA)** with an EMS division within the U.S. Department of Transportation. The National Traffic and Motor Vehicle Safety Act of 1966 provided the coordination and financing for states to develop highway safety programs.

Transportation

Horse-drawn ambulances similar to those used by the military in the Civil War began to appear as hospital-based units in the 1860s and became motorized units at the turn of the 20th century. Most units remained hospital-based until World War II limited the manpower available to provide staffing; the responsibility then shifted to other groups (Page, 1978). In cities, the responsibility was frequently assumed by existing fire department personnel, whereas in rural areas the service might be provided by volunteers associated with existing volunteer fire departments or newly formed independent units.

In 1928, Julian Stanley Wise founded the Roanoke (Virginia) Life Saving and First Aid Squad. This was the first volunteer rescue squad in the United States. Similar units developed in New Jersey. Some were spin-offs from fire departments; others were independently formed units.

Several private ambulance services also developed during this time, some providing only routine medical transport and others providing both emergency and routine transport. In many areas of the country, the service was assumed by the local funeral home, which could, by making minor modifications, readily turn a hearse into an ambulance. In 1966, more than 50% of the ambulances in the United States were run by funeral directors (Beebe & Funk, 2001). In many communities, the hearse

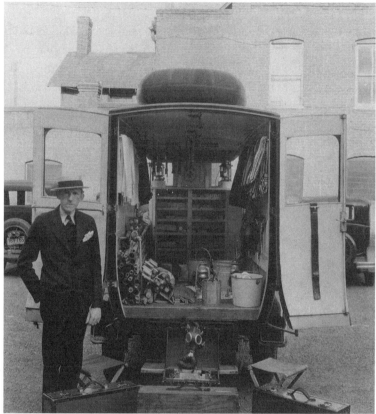

Courtesy of the National Emergency Medical Services Museum.

Figure 2-7 Julian Wise.

was the only available vehicle capable of transporting a prone body. Funeral directors were also readily available to respond to emergencies. Hearses could be easily converted to carry a stretcher; a magnetic red light was easily placed on the roof. Even though funeral directors provided a transport vehicle, most had little, if any, training in first aid.

The training of personnel was basic first aid at best and the emphasis was on speed, as in the phrase "scoop and swoop." Because the attendant did not provide much care, there was no need for interior working space, and the units were usually built along sleek lines that emphasized comfort and style rather than utility. They were the grandest vehicles many attendants had ever driven, and it was with some resistance that they parted with them after prehospital care techniques made a different configuration imperative. By the end of the 1960s, increasing numbers of ambulances had van-type chassis and their attendants had been trained according to the **Emergency Medical Technician-Ambulance (EMT-A) standards** established by the NHTSA.

Military

During this period, the U.S. military participated in five major conflicts that influenced the development of modern EMS. The first was the American Civil War. Battlefield casualties during the Civil War often were not collected until weeks after an engagement, and many men died where they had fallen, days after being injured. Through the efforts of the Sanitary Commission and individuals such as Clara Barton, attempts were made to provide relief to wounded soldiers on both sides of the conflict. Attempts by the Union Army to provide for wounded troops resulted in the first use of ambulances in the United States (Beebe & Funk, 2001).

Improvements in medical care and ground transport helped to reduce mortality in World War I and World War II, but many soldiers still died because of delays in proper treatment. World War I saw the introduction of new, deadlier weapons such as the machine gun, tank, and poison gas. World War I was also the first major conflict served by members of the International Red Cross working under the Treaty of Geneva (Pickett, 1923).

During World War II, professional soldiers functioning as medics provided immediate care to wounded comrades. Pain control using morphine and fluid replacement with plasma were common

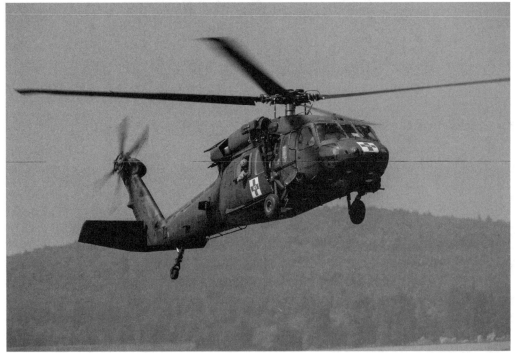

© Stocktrek Images/Getty.

Figure 2-8 Army Medivac helicopter.

practices. However, rapid evacuation of the wounded to surgical field hospitals still was not common-place in the military.

The Korean Conflict of the 1950s saw the introduction of Mobile Army Surgical Hospitals (MASH) and the rapid evacuation of the wounded using helicopters to MASH and treatment hospitals based in battle areas. By the time of the Vietnam War, the use of helicopters for the evacuation of the wounded was well established. It is frequently pointed out that because of this system, an injured soldier in Vietnam was far more likely to survive than was his American counterpart who had been in a serious automobile crash back home.

Cardiac Care

Efforts to revive victims of heart attacks and other sudden-death occurrences continued in this era, culminating in 1960 in the development of modern cardiopulmonary resuscitation (CPR) using mouth-to-mouth ventilation and chest compression. The technique was the result of the combined efforts of doctors and researchers James Elan and Peter Safar, who were investigating the effectiveness of mouth-to-mouth resuscitation at Baltimore City Hospital; and James Jude, Guy Knickerbocker, and William Kouwenhoven, who developed the method of external cardiac massage at Johns Hopkins Hospital.

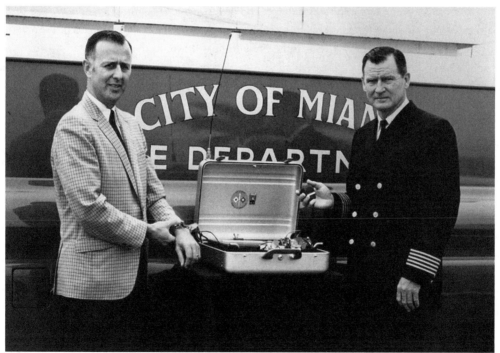

Courtesy of Eugene L. Nagel and Miami Fire-Rescue Department.

Figure 2-9 Dr. Eugene Nagel developed the first unit manned by firefighters trained in the use of defibrillators, the precursors to the paramedics of today.

The combined technique was first used successfully in a prehospital setting by Baltimore City firemen in 1960 (Eisenberg, 1957).

During this era, the importance of **ventricular fibrillation** in heart attacks was discovered, as was the ability to **defibrillate** the heart using electrical shock. First employed in hospitals using an open-chest technique, electric defibrillators were later refined to defibrillate without opening the chest and then redesigned to allow portability. In Belfast, Northern Ireland, Dr. Frank Pantridge, along with his resident Dr. John Geddes, developed the first **mobile intensive-care unit** in 1966. Their modified ambulance carried a standard hospital defibrillator that could be moved into a residence and plugged into a wall circuit or operated in the ambulance by using two car batteries (Eisenberg, 1957). Pantridge's idea spread rapidly and several similar programs using physicians and specially equipped ambulances were initiated in the United States. Dr. Eugene Nagel, working with the Miami Fire Department, developed the first unit manned by firefighters trained in the use of defibrillators, the precursors to the paramedics of today.

Government Involvement

Another development that occurred during this era and that would have important ramifications for the future of EMS was the increased role of the federal government in funding health care and developing healthcare policy. Unlike the governments of many of the industrialized countries of Europe, the federal government had taken only a very limited role in health care in the United States. During the depression years of the 1930s, the Roosevelt administration had considered developing a national health program, but it dropped the plans when opposition to socialized medicine threatened to derail other federal social programs.

The first major federal funding for health care occurred in 1946 during the Truman administration with the enactment of the Hospital Survey and Construction Act, better known as the Hill-Burton Act. This legislation provided funds and loan guarantees for the construction and renovation of hospital facilities. Although the act did not directly address medical care, provisions within the legislation required participating hospitals to justify their needs through planning and to guarantee that a portion of their service would be provided without charge to indigent members of the community. The legislation was significant in that it marked the first major involvement of the federal government in healthcare funding.

The next major federal legislation concerning health care came during the Johnson administration (1965) with the enactment of **Medicare** and **Medicaid**. The legislation, which assisted in the funding of health care for elderly and indigent individuals, rapidly established the federal government as the single largest purchaser of health care. It also eliminated the detached and peripheral role that the federal government had taken toward health care in the past. Besides increasing the demand for health services for elderly and poor people, the legislation opened the possibility for the future consideration of other federally supported healthcare programs.

EMS Development

The first efforts to develop a modern EMS system began to take shape during the 1960s when concern over increasing deaths from auto crashes led to a presidential investigation. In 1966, the President's Commission on Highway Safety issued its final report, "Health, Medical Care and Transportation of the Injured," which focused on the problem of highway accidents and led to the National Highway Safety Act of 1966. This legislation in turn established 18 standards for improving highway safety. Standard 11 of the act specifically addressed emergency medical services. This legislation provided both technical support and funds to improve the prehospital care of accident victims. The legislation was significant because it was the first such federal legislation to specifically address EMS, and many of the activities, including standards for ambulances and training, contributed to the future development of EMS systems.

In the same year, 1966, the National Academy of Sciences published *Accidental Death and Disability: The Neglected Disease of Modern Society*, in which it enumerated the magnitude of the problem of trauma in terms of deaths, disability, and costs. The publication, frequently referred to as the "**White Paper**,"

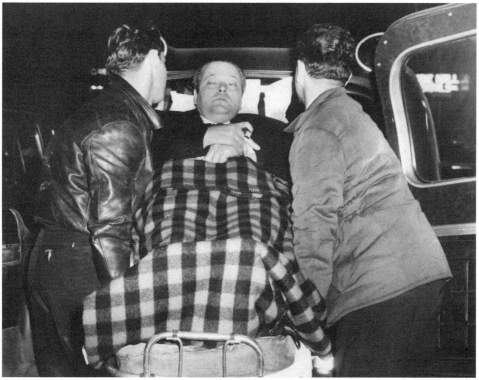

© Bettmann/Getty.

Figure 2-10 Early victims of auto crashes had a reduced chance of survival due to the lack of organized EMS systems.

CONTENTS

Courtesy of United States National Academy of the Sciences.

Figure 2-11 Table of contents for *Accidental Death and Disability: The Neglected Disease of Modern Society,* otherwise known as the "White Paper."

made numerous recommendations regarding training, ambulances, communication, hospital care, record keeping, and research.

Attention to and advancements in coronary care also led to numerous advances in the care of out-of-hospital victims of sudden cardiac death. Building on the work of Pantridge, and with the development of CPR and external defibrillation, **advanced life-support** (ALS) pilot programs were started in various parts of the country. Most significant was the work of Dr. Eugene Nagel with the Miami Fire Department in 1964. Dr. Nagel developed a "portable" field **biotelemetry** unit; in 1967, Miami Fire Department paramedics began functioning. But the field provision of advanced life support was not limited to big-city fire departments and hospitals. In 1968, Dr. Ralph Feichter trained 40 volunteers of the Haywood County Rescue Squad in North Carolina to deliver out-of-hospital coronary care (Page, 1978). This is the first recorded use of volunteers as paramedics.

The importance of advanced life support was also recognized by the American Medical Association at its 1967 Chicago Conference and again in 1969 at the Sixth Bethesda Conference of the American College of Cardiology, which was titled "Early Care for the Acute Coronary Suspect."

In the late 1960s, a pioneering surgeon, Dr. R. Adams Cowley, coined the phrase "**the golden hour**" in reference to the time period during which a seriously injured patient had to receive

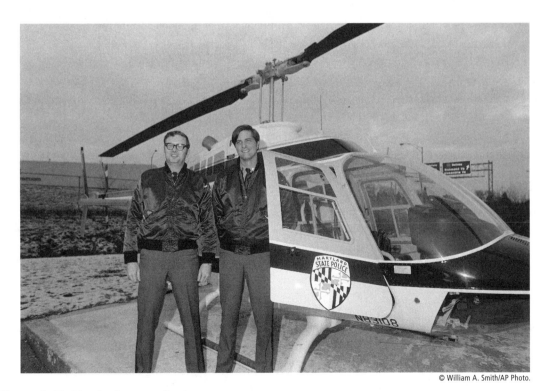

© William A. Smith/AP Photo.

Figure 2-12 Maryland state police jetranger.

definitive care if she or he were to survive. Emulating the military model, Dr. Cowley used Maryland State Police helicopters with a medically trained trooper to bring accident victims to his shock trauma unit at the University of Maryland Hospital. Although successful, the concept of the use of trauma centers and **Medevac** helicopters was not widely accepted until the late 1970s (Franklin & Doelp, 1980).

It was during the 1960s that the first attempt to revise and standardize training for ambulance attendants occurred. In 1966, the U.S. Department of Transportation's EMS Division within the NHTSA issued a request for proposal (RFP) to develop the basic **EMS national standard training curriculum.** In 1969, the EMS Committee of the National Academy of Science-National Research Council (NAS/NRC), published *Training of Ambulance Personnel and Others Responsible for Emergency Care of the Sick and Injured at the Scene and During Transport.* This document was the first of a series of publications that addressed the need for specialized training of EMS personnel. It also identified the need to better equip ambulances.

Modern Era (1970–2000)

By 1970, both the technology and the medical knowledge to develop EMS systems existed, but only the military on the battlefield had developed an effective response. Whether a person lived or died as a result of an accident or a heart attack depended very much on luck and where the person was at the time.

Most hospitals operated emergency rooms as adjuncts to their main operations, without full-time directors and staffed by whoever might be available, frequently the least trained of their medical staff. Even many large hospitals closed their operating rooms after 11:00 p.m.. Patients requiring emergency surgery had to wait until morning. If a person was seriously injured and needed the care of a specialist such as a neurosurgeon, and was taken to a small community hospital, he or she might wait there for days or be transferred too late to be saved.

If a person had a heart attack, family members might watch in horror, not knowing how to summon help or what to do until help arrived. The responding ambulance attendants might know CPR, but the patient would be very lucky if they could defibrillate. Meanwhile, families sat before their television sets watching a television drama called *Emergency!* based on the exploits of Los Angeles County Fire Department paramedics. Conceived as entertainment television, *Emergency!* introduced the entire country to the concept of EMS and made "paramedic" a household word.

1970s

Several groups and individuals were working for change. The White Paper and the Highway Safety Act legislation had a catalytic effect in identifying the problems and engaging professionals to develop solutions. Within the U.S. Department of Health, Education, and Welfare (DHEW), the Division of Emergency Medical Services (DEMS), which had initially been formed to prepare medical services in case of a nuclear attack, became a focal point for change. Working with the American Academy of

Orthopaedic Surgeons and the American College of Surgeons, DEMS assisted in organizing several national conferences on EMS (Boyd et al., 1983). At the conclusion of the second national conference held in December 1971, a telegram was sent to President Richard M. Nixon urging him to take action to improve emergency medical services. In his subsequent State of the Union Message in January 1972, President Nixon announced that he was directing the DHEW "to develop new ways of organizing emergency medical services and providing care to accident victims" (Boyd et al., 1983). As a result, in June 1972, the DHEW initiated five EMS demonstration projects and two EMS communication programs in states and regions around the country. President Nixon firmly believed that EMS was a state and local responsibility and that the role of the federal government should be limited to technical support and guidance. The demonstration projects were intended to develop various approaches that could be copied, but it would be the responsibility of the states and local areas to adopt and fund their own projects (Boyd et al., 1983).

Congress had other ideas, however. As advocates for improving emergency care had pointed out, a medical breakthrough was not necessary. Improvements could be made immediately, across the nation, if start-up funding was made available. In early 1973, both the House and the Senate adopted comprehensive legislation to fund nationwide EMS development. Also included in the bill at the last minute was an amendment to continue the operation of eight U.S. Public Health Service hospitals that the Nixon administration had sought to close. President Nixon objected to both the EMS provision, which he thought inappropriate and excessive, and the continued federal funding of the hospitals. As a result, he vetoed the bill in August 1973 (Boyd et al., 1983). Congress was still committed to the program, however, and after narrowly failing to override the president's veto, it adopted new legislation that did not include any provision for the Public Health Service hospitals. Persuaded that another veto would be overridden, President Nixon signed the Emergency Medical Services Systems Act of 1973 (Pub. Law No. 93-154) into law on November 16, 1973 (Boyd et al., 1983). The law was designed to take a systems approach to EMS through the development of regional programs. It differed from the Highway Safety Act, which had primarily focused on prevention and the prehospital care of accident victims, in that it also addressed hospital care and rehabilitation of an expanded list of emergency medical conditions. Classified as a categorical-project-grant program, it offered matching funds on a competitive basis to regional EMS organizations that addressed the 15 components of an EMS system across seven emergency medical areas. The components and medical areas, which were illustrated in chapter 1, are shown in **Table 2-1**.

Regions were essentially offered five years of funding proceeding from planning (one year) to basic life support (two years) and then advanced life support (two years). Separate grants were also offered for research. Regional development funds could be used across a broad spectrum of categories, including training, equipment, supplies, and travel. Regions were encouraged to use Highway Safety Act funds in appropriate categories to augment the EMS funding. Development and expenditures were closely monitored by DEMS (the federal lead agency headed by Dr. David Boyd) and by the regional DHEW offices. These agencies provided technical assistance and encouragement, as well as the grant funding for compliance in following the guidelines.

Table 2-1 The Components and Emergency Medical Areas Outlined in the EMS Systems Act of 1973

Component	Emergency Medical Area
Communications	Major Accidental Trauma
Manpower	Burn Injuries
Training of Personnel	Spinal Cord Injuries
Use of Public Safety Agencies	Acute Coronary Care/Heart Attacks
Transportation	Poisonings
Mutual Aid Agreements	High Risk Infants and Mothers
Facilities	Behavioral and Psychiatric Emergencies
Accessibility of Care	
Critical Care Units	
Transfer of Patients	
Standard Medical Record Keeping	
Independent Review and Evaluation	
Consumer Information and Education	
Consumer Participation	
Disaster Linkage	

The original legislation was enacted for three years and was renewed with some modification for two additional three-year terms. However, the last renewal was curtailed by President Ronald Reagan's Omnibus Budget Reconciliation Act of 1981, which effectively ended the program. In all, approximately $300 million had been appropriated for the establishment and improvement of EMS delivery systems (NHTSA, 1996). In retrospect it is clear that the program brought about dramatic and fundamental change in EMS. Early planning by DEMS had envisioned a total funding level of approximately $500 million in order to fully establish a nationwide system (Boyd et al., 1983). We can only speculate as to what further progress could have been made if the program had not ended so abruptly.

Despite the difficulties, the program unquestionably spurred the development of EMS systems on a national basis. By 1981, some 303 EMS regions, covering the entire country, had been established and were taking some actions to improve EMS (Boyd et al., 1983). Every region had an EMS council made up of representatives of the major organizations for EMS delivery within their region. Through a series of national meetings sponsored by DEMS, local leaders were able to share their experiences and bring back ideas that had been successful in other regions. The federal program guidelines provided the goals and the monetary incentives to accomplish them. It was up to the regional councils to determine what steps to take to reach these goals. Failure to reach consensus on any specific component, as defined by the federal program guidelines, meant jeopardizing the entire funding, so there was strong incentive to reach agreement. A region could not request funds to equip and train paramedics without also taking steps to categorize their hospitals.

The legislation had been passed in Congress with broad support from the medical community, but opposition developed as some of the more difficult aspects of development had to be addressed. The designation of specialty referral centers, particularly trauma centers, became one of the major areas of contention. Designating one hospital in an area as the trauma center meant that other hospitals would be bypassed by the seriously injured patient being transported to definitive care. This struck at the heart of local medical pride and was seen as a financial threat to the bypassed hospitals. Opposition grew against the concept and the process of designation, resulting in several lawsuits. In other regions, the process of designation was delayed or so modified that the requirement had little effect in changing delivery patterns or improving care. An article in *Time* magazine several years after the program had ended pointed out that only two states had successfully established a statewide trauma system.

Another area of conflict developed between the EMS regions and their state governments. The federal program had deliberately bypassed state health departments in favor of regional organizations. Consequently, many people in state government felt that the federal program had interfered with state authority and prerogatives and so favored legislation that would give the states greater discretion.

The 1970s also were a time of great expansion for EMS training. In 1971, the first national curriculum for training of emergency medical technician-ambulance (EMT-A) workers was adopted. By 1977, a revision of the original EMT-A was needed and approved by the NHTSA.

In 1970, the NAS/NRC EMS Committee appointed a task force to examine the training of "advanced" EMTs through a proposed 480-hour program. Although ALS was being provided by specially trained firefighters and EMTs outside the hospital, the first legal recognition of ALS providers came with California's passage of the **Wedworth-Townsend Paramedic Act**. This law was the first legal recognition of paramedics and served as model legislation for other states. As more and more local paramedic programs developed, the NHTSA recognized a need for standard training similar to that of the EMT. A contract for the development of a national standard curriculum for the **Emergency Medical Technician-Paramedic** was developed in 1975. The final curriculum was presented to the NHTSA for acceptance in 1976.

1980s

As stated earlier, EMS programs initiated and funded under the EMS Systems (EMSS) Act of 1973 effectively came to an end with the enactment of the Omnibus Budget Reconciliation Act of 1981. Funding for the program was combined with other federal preventive healthcare programs, reduced in total, and then distributed to the states as block grants to be used as they deemed appropriate. Compliance with federal program guidelines was eliminated and the federal lead agency, DEMS, was abolished. The legislation was not specifically targeted at EMS but included a number of federal grant programs that had developed over the years. The action reflected the Reagan administration's concern both for reducing the federal budget and for limiting the role of the federal government in what had traditionally been state and local functions.

The budget legislation was particularly serious for EMS because of the dependence that had developed between the federal program and the regional EMS agencies for both funding and leadership.

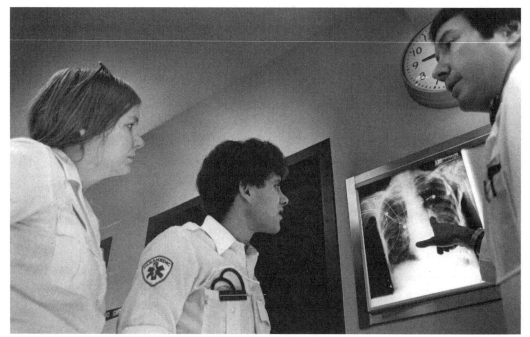

© The Denver Post/Getty.

Figure 2-13 Early paramedic education class.

While the regional structure made sense operationally, it lacked the traditional political structure to replace the lost federal funds. As a result, many of the regional offices collapsed as state and local governments decided that they were unable or unwilling to support the regional infrastructure. While much of the development toward an effective system had occurred because of the federal insistence on standards, their efforts had also provided a forum for an exchange of ideas with national EMS leaders and among managers of developing regional programs. Suddenly this national consensus-building structure was gone, along with the funding.

A successful federal legislation began almost unnoticed in 1984 when the **Emergency Medical Services for Children (EMS-C)** program was established. The program, which is directed by the Maternal and Child Health Bureau within the U.S. Department of Health and Human Services (DHHS, the successor to DHEW), focuses on the special needs of children in EMS. Funding for the program has continued to grow and now represents the largest federal funding commitment to EMS since the end of the EMSS Act in 1981 (NHTSA, 1996). While its focus is children, many of the projects also benefit EMS in general.

While EMS funding was the first priority, national leadership and consensus-building were also important, and the DOT's NHTSA emerged as the lead federal agency for EMS development. During the EMSS Act period, the agency had been placed in a subordinate role, but the agency has gradually increased both its perspective and its role in EMS development since that time. Although direct matching funds for prehospital EMS projects have significantly decreased, the agency has sponsored a number of broader projects to encourage the adoption of standards and the strengthening of EMS systems.

The training of EMS providers continued to evolve during the 1980s. The basic training course for EMTs was expanded to 110 hours in 1983. In 1989, the NHTSA put out a request for proposal to again revise the basic curriculum. Perhaps the most significant training development of the 1980s was the introduction of **EMT-Intermediate (EMT-I)**. Not all states were able or willing to train all of their EMS personnel to the paramedic level. The EMT-I was seen as a means to provide ALS at a minimum level and with a training schedule more conducive to volunteers and rural providers. In 1980, the National Registry of Emergency Medical Technicians recognized EMT-I. The national acceptance of EMT-I took an approach in reverse to that of the basic and paramedic curricula. Various local programs were developed that later were recognized by the NHTSA. In 1982, the NHTSA sponsored a study of EMT-I in conjunction with the National Council of State EMS Training Coordinators. A curriculum was developed in 1983 and approved by the NHTSA in 1985.

1990s

In the immediate aftermath of the end of the federal EMS program, there was a general feeling of pessimism and failure, but too much progress had been made for a complete collapse of the system. Standards for training, equipment, and operations, though they were no longer enforced by the federal government, had been incorporated into day-to-day operations. The concept of a systems approach to EMS was ingrained in the minds of EMS administrators, and no one was advocating a return to the pre-system status. Several strategies developed at the state and national levels as administrators sought to make the best of the new conditions. The first concern was funding, and two basic initiatives developed. The first was to create a mechanism for the states to replace some of the federal funds and the second was to reintroduce federal legislation that would at least support portions of the system.

Many state and local governments began or continued to support EMS development through general tax funds, but several states also enacted special taxes to support EMS. Virginia gained nationwide recognition with its One for Life Program, which added one dollar to its vehicle registration fee and earmarked the new revenue for EMS development. The program has been copied by several other states at varying levels of taxation. A variation that has been used by several states involves adding an extra fine to vehicle moving violations.

The results of efforts to reintroduce federal EMS legislation have been mixed. A few years after the cessation of the federal EMSS Act, a U.S. Government Accountability Office (GAO) report indicated that, while states had in part replaced the federal funding, there were three problematic areas that needed to be addressed: statewide trauma center planning, rural EMS, and completion of the 9-1-1 system. With support from several agencies and organizations, including the American Hospital Association, which lobbied for funds to reimburse trauma hospitals for uncompensated care, the

Trauma Care Systems Planning and Development Act was enacted in 1990. To develop the program, a new organization was created within the federal Department of Health and Human Services (the successor agency to HEW) called the Division of Trauma and EMS (DTEMS). Charged with addressing those areas identified by the GAO, the agency was hampered from the start by delays in funding. When funds were finally appropriated at the level of approximately $5 million per year, they were so paltry that only the state trauma-planning portion could be addressed in any detail. Without funding to encourage participation and compliance, the planning effort did little more than create a paper exercise. The half-hearted effort ended with the loss of appropriations and the disbanding of DTEMS in 1995 (*EMS Agenda for the Future*, 1996).

The 1990s were a time of great change for EMS training and education. Changes in the nature of EMS and the proliferation of state variations in provider training led to the convening of the National EMS Training Blueprint Task Force in 1992. The task force identified four levels of EMS provider and standardized the knowledge and skills necessary for each level in its final document, the *National EMS Education and Practice Blueprint*. Building on the recommendations of the Blueprint Task Force, the NHTSA again called for the revision of the EMT curriculum. The resultant national curriculum for basic EMT changed the formal designation of the EMT from EMT-Ambulance (EMT-A) to **EMT-Basic (EMT-B)**. The curriculum also made a fundamental change in the approach used to train EMT-Bs. As a result of the change to EMT-B, the paramedic curriculum was also revised and accepted in 1998.

Perhaps the most significant development of the 1990s was the creation of the *EMS Agenda for the Future* in 1995 and 1996. This national consensus document recognized the **14 attributes** considered essential to a well-functioning EMS system. It called for increased emphasis on education and research in EMS as well as integration of EMS into the national healthcare system. As a result of the *EMS Agenda for the Future*, the process of developing individual agendas for each of the 14 attributes began, with provider education the first area to be addressed. The close of the 20th century saw EMS leaders, regulators, and educators working together to develop the *EMS Education Agenda for the Future*.

Twenty-First Century

As EMS moved into the next millennium, its efforts to grapple with many of the same issues that had shaped its past were overshadowed by the devastating events of the September 11, 2001, attacks on the United States. Changes in healthcare funding and insurance reimbursement remain a major area of concern. Economic changes have had a profound effect on the delivery of EMS by private, for-profit providers, with a number of major consolidators either going out of business or being forced to sell off their assets. As a result, fire department-based EMS has experienced a resurgence with renewed interest and support from fire service leaders.

The role of the NHTSA changed as a result of increased cooperation with the EMS-C program administered through the Maternal and Child Health Bureau of the DHHS Public Health Services, Health

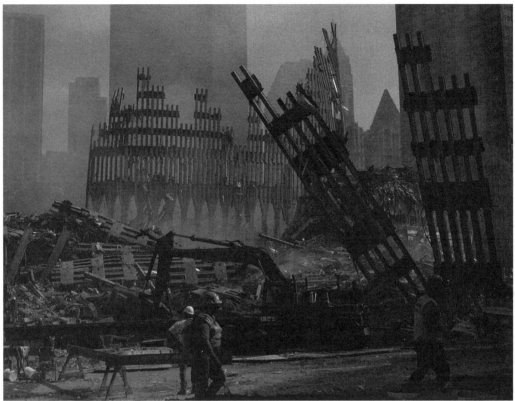

© Larry Bruce/Shutterstock.

Figure 2-14 World Trade Center collapse of September 11, 2001.

Resources and Services Administration. Maternal and Child Health and the NHTSA signed a memorandum making each full partners in the role of a national lead agency for EMS. The *EMS Education Agenda for the Future* was accepted by the NHTSA and the EMS community in 2000.

September 11, 2001

Although tragic, the incidents that occurred on September 11, 2001, have had a positive effect on EMS. Not only did they highlight the importance of EMS response in a national emergency, they also stimulated federal support for emergency response in general. The creation of the **Department of Homeland Security (DHS)** and its grant funding to develop emergency response infrastructure provided badly needed dollars to states and communities. Unfortunately, because EMS was not considered separate from the "fire service," it received a disproportionately low amount of funding compared to other emergency services. Furthermore, EMS provided by private agencies under contract to municipalities received little if any grant funding, even though such services are the primary providers of EMS in a disaster or national emergency.

Perhaps the greatest effect that the events of September 11, 2001, had on EMS and emergency response was the creation of the DHS by the Homeland Security Act of 2002 (Pub. Law No. 107-296), which combined numerous federal law enforcement and emergency management agencies into one entity. Although slow in melding the various agencies and missions into one coherent, functioning federal agency, the DHS has now become the federal focal point for funding, regulation, and policy related to emergency response to national emergencies.

Institute of Medicine Reports

On June 14, 2007, the Institute of Medicine of the National Academies released a report entitled *Emergency Medical Services at the Crossroads*, one of three reports examining the full scope of emergency care in the United States. This extensive, multiyear study highlighted 20 recommendations to improve the EMS system as a whole, many of which were reminiscent of the original "White Paper" (system finance, communications, etc.) and the *EMS Agenda for the Future* (national standards for training and credentialing). Interesting additions included the call for establishment of a lead federal agency for emergency and trauma care, attempts to regionalize EMS, and the need for EMS research. While it is too early to tell what impact the IOM report may have on EMS, the changes are likely to be substantial.

Katrina and Disaster Response

Hurricane Katrina made landfall on August 29, 2005, as a category 3 hurricane in an area stretching from New Orleans to Biloxi, Mississippi, resulting in more than 2,500 casualties and $81.2 billion in financial damage. Collapse of the levees in New Orleans along with a 27-foot storm surge in Mississippi left communities with little or no basic services and posed a great challenge to the EMS system. With very little prior support or formal arrangements, hundreds of providers in hundreds of ambulances converged on the area to support thousands of people in need. This type of massive, sustained response was previously unheard of but would set the stage to prove the need for a **national response system** to both natural and manmade emergencies.

Because of the highly criticized federal response to Katrina, the Post-Katrina Emergency Management Reform Act of 2006 directed the DHS to make significant changes in the policies and procedures for future response to national emergencies. Subsequently, federal response to more recent natural disasters, such as Hurricane Ike in 2008, were better prepared and coordinated. More information on the DHS and disaster response can be found in chapter 12.

Emergency Medical Direction in the Federal Government

Starting in the mid-1990s, a number of emergency medicine physicians were appointed to leadership positions in those government agencies that had EMS programmatic elements. Most significantly, Dr. Richard Martinez became the NHTSA Administrator; it was during his tenure that the

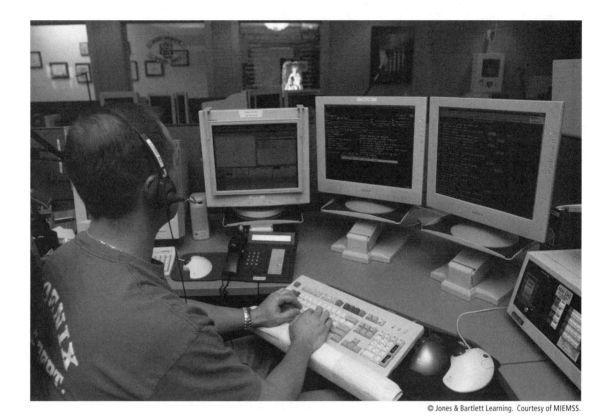

© Jones & Bartlett Learning. Courtesy of MIEMSS.

Figure 2-15 9-1-1 dispatch centers play an integral role in the coordination and delivery of EMS.

EMS Agenda for the Future was drafted. Dr. Jeff Runge succeeded Dr. Martinez in 2001 and continued the programmatic growth of the NHTSA Office of EMS, particularly in developing the series of Agenda for the Future documents. Congress created the **Federal Interagency Committee on EMS (FICEMS)** under the administrative leadership of Dr. Runge's EMS office. When DHS Secretary Michael Chertoff recognized that the DHS needed emergency medical expertise to address issues related to significant public health emergencies such as pandemic flu, he created the position of **Chief Medical Officer (CMO)** and recruited Dr. Runge to the position. Now, the CMO heads the DHS Office of Health Affairs, staffed with a number of emergency physicians. At the DHHS, the Assistant Secretary of Preparedness and Response has appointed a number of emergency physicians to lead the National Disaster Medical System (NDMS) and other health-related emergency response capabilities. President George W. Bush appointed Dr. Richard Carmona, a former paramedic, emergency physician, and trauma surgeon, as the U.S. Surgeon General who served from 2002–2006.

FICEMS/NEMSAC

While it is generally accepted that EMS needs a lead agency at the federal level, no such agency currently exists. There are several federal agencies that have EMS programs, the most prominent being the NHTSA. Although these federal programs have tried to cooperate and coordinate their activities, Congress recognized the need to strengthen the coordination and to create some accountability to Congress. In 2005, the U.S. Department of Transportation was reauthorized; that legislation, known as SAFETEA-LU, contained a provision that authorized the establishment of the Federal Interagency Committee on EMS (FICEMS). The committee has assistant-secretary-level members chosen by the secretaries of the DOT, the DHS, and the DHHS, as well as other federal agencies that have EMS programs such as the Centers for Disease Control and Prevention, Centers for Medicare and Medicaid Services, and the Federal Communications Commission. FICEMS is supported by staff from many agencies that do issue development in five key areas: EMS system assessment, disaster preparedness, medical oversight, data and research, and 9-1-1.

The NHTSA Office of EMS, which has administrative responsibilities to support FICEMS, recognized the need to get direct input from nonfederal EMS leaders to support the programmatic work of FICEMS. In 2007, the **National EMS Advisory Council (NEMSAC)** was created as a federal advisory committee to the Secretary of Transportation. Twenty-four individuals representing every component and perspective of EMS were selected by the secretary to serve on NEMSAC. NEMSAC initially chose to work and make recommendations on issues in the five following areas: safety, EMS finance, systems, analysis-oversight-research, and education and workforce. The FICEMS meets twice per year in Washington, D.C., with NEMSAC meeting four times per year.

Ambulance Fee Schedule

In one of the provisions of the Balanced Budget Act of 1997 (BBA 97), Congress put ambulance service on a Medicare **fee schedule** (a form of prospective payment). Ambulance service was the last medical provider group to be placed on a fee schedule. The American Ambulance Association advocated that the rulemaking related to the fee schedule (AFS) should be conducted as negotiated rulemaking in which EMS stakeholders would work with the Centers for Medicare and Medicaid Services (CMS) to hammer out a consensus on the structure of the fee schedule. The list of stakeholders included the American Ambulance Association, International Association of Fire Chiefs, American Hospital Association, International Association of Fire Fighters, National Volunteer Fire Council, National Association of Counties, and Association of Air Medical Services. Negotiations began in 1999 and concluded in 2000. The fee schedule was introduced in 2003 and was fully implemented by 2010.

Because the AFS was a result of BBA 97, Congress ruled that no additional spending was authorized other than that produced by volume. Therefore, the rates established by the fee schedule were never tied to the cost of providing ambulance service. All EMS provider groups indicated that the new AFS was inadequate. In 2003, Congress authorized the GAO to study the cost of ambulance service and the adequacy of the Medicare ambulance fee schedule. This study was released in 2007 and indicated that the average reimbursement by Medicare was 6% below the average cost of providing ambulance service. Almost all other healthcare providers had a positive Medicare margin, compared to the negative margin that existed for ambulance services. Because of this inequity, the economics of delivering ambulance service were greatly affected.

EMS Caucus

From time to time, members of Congress form issue caucuses to support various causes and interests. A caucus is a group of senators and representatives who work together to support legislation supportive of that issue. Until 2008, EMS did not have such representation in Congress. In the fall of 2008, members of Congress came together to form the Congressional EMS Caucus. The formation of a caucus enhances the chances of favorable EMS legislation being passed in Congress.

Provider Levels and Training

Following the development of the *EMS Agenda for the Future*, the *EMS Education Agenda for the Future* brought about significant changes in the training of EMS personnel. The agenda moved EMS training to be more in line with the approach used by other allied healthcare providers. The development of an EMS core content and scope of practice resulted in new provider levels and moved EMS education from being based on a fixed national standard curriculum to dynamic EMS educational standards. This change would allow educational institutions to be more responsive to changes in medical protocols and educational approaches.

Other Developments

In addition to the developments cited above, several other significant trends have affected EMS since 1970. A question often posed today is, "What group is best capable of providing prehospital ambulance service?" In the 1970s and early 1980s, emergency ambulance service was almost entirely provided either by career municipal services, usually associated with fire departments, or by volunteer units that were also frequently based in fire departments. Typically, an urban fire department (or in some cases a separate municipal service) would be responsible for the city. The suburbs would be serviced by a combination of career and volunteer services and the remaining rural areas would be covered by volunteers. Funding for these units was usually provided by general tax support for the career services and by donations and local subsidies to the volunteers. Patients were seldom billed for care or transportation. Private ambulance services provided emergency care in some areas, but federal funding had not been intended for the private sector. Consequently, many of the private providers found that they could not meet the new standards for training and equipment and either went out of business or were limited to routine transports of subcritical patients. In other areas, private ambulance services were prohibited by local governments from providing emergency care.

Because of the increased costs of training and equipment, by 1985, increasing numbers of both municipal and volunteer organizations began charging patients for services to augment the funds already provided. As the practice became more widespread, the role of the private ambulance service provider was reconsidered. Municipal services are inherently reliable, but like most governmental operations, also inherently inefficient. Because of changing social dynamics, volunteer services often lacked the personnel necessary to make a timely response. Based on the concepts of **system status management** developed by Jack Stout, a pioneer in the economics of prehospital care, private ambulance services reentered the emergency care marketplace. At the same time, the fire service showed increased interest in providing EMS service. This heightened interest from the fire service has benefited some communities and resulted in tensions in others over the proper agency to provide EMS service. Thus, the question of who should provide EMS remains unresolved and contentious.

CPR has also undergone changes during this period, with increased emphasis on the chain of survival advocated by the American Heart Association. This concept—early access, early CPR, early defibrillation, and early advanced care—reinforces the importance of early intervention with CPR and defibrillation. Small automatic defibrillators that require limited training are routinely used by early responding fire and police units, and advocates envision a time when such devices will be as commonplace as fire extinguishers in offices, stores, and even homes.

Star of Life

To conclude the discussion of the history of EMS, it is appropriate to mention the Star of Life that has become both a national and an international symbol of EMS service and hospital emergency rooms. Prior to adoption of the Star of Life, a red cross, the same symbol used by the International and American Red Cross, was used on military and civilian ambulances. With the development of federal standards for ambulance vehicles, some services displayed an Omaha orange cross as an alternative. The Red Cross officially objected to the use of the red-colored cross, so a need developed to find a nationally accepted symbol for EMS. Leo R. Schwartz, then chief of the EMS Branch of the NHTSA, designed a symbol based on the American Medical Association's medical identification symbol (Medic

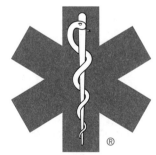

Courtesy of National Highway Traffic Safety Administration.

Figure 2-16 Diagram of Star of Life.

Alert) that also incorporated the staff of Aesculapius, the symbol for healing. The six-sided blue cross displayed on a white background was trademarked as a certification mark by the NHTSA in 1977 for 20 years and its use and display was restricted to vehicles that met the U.S. DOT standards or personnel trained to DOT standards. With the expiration of the trademark in 1997, the use of the symbol has become more widespread and less controlled, appearing on vehicles, personnel, and merchandise not directly associated with EMS.

Each arm of the star has a specific meaning related to the basic functions of EMS. Starting at the top and moving clockwise, the functions associated with the cross are detection, reporting, response, on-scene care, care in transit, and transfer to definitive care.

WRAP UP

Summary

EMS systems are not naturally occurring phenomena. In our mixed-market economy, they are particularly susceptible to being pulled apart by special interests. As stated at the beginning of this chapter, the basic tenet of EMS is that patients will be treated by the right people, in the right place, and at the right time. Over the last 50 years, enormous progress has been made toward this goal; EMS professionals must be educated and vocal advocates to ensure that this trend continues and improves.

Key Terms

advanced life support (ALS)

allied healthcare

alms houses

antiseptic techniques

Basic and Advanced Red Cross First Aid

biotelemetry

cadavers

cardiopulmonary resuscitation (CPR)

Chief Medical Officer (CMO)

city dispensary

core content

defibrillate

Department of Homeland Security (DHS)

educational standards

Emergency Medical Services at the Crossroads

Emergency Medical Services for Children (EMS-C)

Emergency Medical Technician-Ambulance (EMT-A) standards

Emergency Medical Technician-Paramedic (EMT-P)

EMS Agenda for the Future

EMS Education Agenda for the Future

EMS national standard training curriculum

Emergency Medical Technician-Basic (EMT-B)

Emergency Medical Technician-Intermediate (EMT-I)

evacuation

Federal Interagency Committee on EMS (FICEMS)

fee schedule

first aid clubs

first responder

14 attributes

general anesthetics

general hospitals

"the golden hour"
heroic medicine
humoral theory
issue caucuses
Medevac
Medicaid
Medicare
Mobile Army Surgical Hospitals
  (MASH)
mobile intensive-care unit
mortality rates
mouth-to-mouth ventilation

National EMS Advisory
  Council (NEMSAC)
National EMS Education and
  Practice Blueprint
National Highway Traffic
  Safety Administration
  (NHTSA)
national response system
outpatient departments
prehospital
preplanning
respiratory arrest

restorative
resuscitation
resuscitation squads
scope of practice
system status management
trepanning
triaged
ventricular fibrillation
Wedworth-Townsend
  Paramedic Act
"White Paper"

Review Questions

1. List at least two individuals who influenced the development of emergency care in the preindustrial era.
2. Discuss the importance of war in the development of EMS.
3. What is the "White Paper" and what effect did it have on the development of modern EMS?
4. Discuss the role of traffic safety in the development of modern EMS.
5. What has the *EMS Agenda for the Future* contributed to modern EMS?

Additional Resources

Beebe, R. D., & Funk, D. (2001). *Fundamentals of emergency care.* Albany, NY: Delmar Thomson Learning.

Boyd, D. R., Edlich, R. F., & Micik, S. (1983). *Systems approach to emergency medical care.* Norwalk, CT: Appleton-Century-Crofts.

Brunner, G. (Ed.). (1999). *The* Time *almanac.* Boston: Information Please.

Eisenberg, M. S. (1957). *Life in the balance.* New York: Oxford University Press.

Franklin, J., & Doelp, A. (1980). *Sock trauma.* New York: St. Martin's Press.

King, D. (1997). *Sea of words* (2nd ed.). New York: Henry Holt & Co.

National Highway Traffic Safety Administration & Maternal and Child Health Bureau. (1996). *Emergency medical services agenda for the future* (DOT HS 808 441). Washington, DC: U. S. Government Printing Office.

Ohio Trade and Industrial Service. (1959). *Emergency rescue squad manual*. Columbus, OH: Ohio State University.

Page, J. O. (1978). *Emergency medical services* (2nd ed.). Boston: National Fire Protection Association.

Picken, S. E. (1923). *The American National Red Cross: Its origin, purposes, and service*. New York: The Century Co.

Rothstein, W. G. (1987). *American medical schools and the practice of medicine*. New York: Oxford University Press.

Roush, W. R. (1994). *Principles of EMS systems* (2nd ed.). Dallas, TX: American College of Emergency Physicians.

Starr, P. (1982). *The social transformation of American medicine*. New York: Basic Books.

3

Human Resources

Objectives

Upon completion of this chapter, the reader should be able to:

- Briefly state the historical development of current prehospital provider levels.

- Identify prehospital providers involved in the delivery of EMS.

- Identify hospital-based providers involved in the delivery of EMS.

- List examples of specialized EMS providers.

- State the role of allied health professionals in providing EMS.

- State the role of telecommunicators and emergency medical dispatchers in an EMS system.

- Identify sources of EMS providers.

Historical Background

Before the development of modern emergency medical services (EMS) in the 1970s, transport vehicles were often staffed with only a driver, and little, if any, care was provided at the scene or during transport. The normal mode of operation was what has come to be known as "swoop and scoop." Services that maintained trained attendants most often utilized **American Red Cross Standard and Advanced First Aid** as the required training level. As noted in *Accidental Death and Disability: The Neglected Disease of Modern Society:*

> *There are no generally accepted standards for the competence or training of ambulance attendants. Attendants range from unschooled apprentices lacking training even in elementary first aid to poorly paid employees, public-spirited volunteers, and specially trained full-time personnel of fire, police, or commercial ambulance companies. Certification and licensure of attendants is a rarity. (National Academy of Sciences, National Research Council, 1966)*

Not only were ambulances inadequately staffed, as shown in **Figure 3-1**, but upon arrival at the hospital, the patient may not have fared any better. Many hospital **emergency departments** (EDs) were little more than receiving areas for seriously injured patients or "charity" patients who lacked the means to visit a family doctor. Known frequently as "**accident rooms**," the role of the ED had been changing since World War II. A mobile society and the demise of the local family doctor who made house calls resulted in more Americans using the ED as their primary source of health care.

Early EMS-system research and legislation identified the need to not only have well-trained and certified ambulance attendants but also to categorize and accredit EDs. Building on the work of Cowley, related to trauma systems, and Boyd, who developed the 15 components, the concept of a system approach to trauma care developed. With the evolution of more sophisticated EDs and **trauma centers**, the need for specially trained physicians, nurses, and other allied health professionals emerged, eventually leading to the current levels of EMS professionals.

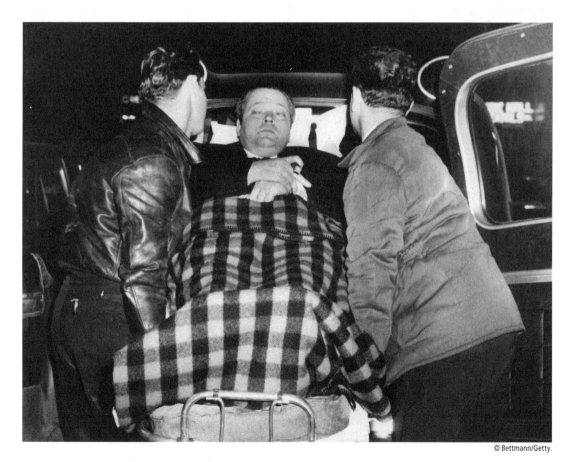

© Bettmann/Getty.

Figure 3-1 Old Early ambulance with crew.

Prehospital Providers

Today, the standard for ambulance attendants is the emergency medical technician (EMT). Advanced care is provided by the paramedic. Other provider levels include advanced EMT (AEMT) and emergency medical responder (EMR). Although defined by a national scope of practice and national EMS educational standards, regional and state variations have resulted in different levels of prehospital providers in some areas. This chapter will focus on the provider levels identified in the national scope of practice.

Emergency Medical Responder

In 1973, the U.S. Department of Transportation (DOT) recognized the need to develop a basic EMS course for law enforcement officers. Police officers are often the first to arrive at the scene of automobile crashes. Before this time, law enforcement personnel were trained in American Red Cross (ARC) first aid or had no training at all. The course developed by the DOT was called Crash Injury Management for Law Enforcement Officers, or CIMFLEO. The course was made available to jurisdictions across the nation through federal grants to training agencies. The CIMFLEO course was 40 hours long and covered basic airway management, CPR, bleeding control, and shock management. It also contained a module on basic automobile extrication using minimal hand tools.

As the training of law enforcement personnel progressed, the fire service realized a similar need for EMS training for firefighters. Although many fire departments provided EMS, not all department personnel were trained to provide even rudimentary first aid. This was especially true of engine company personnel. If an engine company arrived at the scene of an automobile crash before an ambulance, the crew could do little more than comfort the injured. Rather than requiring personnel to complete the more extensive EMT course that was designed for ambulance personnel, a need for a firefighter first-responder course was recognized. This need led to the revision of the CIMFLEO course into the Firefighter First Responder (FFFR) curriculum. Realizing that firefighters were not the only first responders, the course evolved into simply first responder. Now a basic emergency care course was available to personnel such as highway workers, school personnel, camp counselors, the military, and industrial workers.

With the increased focus on first responders following the events of September 11, 2001, and the formation of the Department of Homeland Security (DHS), the term "first responder" became generic for anyone who responds initially to an emergency or disaster situation. To directly address the needs and responsibilities of those first responders who are specifically trained to respond to everyday medical and trauma incidents, the national scope-of-practice model identified the provider level of emergency medical responder (EMR). Thus, the first responder as originally envisioned is now the EMR.

The EMR is described as an individual who is trained to provide initial life-saving assessment and intervention utilizing minimal specialized equipment. EMRs are trained to initiate on-scene stabilizing care and assist other EMS providers (see **Figure 3-2**); in almost all states they are not recognized as a level of certification that would staff an ambulance as the primary patient-care

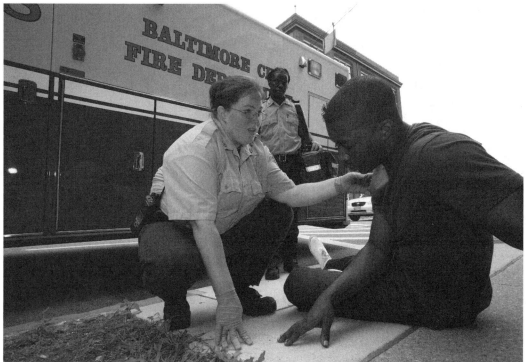

© Jones & Bartlett Learning. Courtesy of MIEMSS.

Figure 3-2 Emergency Medical Responders (EMR) on scene.

provider. Initial course length is 48–60 hours and includes classroom and laboratory training. The *National EMS Scope of Practice* defines the EMR thusly:

> *The primary focus of the Emergency Medical Responder is to initiate immediate life-saving care to critical patients who access the emergency medical system. This individual possesses the basic knowledge and skills necessary to provide lifesaving interventions while awaiting additional EMS response and to assist higher level personnel at the scene and during transport. Emergency Medical Responders function as part of a comprehensive EMS response, under medical oversight. Emergency Medical Responders perform basic interventions with minimal equipment.*

Emergency Medical Technician

The emergency medical technician, or EMT, is the minimal level of training for ambulance personnel. Originally designated EMT-A for ambulance, EMT certification has evolved from a 72-hour course developed by the DOT, to a 110-hour program of basic EMS instruction known as EMT-B (or EMT Basic), to today's EMT. The EMT is trained to assess the ill or injured patient and provide treatment based on assessment findings. This is the minimal level of training required to provide care for a patient on an ambulance in most states. **Certification** requires completion of a course based on the National EMS Education Standards and successful completion of an approved examination, which usually consists of a written and **practical examination**. The initial 150–190-hour course includes **didactic**, laboratory, **clinical**, and **field instruction**. Students are required to assess a minimum of 10 patients either in a clinical or a field setting. The *National EMS Scope of Practice* defines the EMT thusly:

> *The primary focus of the Emergency Medical Technician is to provide basic emergency medical care and transportation for critical and emergent patients who access the emergency medical system. This individual possesses the basic knowledge and skills necessary to provide patient care and transportation. Emergency Medical Technicians function as part of a comprehensive EMS response, under medical oversight. Emergency Medical Technicians perform interventions with the basic equipment typically found on an ambulance. The Emergency Medical Technician is a link from the scene to the emergency health care system.*

Advanced Emergency Medical Technician

The need for a specialized provider with training above the level of the EMT but less than that of the paramedic has been recognized for some time. Although many reasons exist for such a level of certification, one of the most common has been the need to provide some level of advanced life support (ALS) response in rural communities that cannot support or provide paramedic education and response. The concept of an "intermediate" level of provider has also been embraced by some urban EMS systems as a way to provide basic ALS care with a minimal investment in personnel training. But a fundamental reason for creating the AEMT was the recognition that, except for ALS providers in very busy systems, most paramedics do not regularly use all the skills for which they have been trained, which leads to skills degradation. The training of the AEMT is designed to provide a basic set of skills that can be used to manage the majority of ALS responses. As defined in the *National EMS Scope of Practice*:

> *The primary focus of the Advanced Emergency Medical Technician is to provide basic and limited advanced emergency medical care and transportation for critical and emergent patients who access the emergency medical system. This individual possesses the basic knowledge and skills necessary to provide patient care and transportation. Advanced Emergency Medical Technicians function as part of a comprehensive EMS response, under medical oversight. Advanced Emergency Medical Technicians perform interventions with the basic and advanced equipment typically found on an ambulance. The Advanced Emergency Medical Technician is a link from the scene to the emergency health care system.*

Personnel fulfilling this intermediate level have had many different titles and scopes of practice over the years, dictated by state regulations and requirements, including cardiac rescue technician, coronary care technician, EMT-II, EMT-Advanced, and shock trauma technician. Prior to the recognition of AEMT, the National Registry provided testing for "Intermediate 88" and "Intermediate 99" educational programs, depending on which version of the National Standard Curriculum was used.

Paramedic

The paramedic (shown in **Figure 3-3**) is the primary provider of ALS. In addition to having the knowledge of an EMT and AEMT, the paramedic possesses knowledge of **pathophysiology** and the **disease process**. As defined in the *National EMS Scope of Practice*:

> *The Paramedic is an allied health professional whose primary focus is to provide advanced emergency medical care for critical and emergent patients who access the emergency medical system. This individual possesses the complex knowledge and skills necessary to provide patient care and transportation. Paramedics function as part of a comprehensive EMS response, under medical oversight. Paramedics perform interventions with the basic and advanced equipment typically found on an ambulance. The Paramedic is a link from the scene into the health care system.*

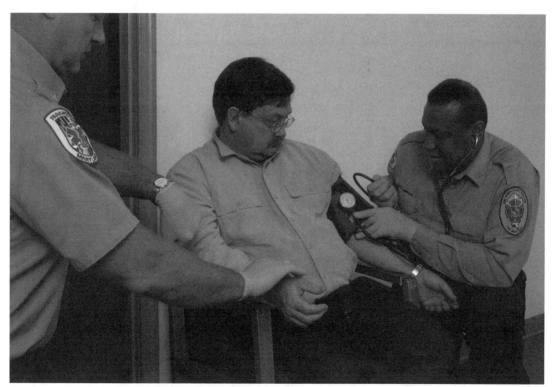

© Jones & Bartlett Learning.

Figure 3-3 In addition to having the knowledge of an EMT and AEMT, the paramedic possesses knowledge of pathophysiology and the disease process.

Preparation for becoming a paramedic involves approximately 2,000 hours of classroom and laboratory instruction along with extensive clinical and field experience. Before enrolling, the student should have knowledge of basic anatomy and physiology as well as preparation in mathematics, reading, and writing.

Specialized Prehospital Providers

In addition to the traditional EMTs and paramedics, there are other prehospital providers trained to provide care to special patient populations. In most cases, these providers are paramedics who have received advanced or special training.

Flight Paramedics and Nurses

Recognizing the need to transport severely injured victims promptly to a trauma center, and building on the experience of the military with helicopter medical evacuation, many hospitals and emergency medical services operate air medical units (**Figure 3-4**). Utilizing helicopters for on-scene response, **air medical units** are typically staffed by either a **flight paramedic** or a **flight nurse**, or a person trained as both a flight paramedic and a flight nurse. Pilots are also specially trained for air medical operations.

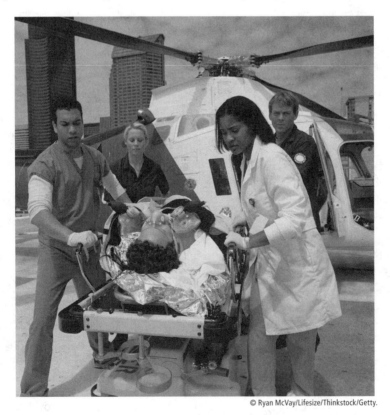

© Ryan McVay/Lifesize/Thinkstock/Getty.

Figure 3-4 Many hospitals and emergency medical services operate air medical units.

Training of flight paramedics and nurses is based on the *Guidelines for Air Medical Crew Education* developed by the Association of Air Medical Services (AAMS), which builds on the knowledge and skills obtained in paramedic and nursing education programs. In addition to the medical knowledge required by the guidelines, air medical crew members receive training in aircraft safety and orientation, communications, rules and regulations, survival, search and rescue, and air medical crew fitness. Crews engaged in **interfacility transports** may also be trained and certified in critical care transport. Flight crew members also adhere to standards established by professional organizations such as the Air Medical Physician Association (AMPA), Air and Surface Transport Nurses Association (ASTNA), and the International Association of Flight Paramedics (IAFP). The ASTNA provides certification examinations in cooperation with the Board of Certification for Emergency Nursing to credential certified flight registered nurses (CFRN) and certified transport registered nurses (CTRN). The ASTNA also provides credentialing for ground critical care transport nurses. For paramedics, the IAFP provides credentialing as a certified flight paramedic (FP-C) in conjunction with the Board of Critical Care Transport Paramedic Certification (BCCTPC).

Critical Care Transport Specialists

The special needs of patients requiring transport between hospitals have led to the development of critical care transport specialists, who are usually paramedics or nurses having additional training in critical care topics. Federal legislation known as **EMTALA**, the Emergency Medical Treatment and Active Labor Act, commonly referred to as "**COBRA**" because of the title of the original legislation containing the act, requires that the level of care being provided to a patient be maintained during transport to, and after arrival at, the receiving facility. To comply with the COBRA requirements, transport services would utilize a nurse from either the sending or the receiving facility to accompany the patient. Although a workable solution, there were many logistical and clinical problems inherent in this approach. Training paramedics and nurses specifically for this role and having them employed by the transport service has eliminated many of those problems. The need for critical care transport has been recognized by the **Centers for Medicare and Medicaid Services** and is reimbursable through healthcare insurance. The need for critical care transport will become even more important with the change to Accountable Care Organizations (ACO) and Medicare Shared Savings Programs (MSSP) as the Affordable Care Act is implemented. Both the ASTNA and IAFP provide training and credentialing for critical care transport nurses and paramedics.

Community Paramedic

In order for ACOs to provide coordinated high quality care, they need to develop a patient care system that is both efficient and value added. One way to accomplish this is to link healthcare providers together into a coordinated network of care. An example of such a network would be a hospital, an EMS service, and a long-term care facility. In such a system, the role of the paramedic is expanded beyond just staffing ambulances. Using advanced training and telemedicine, paramedics provide routine and acute care to residents of a long-term care facility, thus reducing the need or frequency of hospital transports. Hospital outpatients could likewise be evaluated and treated in conjunction with physician consultation via telemedicine. This approach both saves cost as hospital transport is eliminated and adds value to the healthcare system. To meet this increased role of the paramedic, the **community paramedic** concept was developed. Community paramedics are experienced paramedics who have undergone additional training in patient assessment, lifestyle counseling, and preventive services as well as in the technical aspects of telemedicine and advanced patient sensors.

Wilderness EMT

Wilderness medical training is given to the wilderness EMTs to meet the special challenges of extreme environments. The training focuses on extended patient management, availability of limited equipment, and extreme environments such as mountains, rural areas, and oceans. Courses are based on the National EMS Education Standards and are offered at the basic and ALS levels.

Specialized Response Providers

Special response teams exist in many fire departments and law enforcement agencies. Medical care for personnel as well as victims is an integral part of their operations. Many teams either require their members to be cross-trained as EMTs or paramedics or to utilize EMS personnel as part of the team. EMS personnel receive additional training in aspects of emergency care related to the mission of the team. Examples of such specialized personnel include SWAT teams, hazardous material specialists, and tactical rescue team EMTs and paramedics. Physicians may also be involved in high-risk mission teams.

Hospital-Based Providers

Once a patient arrives at the hospital, the provision of emergency medical care is continued by a team of highly trained medical professionals. In some systems that utilize a hospital-based EMS system, the paramedic may continue to provide care while the patient is in the emergency department. If the patient needs advanced care due to severe injury, he or she may be transferred or taken directly to a trauma center staffed by another group of specialists.

Nurses

Nurses continue to play an important role in the EMS system beyond their function in an emergency department (**Figure 3-5**). They serve in all aspects of EMS. Nurses may function as prehospital providers, ALS providers, critical care transport team members, educators, or system coordinators and as flight, trauma, critical care, and pediatric nurses. Nurses were one of the first groups of medical professionals to take an active role in the training of paramedics. Additionally, the broad-based, patient-centered nature of nursing education and practice makes nurses well suited to the many aspects of an EMS system. In the emergency department, nurses are often the first staff member encountered by prehospital providers.

They not only provide a link between the field and the hospital, but they can also play a vital role in providing feedback and support to field personnel. In some systems, specially trained nurses are permitted to provide direct medical control to prehospital providers.

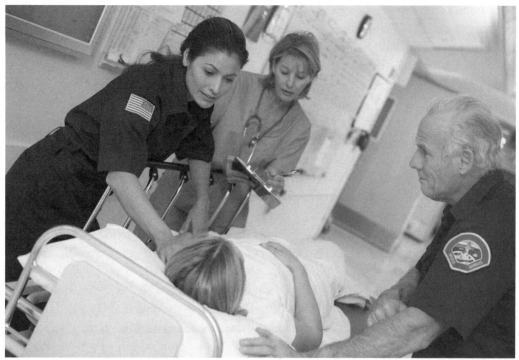

© Monkey Business Images/Shutterstock.

Figure 3-5 Nurses and physicians are an integral part of the EMS system.

In 1970, the Emergency Nurses Association (ENA) was founded to advance emergency nursing practice. The ENA provides education as well as advocacy for the interest of all nurses involved in the delivery of emergency care. Through the *Journal of Emergency Nursing* and educational courses such as the Trauma Nursing Core Course, Emergency Nursing Pediatric Care, and Advanced Trauma Nursing, the ENA provides a wide range of educational opportunities for nurses.

Physicians

Physicians play a critical role in the delivery of EMS. They provide not only specialized medical care but also the **medical direction** necessary for all other levels of providers to function. Historically, physicians have been considered the first EMS responders. Until after World War II, physicians would visit patients at home, an event commonly known as a "house call." Hospital-based ambulances routinely included an intern or resident as part of the crew. Physicians still respond on ambulances as primary crew members in many European and South American countries. In rural communities, it was not uncommon for the "town doc" to be summoned to major automobile crashes or in farm and industrial accidents. Some rural physicians even ran their own small community hospitals. Emergency department physicians are not the only physicians routinely involved in EMS. The first paramedic units were formed to provide out-of-hospital care for victims of sudden cardiac death. Building on the work of EMS pioneers such as Eugene Nagle, a cardiologist who was also an electrical engineer, cardiologists continue to be involved in EMS education, protocol development, and system design.

One of the first textbooks used for EMT training was *Emergency Care and Transportation of the Sick and Injured* (AAOS, 1971). The book had an orange cover and became known as the "orange book." The American Academy of Orthopaedic Surgeons (AAOS) worked to develop an educational program and lesson guides for EMT training. Its efforts were instrumental in the development of a national standard curriculum. The AAOS continues to provide review and input into the development of EMS training curricula.

A major portion of EMS activity is directed toward the trauma patient. Definitive care of serious trauma injuries usually requires surgical intervention. In a manner similar to the AAOS, the American College of Surgeons (ACS) continues its involvement in EMS. The ACS recognizes trauma as a surgical disease. Its Committee on Trauma works to establish standards for the care of the trauma patient. The ACS also developed Advanced Trauma Life Support (ATLS), a course designed to allow surgeons to assess and treat trauma patients in a systematic manner during the critical first hour after a traumatic event.

Central to the care of trauma victims is the concept of the trauma center. As the trauma center concept expanded, the specialized nature of physicians working in the centers also evolved. Surgeons specializing in trauma victim resuscitation are known as **traumatologists**. The specialty of trauma surgery was developed. Nonsurgical physicians dealing with the continued care of critical patients are called **critical care intensivists**.

In addition to the physician roles described earlier, members of almost all medical specialties provide consultation and support to EMS systems. The physician is the central core from which all other provider levels extend. Without physician authority and oversight, an EMS system would not be able to provide the sophisticated care now commonly expected of such systems. (See chapter 6.)

Allied Health Professionals

An EMS system could not function, and proper patient care could not be delivered, without the assistance and cooperation of numerous **allied health professionals**. For example, consider a patient transported to an ED with a simple fracture. An x-ray technician will be needed to take x-rays. An ED technician records vital signs. A surgical **physician assistant** applies the cast after the orthopedist has set the fracture. For a medical patient, other allied health professionals may include medical lab technicians, ECG technicians, and respiratory therapists. In addition to their hospital-based roles, some allied health professionals assist with the interhospital transfer of critical patients. Critical care transport teams may include a respiratory therapist to manage ventilator-dependent patients.

Other Providers and System Personnel

The delivery of prehospital emergency care involves not only personnel who provide direct patient care, but also personnel who provide valuable support functions that are critical to the system's operation.

...municators (shown in **Figure 3-6**) provide a vital link ...t years, the role of the telecommunicator has expanded ...e resource and advocate for the caller in distress. Back ...r the telephone operator, who would connect the caller ...ital. If the caller could not give a good location or ...needs to dial 9-1-1 to be connected to a telecommuni- ...also will provide **prearrival instructions** and remain ...rrect address is ensured through an **enhanced 9-1-1**

...g and certification. Organizations and private compa- ...and materials. Basic telecommunicator courses are ...opics such as roles and responsibilities, telephone ...CAD) systems, and fundamentals of call handling. ...are also available online.

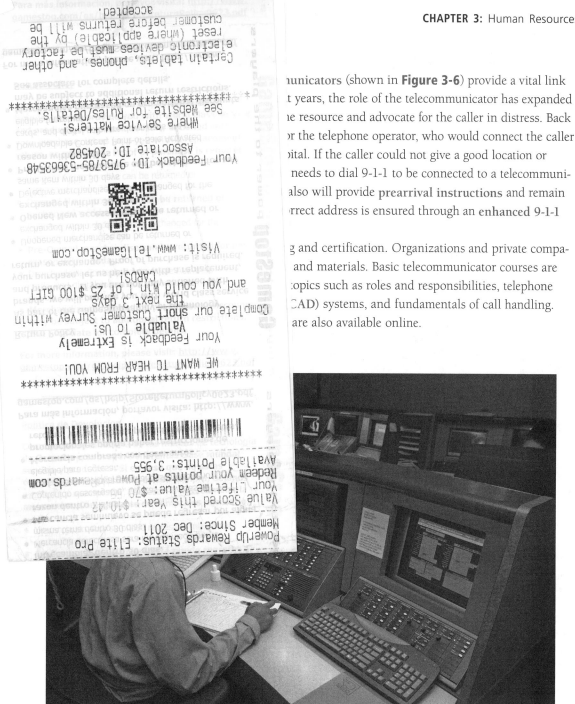

© Jones & Bartlett Learning. Courtesy of MIEMSS.

Figure 3-6 Telecommunicators provide a vital link between the public and EMS.

Emergency Medical Dispatcher

Once a call for EMS assistance has been received by the **call taker** (telecommunicator), it may be transferred to the **emergency medical dispatch (EMD)** dispatcher. The call taker may also serve the dual function of EMD dispatcher. Through a systematic caller interrogation, the EMD dispatcher can determine the nature of the caller's distress. This information is matched to a protocol that provides the dispatcher with scripted prearrival instructions for the caller. This approach provides greater assistance and assurance to the caller. Under the old system, the dispatcher would record the caller's name and location and then hang up. The EMD dispatcher is now able to more accurately determine the proper EMS resources to send, thus improving system efficiency.

Firefighters

In many areas, the fire department also provides EMS service. However, there are still a significant number of fire departments that do not provide these services. Even though they do not provide formal EMS service, these fire departments are often called upon to assist EMS units. The fire department may routinely send a unit as a first responder. This may occur in departments with EMS service if no units are immediately available to respond or will be delayed. Training of firefighters in EMS runs the gamut from paramedic to no formal training. The typical training level for non-EMS fire personnel is EMR. As a minimum, many departments require proficiency in CPR. These minimal training levels allow personnel to provide basic life-saving support until an EMS unit arrives.

Changes in demand for fire department services, coupled with a renewed interest in EMS and budgetary restrictions, have resulted in various approaches to combine traditional firefighting activities with EMS delivery. One such approach is the **paramedic engine company**. A paramedic cross-trained as a firefighter is assigned to an engine company. On medical calls requiring ALS, the engine is dispatched along with a transport unit. The paramedic goes to the hospital in the ambulance and the engine can remain in service. If a fire call is received, the paramedic functions as part of the engine crew. This approach provides greater flexibility and more efficient utilization of specially trained personnel.

Police Officers

Not often thought of as EMS responders, police officers play a vital role in the delivery of EMS. The most obvious role is that of a first responder. Because of the nature of police work, officers are often the first on the scene of incidents requiring EMS. Most police departments provide minimal first aid kits for patrol cars and require officers to be trained to the EMR level. In some areas of the country, the police play a much greater role in EMS. Select police officers are trained to the paramedic level and provide ALS upgrades to local ambulance services. Like paramedic engine companies, this approach also provides greater flexibility and utilization of public safety personnel.

EMS Managers

Although not directly involved in patient care, EMS managers provide management and administration services without which the effective and efficient delivery of EMS services would not be possible.

The role and function of EMS managers varies greatly by system design, type, and size. Common titles associated with EMS managers are supervisor, shift supervisor, coordinator, manager, director, administrator, chief medical officer (CMO), chief operating officer (COO), and chief executive officer (CEO). In the fire service, typical rank titles such as battalion chief, assistant chief, and deputy chief may be applied to personnel assigned to supervise and manage EMS operations.

EMS managers may or may not have or maintain prehospital certification or licensure, depending on their level of involvement in the system and their position in the management hierarchy. Community and four-year colleges provide an educational pathway for EMS managers utilizing the EMS management curriculum model developed through the **Fire and Emergency Services Higher Education (FESHE) project** of the U.S. Fire Administration. The American Ambulance Association (AAA) sponsors the **Ambulance Service Manager** course. The National EMS Management Association (NEMSMA) provides professional affiliation for EMS managers.

EMS Educators

Like EMS managers, EMS educators (see **Figure 3-7**) are not directly involved in patient care, but they are integral to the functioning of EMS systems. Most of the personnel listed earlier would not

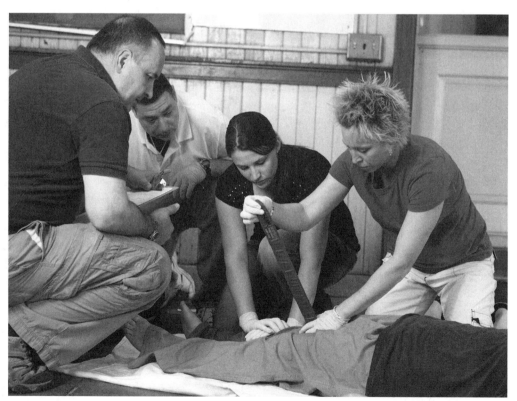

© Jones & Bartlett Learning. Photographed by Darren Stahlman.

Figure 3-7 EMS educators are integral to the functioning of EMS systems.

be able to function if it were not for the efforts and involvement of educators providing classroom, laboratory, clinical, and field training and education. EMS educators provide initial certification training as well as professional and continuing education in various settings and through different modalities.

Basic training for EMS educators varies by state, but the *2002 Guidelines for Educating EMS Instructors* prepared by the National Association of EMS Educators (NAEMSE) for the EMS Office of the NHTSA provides the basis for most instructor training courses.

Sources of Providers

In general terms, prehospital providers can be placed into two groups: volunteer and career. This classification is based upon the nature of the organization for which they work and their status within that organization. However, this dichotomy is not absolute. It is possible for a provider to be a volunteer with one organization and work in a career position with another. There are also providers who are paid on call. This means that they receive compensation only when they respond to a call. For all other activities, they are essentially volunteers.

Volunteer Providers

Volunteers are a significant source of EMS providers. These uncompensated providers deliver all levels of EMS from EMR to paramedic. Volunteers are most often found in rural and suburban areas. However, some significant urban areas are still served by volunteer providers, often with support from paid personnel. In addition to providing emergency response, volunteers are often required to participate in fundraising activities to support their organizations.

Although volunteer providers receive no monetary compensation, they receive many intangible rewards, the most important being a sense of having provided service to their community. To increase recruitment and retention of volunteers, other rewards such as nominal stipends for call response, insurance coverage, reduction or elimination of fees and taxes, worker's compensation eligibility, and length of service awards (retirement) are provided (**Figure 3-8**).

Training and education requirements for volunteers mirror those of career personnel. In **combination departments**, volunteers are often indistinguishable from career staff. State certification requirements for EMS providers are the same for volunteers and career employees. By not distinguishing among providers, the professionalism of all providers is maintained, as is respect among providers. One area in which providers do differ, however, is in the format of training programs. Training for volunteers is often spread out over a longer time period and is offered on weekends and evenings.

A constant area of concern for volunteer organizations is the retention of members. Increased training standards and workplace regulations require volunteer personnel to give more time just to be able to respond to emergency calls. It is not unusual for a new member to take a year's worth of training

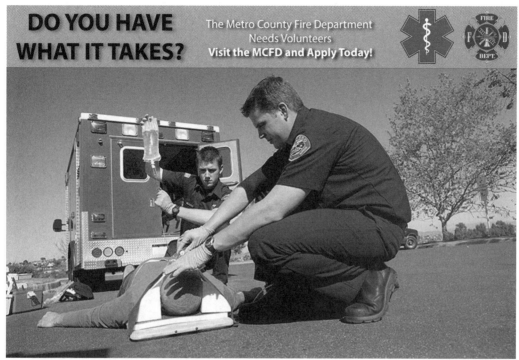

© Air Images/Shutterstock.

Figure 3-8 Volunteer recruitment poster.

before being able to respond to an actual call. This presents a challenge to the organizational leadership to keep the member motivated.

As a member's family or work situation changes, his or her ability to volunteer may also change, leading to conflicts at home, at work, and within the volunteer organization. To maintain sufficient volunteers, organizations must engage in recruitment efforts. Although a necessary activity, it is nonetheless another demand placed upon volunteers.

Career Providers

Career providers include all providers whose primary job is to provide service. Employees of fire departments, hospitals, and commercial ambulance providers would be included in this category. Because career personnel do not have to be concerned with earning a living as well as volunteer organizational and fundraising issues, they can focus more directly on the job of providing EMS. In some areas, the provision of ALS is limited to career personnel due to the training and skill proficiency requirements.

Career providers not only face the demands of providing prehospital care but also are subject to the stresses and demands found in any workplace environment (**Figure 3-9**). These may include unionization, pay disputes, discrimination, management issues, and workplace safety. Career providers often

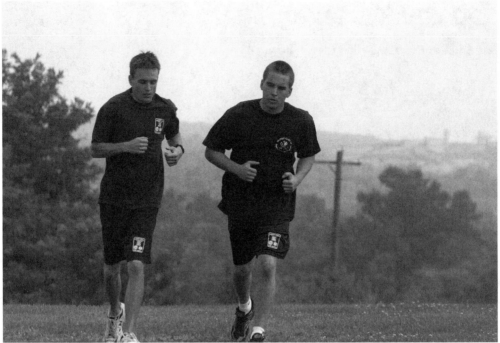

© Jones & Bartlett Learning. Courtesy of MIEMSS.

Figure 3-9 Physical fitness training can help combat stress.

work in **high-volume systems**; thus they have the opportunity to practice their skills more frequently than in traditional volunteer systems. However, working in an understaffed, high-demand system could lead to provider **burnout**. Because EMS is their livelihood, career providers cannot just slow down or quit. This often leads to conflict and increased stress.

In suburban areas surrounding large urban centers, career personnel employed by the urban municipality have been a source of trained volunteers. This trend continues in many areas, but increased demands by unions and labor regulations have had an impact on this source of volunteer providers. Likewise, family and financial demands often require career personnel to have second jobs, thus limiting their availability to volunteer.

WRAP UP

Summary

An EMS system cannot function without a human element. Building on the tradition of early first aid providers, the prehospital provider of today is recognized as a trained and skilled provider of emergency care. National standard curricula ensure consistency in the education of EMS personnel. The role of the prehospital provider is recognized through statewide certification and licensure requirements and legislation.

No matter how well trained or highly skilled, the prehospital provider alone cannot meet all the needs of the sick or injured. Prehospital providers work in coordination with hospital-based providers in a system approach to the delivery of EMS. Hospital providers have a long tradition of EMS involvement as providers, educators, and medical directors.

EMS providers come from varied backgrounds and work in a variety of system configurations. Some are dedicated volunteers while others are employed full time in EMS. Regardless of their status, all EMS providers face numerous challenges working in the profession. This can lead to stress and, in severe cases, traumatic stress. It is important for providers to be aware of their own well-being and to recognize when help is needed.

Key Terms

2002 Guidelines or Educating EMS Instructors

accident rooms

Accountable care organization (ACO)

Advanced EMT (AEMT)

air medical units

allied health professionals

ambulance service manager

American Red Cross Standard and Advanced First Aid

assessment

automobile extrication

burnout

call taker

career providers

Centers for Medicare and Medicaid Services

certification

clinical

Consolidated Omnibus Budget Reconciliation Act (COBRA)

combination departments

community paramedic

computer-aided dispatch (CAD)

Crash Injury Management for Law Enforcement Officers (CIMFLEO)

critical care intensivists

didactic

disease process

emergency departments

emergency medical dispatch (EMD)

emergency medical responder (EMR)

emergency medical technician (EMT)

EMTALA

engine company personnel

Enhanced 9-1-1 system

field instruction

Fire and Emergency Services Higher Education project (FESHE)

Firefighter First Responder (FFFR)

flight nurse

flight paramedic

Guidelines for Air Medical Crew Education

high volume systems

interfacility transports

laboratory training

medical direction

National EMS educational standards

paramedic

paramedic engine company

pathophysiology

physician assistant

practical examination

prearrival instructions

scope of practice

telecommunicators

trauma centers

traumatologists

volunteers

wilderness medical training

Review Questions

1. What are the four levels of prehospital provider and how do they differ?
2. Name three types of hospital-based providers who are routinely involved in the EMS system.
3. How does a wilderness EMT differ from an EMT?
4. Defend the position that emergency medical dispatchers should be considered EMS providers.
5. List at least three sources of EMS system providers.
6. State the role of the medical director in an EMS system.
7. Which national consensus document defines the four levels of prehospital providers?

Additional Resources

American Academy of Orthopaedic Surgeons. (1971). *Emergency care and transportation of the sick and injured*. Menasha, WI: George Banta Co.

National Academy of Sciences, National Research Council. (1966). *Accidental death and disability: The neglected disease of modern society* (p. 73). Washington, DC: Author.

4

Educational Systems

Objectives

Upon completion of this chapter, the reader should be able to:

- Outline the historical development of EMS education in the United States.

- Identify the major components of the *EMS Education Agenda for the Future* and the purpose of each.

- Identify the structure and parts of the National EMS Education Standards.

- State the function of the National Registry of EMTs.

- List six settings for EMS education and training.

- Identify specialized courses developed to meet the needs of special clinical populations.

- State the role of continuing education in EMS provider recertification.

- State the role of accreditation in EMS education and training.

- State the role of technology in the delivery of asynchronous learning.

Introduction

The education of prehospital providers in the United States can be traced back to the 1890s and the mining towns of Pennsylvania. To provide care for injured miners, towns formed first aid clubs as shown in **Figure 4-1**. Some of the original instruction was provided by members of the St. John's Ambulance Association of England, because such training did not exist in the United States. As more and more towns developed first aid clubs, contests in first aid were held between the towns. In 1908, members of the executive committee of the American Red Cross (ARC) observed a first aid contest. This led to the organization of the ARC First Aid Bureau. To assist the ARC in developing a national first aid course, Colonel Charles Lynch was detailed from the U. S. Army. In 1910, Lynch wrote the first in a long series of Red Cross first aid textbooks.

Until the early 1970s, **ARC Advanced First Aid** was the de facto standard for ambulance personnel. Although most personnel were trained to this level, there were no standards for ambulance crews, so

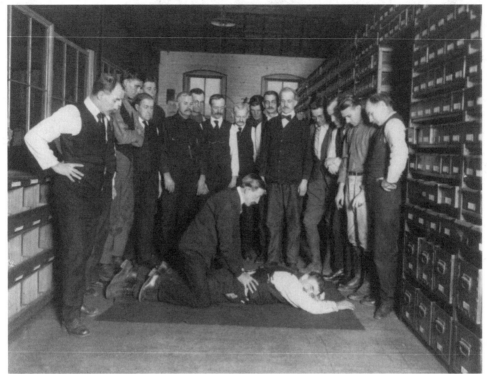

Courtesy of Library of Congress.

Figure 4-1 An early first aid club.

some services responded with personnel who had no formal training or who had received minimal in-house training at the local rescue station. It is interesting to note that ARC first aid manuals from the 1960s state what should be done "until the ambulance arrives," yet these very manuals were the ones being used to train the ambulance personnel.

The publication of *Accidental Death and Disability: The Neglected Disease of Modern Society* (NAS/NRC, 1966) exposed the poor level of training for ambulance providers. The document stated the following:

> *There are no generally accepted standards for the competence or training of ambulance attendants. Attendants range from unschooled apprentices lacking training even in elementary first aid to poorly paid employees, public-spirited volunteers, and specially trained full-time personnel of fire, police, or commercial ambulance companies.*

The EMS Committee of the National Academy of Sciences, National Research Council (NAS/NRC), investigated the training of ambulance personnel. In response, it published *Training of Ambulance Personnel and Others Responsible for Emergency Care of the Sick and Injured at the Scene and During Transport* in 1969. This report outlined basic topics to be covered in a training program for ambulance personnel. The report also called for the establishment of a national training curriculum.

Concurrent with the work of the NAS/NRC, the U.S. Department of Transportation (DOT), as part of an initiative to reduce highway fatalities, released a request for proposals (RFP) to develop a **national standard curriculum** for emergency medical technicians (EMTs). As a result of this federal involvement, an 81-hour national standard curriculum for training of EMTs was adopted in 1970. Revised over the years, this curriculum became the EMT-Basic National Standard Curriculum, last revised in 1994. Subsequent national standard curriculums were created for the EMT-Paramedic, EMT-Intermediate, and first responder. In 2009, the National EMS Educational Standards replaced the EMT-Basic National Standard Curriculum as the basis for emergency medical services (EMS) education. The National EMS Education Standards were a departure from the more rigid and extensive EMT-Basic National Standard Curriculum, but provide more flexibility to institutions, faculty, and students in the delivery of EMS education.

Controversies in EMS Education

Acceptance of EMT and paramedic training was not universal and immediate. For years, ARC Advanced First Aid had been the standard. Many providers resisted EMT training, viewing it as too complex and too long. A common refrain was "What are they trying to do, make us doctors?" This was especially true among ambulance providers in career departments, many of whom had been providing service for years and were now required to return to the classroom to take new training from doctors and nurses. EMT training also required a more rigorous approach to testing, including practical testing. This was in contrast to the less stringent requirements of many first aid courses. Even to this day, concern over the length of a course is often more of an issue than the course objectives or advantage to the patient.

Another controversy in EMS education is the importance of **skills** in defining **provider levels**. Although the amount of knowledge increases as one moves from EMT to paramedic, providers have historically measured their increased responsibility in terms of the number and nature of new skills that they can perform. The **National EMS Core Content** defines all of the skills available to EMS providers. The skills each level of provider can perform as well as the required knowledge to effectively perform these skills in the field are outlined in the *National EMS Scope of Practice*. As one moves from EMR to paramedic, not only do the number of skills increase but also the level of knowledge as to the "what" and "why" of prehospital medicine, in addition to the "how."

Perhaps the greatest influence on EMS education has been the unfortunate situation of education guiding policy instead of the inverse. In an ideal situation, education would serve to teach students system policy. Instead, education has been used as a tool to force system change and to influence policy and protocols. It is not uncommon for students to learn techniques and medications that are not currently approved in their EMS system, or to learn a certain **protocol** to pass a **certifying examination** only to "unlearn" it to function appropriately in their local system. This is frustrating to students and causes tension between educators and administrators. EMS professionals hope that the implementation of the educational process presented by the *EMS Education Agenda for the Future: A Systems Approach* will resolve this and other current controversies in EMS education.

National Standard Curriculum

Due to federal involvement in the curriculum development process, a series of national standard curricula were developed for EMS provider education. EMS was unique in that it was the only health profession to have a formalized, standard curriculum that was nationally accepted. In other areas of allied health education, standards or guidelines exist for education and training. However, these standards are not an actual curriculum complete with learning objectives and lesson plans.

A national standard curriculum provided a basis for education. Because the curriculum was designed for national acceptance, it provides a foundation upon which states and regions can build local training programs. Many states have developed their own local training curricula, building on the national standard. Some states have even codified the national curriculum as part of their EMS legislation, thus complicating the transition to the new National EMS Standards. The common foundation of a national curriculum, however, was to ensure some degree of commonality between training programs and to provide a basis for national certification and reciprocity (acceptance of training and certification by another jurisdiction). However, because the curriculum was designed for national acceptance, it is in many ways a compromise. It is impossible to write a curriculum that will ideally serve every EMS jurisdiction. Realization of this limitation was one of the impetuses for the development of the *EMS Education Agenda for the Future: A Systems Approach*, which has replaced the national standard curriculum with core content, a practice model, and educational standards.

EMS Education Agenda for the Future

The *EMS Agenda for the Future* identified 14 attributes and indicated a specific agenda should be developed for each. In response, the *EMS Education Agenda for the Future: A Systems Approach* (the cover of which is shown in **Figure 4-2**) was developed for the education systems attribute. A task force of administrators, medical directors, regulators, educators, and providers worked together to develop the *EMS Education Agenda* that was accepted by the National Highway Traffic Safety Administration (NHTSA) in 2000. Full implementation of the *EMS Education Agenda* was projected for 2010; however, this goal has not been met as parts of the agenda are still being implemented. The following five components covering curriculum, testing, and accreditation make up the *EMS Education Agenda*.

National EMS Core Content

In the past, EMS providers were taught using a national standard curriculum based on a *National EMS and Education Blueprint*. Now, the knowledge, skills, and attitudes needed for each provider level are broadly defined in the National EMS Core Content. The core content presents a broad overview of what an EMS provider must know and be able to do. It is broad in focus to allow for state-of-the-art changes as well as state and regional variations. It is also based on research and a practice analysis, neither of which were used to significantly develop the previous national standard curriculum. Because the core content is global in scope, individual provider levels can be defined as they are needed, building on the foundation of the Blueprint. Although new to EMS, the idea of core content has been used in the education of other professions. Information on the National EMS Core Content can be found at www.nhtsa.dot.gov/.

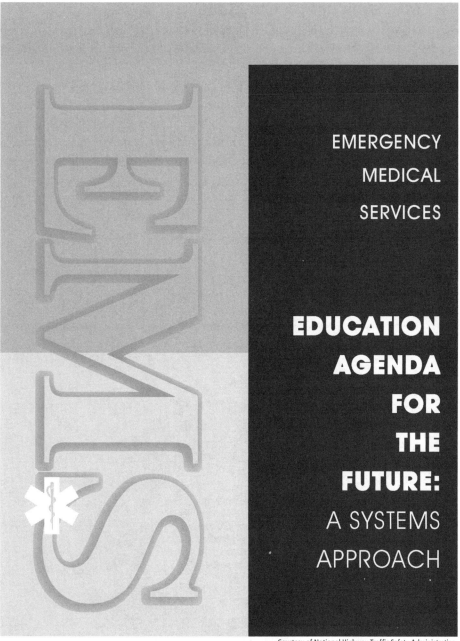

Figure 4-2 EMS Education Agenda for the Future.

National EMS Scope of Practice Model

The *National EMS Scope of Practice Model* was developed from, and replaced, the Blueprint. It defines the levels of EMS providers, the knowledge and skills needed for each provider level, and the entry competencies for each level. The scope is the basis for state scopes of practice and reciprocity. A copy of the *National EMS Scope of Practice Model* can also be found on the NHTSA website.

The scope of practice (SOP) is defined in the document as " … a legal description of the distinction between licensed health care personnel and the lay public and among different licensed health care professionals." In other words, the SOP identifies the levels of EMS providers and their titles, and defines what they can and cannot do medically. However, broad and general activities routinely carried out by all levels of EMS providers (such as lifting and moving patients) are not specifically defined in the SOP as such activities cover many different techniques and approaches and do not have specific medical control requirements (**Figure 4-3**).

For each level of EMS provider, the SOP provides three areas of information. The first is the "Description of the Profession." This narrative describes the role, function, and interaction and autonomy of the provider as well as the education required to be licensed at that level. Next is a listing of the psychomotor (hands-on) skills to be performed by providers at each level. Finally, the SOP lists, in broad terms, the level of knowledge needed to function at a particular provider level.

To assist users in better understanding the *National EMS Scope of Practice*, appendix A (**Figure 4-4**) is provided, which describes the interpretive guidelines for each of the major skill areas.

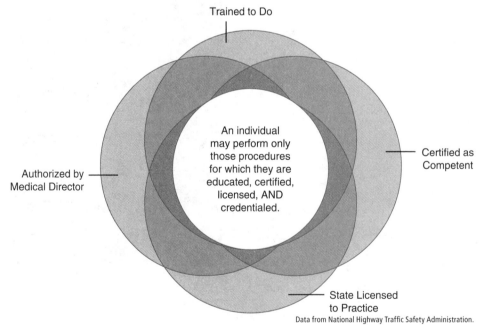

Trained to Do

An individual may perform only those procedures for which they are educated, certified, licensed, AND credentialed.

Certified as Competent

Authorized by Medical Director

State Licensed to Practice

Data from National Highway Traffic Safety Administration.

Figure 4-3 Relationship among education, certification, licensure, and credentialing.

Appendix A: Interpretive Guidelines

The interpretive guidelines are used to help guide the users of this document by providing additional insight into the discussions and deliberations that revolved around the decisions of the Scope of Practice Task Force. These interpretive guidelines represent the collective opinions of the Scope of Practice team in June 2005.

The interpretive guidelines are included to allow future users to apply similar methodology in deciding the appropriateness of new interventions at each provider level. *They are illustrative, and NOT all-inclusive.*

> The interpretive guidelines are intended to guide the development of National EMS Education Standards, National EMS Certification, and National EMS Education Program Accreditation. The interpretive guidelines will also assist State regulatory agencies in developing and further refining their legislation and administrative rules/regulations. ***These guidelines are not intended to appear in practice acts.***

Airway and Breathing Minimum Psychomotor Skill Set

Emergency Medical Responder	Emergency Medical Technician	Advanced EMT	Paramedic
Oral airway BVM Sellick's Maneuver Head-tilt chin lift Jaw thrust Modified chin lift Obstruction–manual Oxygen therapy Nasal cannula Non-rebreather face mask Upper airway suctioning	Humidifiers Partial rebreathers Venturi mask Manually Triggered Ventilator (MTV) Automatic Transport Ventilator (ATV) Oral and Nasal airways	Esophageal-Tracheal Multi-Lumen Airways	BiPAP/CPAP Needle chest decompression Chest tube monitoring Percutaneous cricothyrotomy[2] ETCO$_2$/Capnography NG/OG tube Nasal and oral Endotracheal intubation Airway obstruction removal by direct laryngoscopy PEEP

[2] Percutaneous means access via needle-puncture (or other approved puncture device) and DOES NOT include "surgical" access using a scalpel.

Assessment Minimum Psychomotor Skill Set

Emergency Medical Responder	Emergency Medical Technician	Advanced EMT	Paramedic
Manual BP	Pulse oximetry Manual and auto BP	Blood glucose monitor	EKG interpretation Interpretive 12 Lead Blood chemistry analysis

Figure 4-4 National EMS Scope of Practice, Appendix A: Interpretive Guidelines.

Pharmacological Intervention Minimum Psychomotor Skill Set

Emergency Medical Responder	Emergency Medical Technician	Advanced EMT	Paramedic
Tech of Med Administration -Unit dose auto-injectors for self or peer care (MARK I)	Assisted Medications -Assisting a patient in administering his/her own prescribed medications, including auto-injection Tech of Med Administration -Buccal -Oral Administered Meds -PHYSICIAN-approved over-the-counter medications (oral glucose, ASA for chest pain of suspected ischemic origin)	Peripheral IV insertion IV fluid infusion Pediatric IO Tech of Med Administration -Aerosolized -Subcutaneous -Intramuscular -Nebulized -Sublingual -Intranasal -IV push of D50 and narcotic antagonist only Administered Meds -SL Nitroglycerine for chest pain of suspected ischemic origin -SQ or IM epinephrine for anaphylaxis -glucagon and IV D50 for hypoglycemia -Inhaled beta agonist for dyspnea and wheezing -Narcotic antagonist -Nitrous oxide for pain relief	Central line monitoring IO insertion Venous blood sampling Tech of Med Administration -Endotracheal -IV (push and infusion) -NG -Rectal -IO -Topical -Accessing implanted central IV port Administered Meds -Physician-approved medications -Maintenance of blood administration -Thrombolytics initiation

Emergency Trauma Care Minimum Psychomotor Skill Set

Emergency Medical Responder	Emergency Medical Technician	Advanced EMT	Paramedic
Manual cervical stabilization Manual extremity stabilization Eye irrigation Direct pressure Hemorrhage control Emergency moves for endangered patients	Spinal immobilization Seated spinal immobilization Long board Extremity splinting Traction splinting Mechanical pt restraint Tourniquet MAST/PASG Cervical collar Rapid extrication		Morgan lens

Medical/Cardiac Care Minimum Psychomotor Skill Set

Emergency Medical Responder	Emergency Medical Technician	Advanced EMT	Paramedic
CPR AED Assisted normal delivery	Mechanical CPR Assisted complicated delivery		Cardioversion Carotid massage Manual defibrillation TC pacing

Figure 4-4 *(Continued)*

National EMS Education Standards

The core content and SOP together form the basis for the education of EMS providers. The National EMS Education Standards identify the minimal terminal education objective for students completing training at each provider level. The standards are the closest of the five components to the former national standard curriculum. All educational programs are required to teach to the standards, but how they achieve the **terminal objectives** is not specified. Institutions and instructors may use any approach or technology they like—as long as they produce competent students. This makes changes in both the core content and educational technology, as well as regional and state variations, easier to implement. However, this flexibility requires institutions and regulatory agencies to engage in continued evaluation of the educational process and **student outcomes** to ensure its quality and compliance with the educational program.

For each provider level, a **competency** is provided for each of the major areas of prehospital care. Associated with each competency is an elaboration of knowledge and a description of the **clinical behaviors and judgments**, as shown in **Figure 4-5**.

Because the National EMS Education Standards are a significant departure from the traditional national standard curriculums, the standards contain **Instructional Guidelines** that provide additional information to assist the instructor in the transition to the standards from the national standard curriculum. It is anticipated that future versions of the standards will not contain the instructional guidelines.

One area of controversy that has continually plagued EMS education is the idea of setting a minimum number of **contact hours** for each level of provider. EMS educators argue that competency should be measured by student performance, not the number of hours spent in the classroom (didactic), laboratory, and clinical and field experience. Agencies and jurisdictions, on the other hand, have a need for some range of program hours for planning and budgeting purposes. To address this need, the standards

Format of National EMS Education Standards				
	EMR	**EMT**	**AEMT**	**PARAMEDIC**
Content Area	Competency	Competency	Competency	Competency
Elaboration of Knowledge	Additional knowledge related to the competency	Additional knowledge related to the competency	Additional knowledge related to the competency	Additional knowledge related to the competency
	Clinical behaviors and judgments	Clinical behaviors and judgments	Clinical behaviors and judgments	Clinical behaviors and judgments
	Educational Infrastructure	Educational Infrastructure	Educational Infrastructure	Educational Infrastructure

Reproduced from National Highway Traffic Safety Administration.

Figure 4-5 National EMS Educational Standards: Format.

TABLE 4-1 Suggested Training Hours for Each Level of EMS Provider				
	EMR	**EMT**	**AEMT**	**PARAMEDIC**
Suggested course length in hours	48–60	150–190	150–250	Reference Committee on Accreditation for EMS Professions (CoAEMSP) *Standards and Guidelines*

Suggested training hours for EMS educational programs.

suggest a range of training hours (**Table 4-1**) for each provider level. The standards also provide the flexibility to use various methods of program delivery, including such nontraditional approaches as online or computer-assisted learning.

National EMS Education Program Accreditation

The *EMS Education Agenda* calls for the national accreditation of all EMS training programs to assure students and consumers that the education being provided meets national guidelines. Previously, educational program accreditation was voluntary except in states that required all paramedic education to be accredited by the Committee on Accreditation of Emergency Medical Services Professions (CoAEMSP). National accreditation provides for self-review and peer assessment of educational programs as a means to ensure quality and compliance with national guidelines. However, this remains an area of controversy in the implementation of the *EMS Education Agenda*, because it is possible that some states may assume the role of the accreditation body. There is also a financial cost associated with the current accreditation process that may be burdensome for some small programs. However, the sole national EMS certification body, the National Registry of EMTs, has mandated that it will test for certification only those paramedic candidates who have completed a CoAEMSP accredited program.

National EMS Certification

The states grant the authority—either in the form of certification or licensure—to practice as an EMS provider at any level. Certification is a means to identify people who have demonstrated a minimally acceptable level of proficiency. Certification may be obtained from states or recognized certification bodies. Licensure is authorization from an agency to practice based on the evidence of competency or certification. Currently, the National Registry of EMTs is the only organization providing competency testing at a national level.

The *EMS Education Agenda* calls for the establishment of a single, independent, testing agency providing national EMS certification. This agency would be accepted by all states as certifying minimal competency for all levels of providers. Only graduates of nationally accredited education programs would be permitted to participate in national testing. As with national accreditation, national testing remains controversial because of its impact on the role of states in the certification process and because it would require the acceptance of one national testing agency.

The National Registry of EMTs

As EMT and paramedic training opportunities increased in the early 1970s, the need for a uniform method of evaluating EMTs and paramedics was recognized. Many states had not yet developed formal certification or licensure procedures. Thus the National Registry of Emergency Medical Technicians was formed in 1970 with support from the American Medical Association (AMA). The formation of this national registration body served to increase the recognition of EMTs and aid their acceptance by the medical community. The National Registry, as it is commonly known, is a nonprofit independent non-governmental agency. The National Registry develops standardized examinations for all levels of EMS providers as well as standards for registration and reregistration.

Currently, the National Registry plays an important role in EMT and paramedic education and certification. National Registry registration is used by many states as a means to grant reciprocity. It is also gaining wide acceptance by states as a primary means of EMT and paramedic testing as well as moving to fill the role of a national certifying agency, as specified in the *EMS Education Agenda*. Up-to-date information on states' acceptance of the National Registry can be obtained on the National Registry website: www.nremt.org. Representatives from the National Registry serve on various EMS-related boards and commissions and provide assistance in practice analysis and curriculum development.

CoAEMSP

As the number of institutions providing EMS education continued to grow, a means was needed to measure and ensure program quality. In 1975, the paramedic was recognized by the AMA as an allied health occupation. In 1976, a number of national organizations developed educational standards for paramedic education programs. These standards, or **essentials**, were adopted by the Council on Medical Education of the AMA as the basis for accreditation of paramedic education programs. A Joint Review Committee on Educational Programs for the EMT-Paramedic (JRCEMT-P) was formed to review and recommend programs for accreditation.

In 1994, the JRCEMT-P became part of the **Commission on Accreditation of Allied Health Education Programs (CAAHEP)**, an organization formed following the withdrawal of the AMA from the allied health accreditation process. CAAHEP accredits 18 recognized allied health professions and is recognized as a national accreditation body by the Commission on Recognition of Postsecondary Accreditation (CORPA) and the U.S. Department of Education. In 2000, CAAHEP reorganized its accreditation bodies into Committees on Accreditation (CoA). The JRCEMT-P became the Committee on Accreditation of Emergency Medical Services Professions (CoAEMSP). This name change also signaled the intention of the CoAEMSP to begin providing accreditation for all levels of EMS provider education programs, not just paramedic education. This was in anticipation of the call for a national accreditation contained in the *EMS Education Agenda*.

To become accredited, a program must comply with the CoAEMSP guidelines. After completing a formal application, the applying institution completes an extensive **self-study**. A referee reviews the study and, if it is found to be complete, a **site visit** is authorized. During the site visit, a **program director** and a medical director visit the site and verify compliance with the guidelines. If all reports are acceptable, the institution is granted accreditation for a given term. To remain accredited, the institution must submit yearly progress reports and reapply as required by the CoAEMSP.

Although useful as a means to recognize educational programs that meet a set of nationally accepted guidelines, accreditation has for the most part been voluntary, and is currently only available at the paramedic level. Some states and regions have developed their own accreditation programs similar to the national model, which may be required in addition to or in lieu of national accreditation.

Settings for EMS Education

The delivery of EMS education has traditionally taken place in a wide variety of venues, including healthcare organizations, educational institutions, public safety agencies, and the military. The National EMS Education Standards suggestions for each level of EMS provider are shown in **Figure 4-6**.

In addition, most states and accreditation agencies require that EMS training programs be both state-approved and conducted by an acceptable sponsoring agency. For paramedic programs, the standards approved by the CoAEMSP for program accreditation are often used.

Hospitals

Hospitals are connected to EMS through their emergency departments. Hospitals have long been involved in providing EMS education. During the late 1960s and early 1970s, hospitals were the primary source of experienced healthcare professionals with an interest in EMS. Many hospitals had established nursing and allied health education programs that could provide the personnel and resources required to train EMTs and paramedics. The availability of a hospital in most communities meant that EMS education could be offered to a wide variety of EMS providers. It was in the best

Educational Infrastructure				
	EMR	**EMT**	**AEMT**	**PARAMEDIC**
Educational Facilities	■ Facility sponsored or approved by sponsoring agency ■ ADA-compliant facility ■ Sufficient space for class size ■ Controlled environment	Same as previous level	Same as previous level	■ Reference Committee on Accreditation for EMS Professions (CoAEMSP) *Standards and Guidelines* (www.coaemsp.org)[1]

[1]The *National EMS Education Agenda for the Future: A Systems Approach* calls for national accreditation of paramedic programs. CoAEMSP is currently the only national agency that offers EMS paramedic education program accreditation; it is used or recognized by most states. While the CoAEMSP *Standards and Guidelines* are adopted for the Education Infrastructure section, this does not itself require the program to be CoAEMSP accredited. Recognition of national accreditation is the responsibility of each State.

Figure 4-6 Guidelines for educational facilities at each level of EMS provider.

interest of hospitals to participate in EMS education as they were often the receiving site for patients treated by EMS personnel. In urban areas where hospital catchment areas overlapped, investing in EMS education was often seen as a means to encourage EMTs to transport patients to a participating hospital, thus directly affecting hospital revenue. Some hospitals even started their own EMS services.

Because of the requirement for clinical training in the advanced levels of EMT, hospitals have taken a more active role in this area. However, some institutions do provide classroom space for EMT instruction that is provided by non-hospital-affiliated instructors. Often, hospital-based EMS instruction is coordinated either through the hospital's existing training department or by an EMS coordinator working for the emergency department. Hospitals have even developed paramedic training programs into self-supporting enterprises.

Fire Departments

The history of early EMS is filled with examples of fire departments taking a pioneering role in the development of EMS, especially in the area of advanced life support (ALS). One reason for this involvement was that fire departments were already in place as a means to provide emergency services. Likewise, they had an organizational and training structure that could easily be adapted to support EMS activities.

Fire departments have always placed great emphasis on training. Most fire departments have an identified training staff as well as a training facility. Often referred to as the **academy**, this facility is the focal point for training activities. It is the site for training new recruits, thus the common reference in the fire service of "having gone through the academy." As the fire service expanded its role into EMS, the academy has become the focal point for EMS training activities as well. Various models for the delivery of EMS training by fire academies have evolved. In some departments, EMS training is a division of the training staff. In others, EMS training is a function of the EMS division, but is usually offered in conjunction with the academy staff (**Figure 4-7**).

In suburban and rural fire departments, often fully or partially staffed by volunteers, the provision of EMS training may take many forms. Local jurisdictions may have a centrally located training center that serves the needs of local fire departments. A dedicated training staff or coordinator may be employed, or part-time and volunteer instructors may staff the center. In some states, a statewide training agency provides extension or field courses in the local area, often at centrally located fire stations or training facilities. In rural or less organized locations, the provision of EMS training may be handled by the individual fire departments, using internal company instructors or local resources.

Because of the unique nature of EMS training, fire departments often partner with other agencies to provide the necessary training and field experience. For example, a fire department may enlist the assistance of a nurse from the local hospital to provide instruction while utilizing the hospital as a clinical experience site. Other educational institutions, such as community colleges or technical training centers, may partner with the fire department to provide classroom and instructional infrastructure for effective EMS training.

With the renewed emphasis on national accreditation put forth by the *EMS Education Agenda*, the CoAEMSP has developed standards for fire departments that are recognized by the state as an educational entity to become accredited. Other fire departments seeking such accreditation are establishing

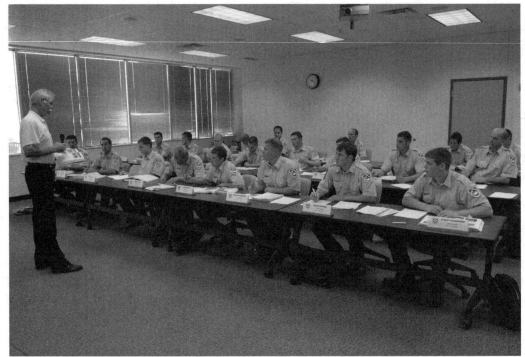

Figure 4-7 Fire department EMS class in session.

relationships with healthcare institutions or colleges to meet the requirements of the CoAEMSP. Some departments are even phasing out their in-house training and contracting with a community college, four-year college, or university to provide all of their AEMT and paramedic training needs.

Technical Centers

The development of EMS fostered the need to provide EMS training to individuals and organizations not traditionally associated with EMS delivery, including businesses, factories, industrial safety teams, organizations, and others who might need to provide on-site emergency care to special populations. As many of the traditional EMS training facilities were unable to meet the needs of such groups, either commercially operated **technical training centers** developed or an EMS curriculum was added at existing institutions. The rise of commercial providers of EMS also spawned the need for stand-alone EMS training operations.

In most states, the provision of technical training by private institutions is closely regulated, and centers and programs are usually required to be accredited. The curriculum usually follows a national standard to provide students with the greatest potential for employment. Most proprietary training centers are eligible for national accreditation if they are recognized as a higher education institution by a regional educational accrediting body.

Community Colleges

Community, junior, and technical colleges play an important role in EMS education, especially at the higher levels of ALS training. Community college offerings fall into two broad categories: credit and noncredit programs. Students enrolled in a credit program not only complete course work leading to certification or licensure, but also receive college credit that can be applied toward a degree or certificate. Noncredit programs are often provided under contract with a fire department, a hospital, or a private provider as a means to provide training for their personnel. This approach eliminates the need for an agency to maintain a dedicated training staff and facility. Faculty for community college programs often come from the ranks of the agency or group for which the training is offered.

The role of the community college in EMS education has increased over the years. With the development of national EMS education standards that require prerequisite instruction in areas such as anatomy and physiology, community colleges are ideally suited to provide program instruction and coordination. The increasing sophistication of EMS education makes the community college an ideal setting for program delivery and is recommended in the *National EMS Scope of Practice* document as the venue of choice for paramedic education. More and more states mandate that paramedic education must take place at the community college level; some even require paramedics to have at least an associate's degree.

Colleges and Universities

Four-year colleges and universities have made a recent entry into the education of EMS providers. Since 1980, a number of institutions have been providing baccalaureate education in emergency health services. In addition, graduate-level programs are now available.

The approach to EMS education in colleges can be grouped in three ways. The first approach is to offer a strictly clinical curriculum leading to a paramedic certification. This is most common among programs offered in conjunction with academic health centers and allied health programs. The second approach is a combination curriculum that provides clinical education along with administrative and management education. Such programs often have agreements with business or management departments to provide the required nonclinical course work. The third configuration is a nonclinical curriculum that does not lead to clinical certification or licensure but prepares EMS providers for leadership positions in EMS agencies.

To facilitate the educational needs of paramedics who have received training outside of a college or university, some colleges provide the means to formally recognize this training. Enrolled students are able to challenge clinical courses for credit via written and practical testing. Students who have completed paramedic training at a site that is accredited by the CAAHEP may also directly receive academic credit from some institutions. Likewise, many public four-year colleges have "2 + 2" articulation agreements (two years of community college plus two years at a four-year college) with community colleges.

This ensures graduates of community college programs admission into the program and allows them to enter with 60 credits toward a degree.

Military

The military has an obvious need to train personnel to serve as medics or corpsmen for providing immediate care to wounded personnel and to staff aid stations, clearing stations, and field hospitals. Additionally, the military must provide basic EMS services to military, dependent, and civilian personnel at larger military installations worldwide. Combat medics are given the designation "91 Whiskey" by the military.

The training of military personnel closely follows the provider levels in civilian EMS. Medics and corpsmen are trained as EMTs, with some receiving AEMT and paramedic level training. Because military personnel are likely to be reassigned on a regular basis, it is not practical to have local certification or licensure. To address the need for certification, the military makes use of National Registry certification. The National Registry even provides special "military style" certification patches for uniforms. Because military personnel have had training equivalent to civilian EMS providers, the military is a ready source of trained providers, both after personnel leave the military and while they are still on active duty. It is not uncommon for military personnel living in a civilian community to volunteer or work part time for EMS services.

A current trend in military medical education and continuing education is the reduction of such training by the military and a reliance on civilian training sources and contractors for general medical education. This is especially true for specialized courses commonly provided to civilian EMS personnel.

Provider Courses

The complexity and length of the initial training course for each level of EMS provider depends on the SOP for that particular level. The four levels of provider are designed to build on the knowledge and skills learned at each level, although completion of one level is not necessarily required for advancement to another. However, each level of provider assumes mastery of the previous level competencies and clinical behaviors. Thus someone enrolling directly into a paramedic program will be required to master the competencies and clinical behaviors of the EMR, EMT, and AEMT levels.

The National EMS Education Standards group the competencies for each level into traditional areas of EMS instruction, with the difference being the breadth and depth of the knowledge and skills required for each level. At the EMR and EMT/AEMT levels, the student is taught an assessment approach to patient care. In this approach, the student is taught to assess the patient in a particular way and order and to respond to findings with a particular response or action. At the paramedic level, instruction takes a more diagnostic approach in that the student is taught to analyze a number of assessment and clinical findings and arrive at a field diagnosis to develop a specific treatment plan. The broad grouping of competencies in the National EMS Education Standards is presented in **Figure 4-8**.

	EMR	EMT	AEMT	PARAMEDIC
Preparatory	Uses simple knowledge of the EMS system, the safety/well-being of the EMR, and medical/legal issues at the scene of an emergency while awaiting a higher level of care.	Applies fundamental knowledge of the EMS system, the safety/well-being of the EMT, and medical/legal and ethical issues to the provision of emergency care.	Applies fundamental knowledge of the EMS system, the safety/well-being of the AEMT, and medical/legal and ethical issues to the provision of emergency care.	Integrates comprehensive knowledge of EMS systems, the safety/well-being of the paramedic, and medical/legal and ethical issues that are intended to improve the health of EMS personnel, patients, and the community.
Anatomy and Physiology	Uses simple knowledge of the anatomy and function of the upper airway, heart, vessels, blood, lungs, skin, muscles, and bones as the foundation of emergency care.	Applies fundamental knowledge of the anatomy and function of all human systems to the practice of EMS.	Integrates complex knowledge of the anatomy and physiology of the airway, respiratory, and circulatory systems to the practice of EMS.	Integrates a complex depth and comprehensive breadth of knowledge of the anatomy and physiology of all human systems.
Medical Terminology	Uses simple medical and anatomical terms.	Uses foundational anatomical and medical terms and abbreviations in written and oral communication with colleagues and other health care professionals.	Same as previous level	Integrates comprehensive anatomical and medical terminology and abbreviations into written and oral communications with colleagues and other health care professionals.
Pathophysiology	Uses simple knowledge of shock and respiratory compromise to respond to life threats.	Applies fundamental knowledge of the pathophysiology of respiration and perfusion to patient assessment and management.	Applies comprehensive knowledge of the pathophysiology of respiration and perfusion to patient assessment and management.	Integrates comprehensive knowledge of the pathophysiology of major human systems.

Figure 4-8 Broad grouping of competencies from EMS Educational Standards.

	EMR	EMT	AEMT	PARAMEDIC
Life Span Development	Uses simple knowledge of age-related differences to assess and care for patients.	Applies fundamental knowledge of life span development to patient assessment and management.	Same as previous level	Integrates comprehensive knowledge of life span development.
Public Health	Has an awareness of local public health resources and the role EMS personnel play in public health emergencies.	Uses simple knowledge of the principles of illness and injury prevention in emergency care.	Uses simple knowledge of the principles of the role of EMS during public health emergencies.	Applies fundamental knowledge of principles of public health and epidemiology including public health emergencies, health promotion, and illness and injury prevention.
Pharmacology	Uses simple knowledge of the medications that the EMR may self-administer or administer to a peer in an emergency.	Applies fundamental knowledge of the medications that the EMT may assist/administer to a patient during an emergency.	Applies to patient assessment and management fundamental knowledge of the medications carried by AEMTs that may be administered to a patient during an emergency.	Integrates comprehensive knowledge of pharmacology to formulate a treatment plan intended to mitigate emergencies and improve the overall health of the patient.
Airway Management, Respiration, and Artificial Ventilation	Applies knowledge (fundamental depth, foundational breadth) of general anatomy and physiology to assure a patent airway, adequate mechanical ventilation, and respiration while awaiting additional EMS response for patients of all ages.	Applies knowledge (fundamental depth, foundational breadth) of general anatomy and physiology to patient assessment and management in order to assure a patent airway, adequate mechanical ventilation, and respiration for patients of all ages.	Applies knowledge (fundamental depth, foundational breadth) of additional upper airway anatomy and physiology to patient assessment and management in order to assure a patent airway, adequate mechanical ventilation, and respiration for patients of all ages.	Integrates complex knowledge of anatomy, physiology, and pathophysiology into the assessment to develop and implement a treatment plan with the goal of assuring a patent airway, adequate mechanical ventilation, and respiration for patients of all ages.

Figure 4-8 (Continued)

	EMR	**EMT**	**AEMT**	**PARAMEDIC**
Assessment	Uses scene information and simple patient assessment findings to identify and manage immediate life threats and injuries within the scope of practice of the EMR.	Applies scene information and patient assessment findings (scene size-up, primary and secondary assessment, patient history, and reassessment) to guide emergency management.	Same as previous level	Integrate scene and patient assessment findings with knowledge of epidemiology and pathophysiology to form a field impression. This includes developing a list of differential diagnoses through clinical reasoning to modify the assessment and formulate a treatment plan.
Medicine	Recognizes and manages life threats based on assessment findings of a patient with a medical emergency while awaiting additional emergency response.	Applies fundamental knowledge to provide basic emergency care and transportation based on assessment findings for an acutely ill patient.	Applies fundamental knowledge to provide basic and selected advanced emergency care and transportation based on assessment findings for an acutely ill patient.	Integrates assessment findings with principles of epidemiology and pathophysiology to formulate a field impression and implement a comprehensive treatment/disposition plan for a patient with a medical complaint.
Shock and Resuscitation	Uses assessment information to recognize shock, respiratory failure or arrest, and cardiac arrest based on assessment findings; manages the emergency while awaiting additional emergency response.	Applies funda-mental knowledge of the causes, pathophysiology, and manage-ment of shock, respiratory failure or arrest, cardiac failure or arrest, and post-resuscitation management.	Applies fundamental knowledge to provide basic and selected advanced emergency care and transportation based on assessment findings for a patient in shock, respiratory failure or arrest, cardiac failure or arrest, and post-resuscitation management.	Integrates comprehensive knowledge of causes and pathophysiology into the management of cardiac arrest and peri-arrest states. Integrates a comprehensive knowledge of the causes and pathophysiology into the management of shock and respiratory failure or arrest with an emphasis on early intervention to prevent arrest.

Figure 4-8 *(Continued)*

	EMR	EMT	AEMT	PARAMEDIC
Trauma	Uses simple knowledge to recognize and manage life threats based on assessment findings for an acutely injured patient while awaiting additional emergency medical response.	Applies fundamental knowledge to provide basic emergency care and transportation based on assessment findings for an acutely injured patient.	Applies fundamental knowledge to provide basic and selected advanced emergency care and transportation based on assessment findings for an acutely injured patient.	Integrates assessment findings with principles of epidemiology and pathophysiology to formulate a field impression to implement a comprehensive treatment/disposition plan for an acutely injured patient.
Special Patient Populations	Recognizes and manages life threats based on simple assessment findings for a patient with special needs while awaiting additional emergency response.	Applies a fundamental knowledge of growth, development and aging, and assessment findings to provide basic emergency care and transportation for a patient with special needs.	Applies a fundamental knowledge of growth, development and aging, and assessment findings to provide basic and selected advanced emergency care and transportation for a patient with special needs.	Integrates assessment findings with principles of pathophysiology and knowledge of psychosocial needs to formulate a field impression and implement a comprehensive treatment/disposition plan for patients with special needs.
EMS Operations	Knowledge of operational roles and responsi- bilities to ensure patient, public, and personnel safety.	Same as previous level	Same as previous level	Same as previous level

Figure 4-8 *(Continued)*

For each level of provider, the course also provides laboratory (skills practice or simulation), clinical (in-hospital), and field (riding an ambulance) instruction. The competencies to be mastered in this area are listed in the standards as "Clinical Behavior/Judgment." These consist of:

- Assessment;
- Therapeutic communications and cultural competency;
- Psychomotor skills;
- Professionalism;
- Decision making;

- Record keeping;
- Patient complaints;
- Scene leadership; and
- Scene safety.

Specialized Courses

Although EMS education is centered on national core content and educational standards, there has been a need for specialized courses that focus on particular patient populations. Stand-alone courses to address the specific needs of the trauma victim, cardiac victim, and pediatric patient have been developed. These "alphabet soup" courses are presented in an intense format usually designed around a weekend program of 16 hours. Textbooks, instructional materials, and instructor training are provided by the sponsoring agency. Students are required to pass a written or practical (or both) test to receive a certificate of successful completion.

Continuing Education and Refresher Training

Prehospital provider education exposes the student to a vast body of knowledge and a variety of skills. The comprehensive nature of EMS requires that the student possess a basic knowledge of a wide variety of medical conditions and complications. However, the length of EMS training programs is insufficient to develop competency in all areas. Additionally, the case mix seen by the average field provider does not provide an opportunity for practice in all areas of EMS. Thus over time, the provider is inclined to forget rarely used knowledge and skills. This natural decay of proficiency is one reason why continuing education and refresher training is required of most certified or licensed prehospital providers.

The field of medicine in general, and of EMS in particular, is constantly changing. New approaches, procedures, drugs, and equipment continually appear. Each new addition requires that the field provider receive training in the new intervention. In order to keep current professionally, the field provider must participate in **continuing education**. Continuing education also provides a means for reviewing areas that quality assurance assessments identify as needing attention.

Continuing education for EMS providers is often part of **recertification** or **relicensure** requirements. Providers are required to complete a minimum number of hours, often in specified topic areas or a formalized refresher course. Additional hours in area(s) of the provider's choice may be required to meet the total hour requirement. Run sheet reviews, case presentations, and rounds are examples of other approaches to continuing education.

Because of the varied nature of continuing education, a system was needed to "collect" continuing education credits and to standardize the value of a continuing education experience. This is provided by the use of **continuing education units (CEU)**. One CEU is awarded for participation in a set number of hours of continuing education. The term "continuing medical education" (CME) is commonly used for physician continuing education. The value of a CEU and approval for a program to offer CEUs are determined by the various professional and regulatory agencies in the EMS field. To standardize

EMS education, the national Continuing Education Coordinating Board for EMS (CECBEMS) was formed, comprising representatives from EMS organizations. The board approves continuing education programs and assigns the number of CEUs to be awarded.

For continuing education to be effective, it must be available to providers in a convenient form. Providers wishing to participate in continuing education may do so through any of the following activities:

- Conferences and expositions
- Local training programs
- Regional or state training programs
- Articles in trade journals
- Subscription videotapes
- Satellite and cable broadcasts
- Commercial training enterprises
- Online educational resources

In contrast to continuing education, refresher training implies a formal, structured educational activity. Participation in a refresher program is often mandated for recertification or relicensure. Typical refresher programs provide an overview of the entire curriculum as well as important skills. A written or practical test (or both) may be associated with such training. The National Registry of EMTs requires biannual refresher training. As an alternative, the National Registry has now started allowing paramedics to prove competency by retaking a cognitive exam and submitting a simple reregistration document.

Technology in Education

There was a time in EMS education when an instructor would just show up at an ambulance station, set up some tables and chairs, pull a few items off the ambulance for demonstration, and be all set to teach. That is rarely the case today. Advances in educational technology as well as the sophistication of prehospital care have changed the approach to education. Longer courses, additional required training, and increased responses are placing greater demands on EMS providers. Any time spent for training must be used efficiently.

Technology plays two major roles in EMS education. First, it assists the instructor in producing course materials and instructional aids. For centuries, teachers wrote on blackboards with chalk; now, this process seems archaic. The availability of learning management systems and easily produced audiovisual aids allow the instructor to produce state-of-the-art course materials. Instructors who do not use the latest technology are almost considered inferior by students—even if the knowledge they impart is sound.

The second role of technology is in the areas of skills instruction and development of critical thinking. Many of the techniques used in EMS are invasive, requiring insertion of a needle or cannula into the body. It is not always practical or ethical to have students perform these skills on one another or on patients who do not have a clear medical need. It is also not possible to present every type of patient or pathology to a student. The alternative is simulation.

Simulation has been used in medical and EMS education for years. Many a student has learned to give an intramuscular injection using an orange: a low-fidelity simulation. And the history of medical education contains numerous accounts of students and physicians "robbing graves" to acquire cadavers for experimentation and learning. One of the earliest examples of simulation in EMS was the development of the CPR mannequin by Asmund S. Laerdal in 1960. It was Laerdal's belief that a realistic-looking mannequin would help people learn CPR (Laerdal, 2000). Now, the inanimate CPR mannequin has been replaced by a simulator that not only gives feedback of student performance but also allows the mannequin itself to respond in different ways. As advanced as this may seem, the potential of **high-fidelity human simulation**, shown in **Figure 4-9**, and virtual reality will surely replace this analog model with an educational experience as real and intense as actual CPR. The future of technology in EMS education is limited only by computer and virtual technology and by instructors' ability to apply it to an educational experience.

High-fidelity simulation now allows simulated patients, in the form of mannequins, to breathe, talk, have a pulse, sweat, cry, and even bleed. New simulators are completely wireless, allowing providers to pick up their simulated patients at a scene, transport them in their ambulance, and hand them off to

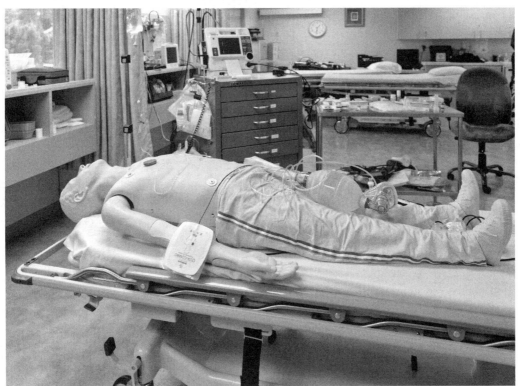

© Carolina K. Smith, M.D./Shutterstock.

Figure 4-9 High-fidelity patient simulation.

their local emergency department. Multidisciplinary training with simulators is growing in popularity, meaning that the same patient with whom EMS trains may also interact with the local police and fire departments, doctors, nurses, and the entire healthcare system.

When coupled with **standardized patients** (actors), mannequins provide a real-life experience that the learner may not otherwise encounter. Mass-casualty incidents can be staged with patients ranging from walking wounded to those needing invasive procedures. Additionally, the realism provided can help build critical thinking, a skill at the core of all EMS. Future education models may also utilize simulation for high-stakes testing, including certification examinations.

Asynchronous Learning

The traditional approach to education is to have students come to the instructor in an environment designed for learning. In EMS education, this approach has been slightly modified with the ability of the instructor to come to a physical location where a group of students is clustered. Now, it is no longer a requirement for students and instructors to assemble in the same physical location. Computer and data transmission technology have provided the means to bring instruction to any student, at any place, at any time. This concept is known by a number of different names, including **distance learning, distance education, distributed learning, technology-enhanced learning**, and **asynchronous learning**.

Asynchronous learning has great potential in EMS education. Many EMS providers are shift workers, making it difficult to have each provider in the same classroom at the same time. Asynchronous learning provides a means to present educational materials to each shift or individual provider at a time most convenient for them. This eliminates the need for overtime shifts and allows for the rapid dissemination of information. Likewise, the student residing in an area not served by an EMS educational site would be able to receive training he or she would not otherwise have access to. Students are not the only ones who benefit from asynchronous learning; instructors and experts can now be available to students around the world to provide the best in EMS and medical education. Acceptance of asynchronous learning by the EMS and medical community is evidenced by the increasing number of online courses, such as Advanced Burn Life Support NOW and BLS Healthcare Provider Online. The National Registry also accepts a limited number of CEUs acquired online.

Mobile Learning Applications

The fact that nearly everyone owns a smartphone has led to a change in both the way education is delivered and the way information is retrieved. Mobile applications now replace large textbooks, drug books, and most reference materials. Channels such as iTunes U can provide supplementary materials for both initial and ongoing education. When coupled with audiobooks, multimedia applications can be an essential component for learning.

Caution is needed, however, as the legitimacy of these applications vary. Some EMS agencies or universities now provide their own applications, and some even provide devices such as tablet computers to each student. Applications must be reliable and kept up to date in order to be useful. Prior to using any online application, students need to research the reliability and authors to ensure that they are learning the correct material.

WRAP UP

Summary

The education of EMS providers has contributed significantly to the development of present-day EMS. Integral to the development of new provider levels and medical protocols have been the development and integration of education. Often, the availability and sophistication of EMS educational programs have led to an expanded scope of practice for EMS providers.

The increasing demand for trained EMS providers has resulted in the need to ensure consistency in the delivery of prehospital education. To meet this goal, the *EMS Education Agenda for the Future: A Systems Approach* has been adopted. This consensus document resulted in the establishment of core content and a practice model to support national education standards. The venues for EMS education are varied, but programs teaching EMS are accredited and participate in national testing.

Because of the ever-changing nature of EMS and medicine, specialized courses are offered to supplement basic training. Additionally, refresher courses for each provider level are offered to ensure proficiency and currency in both provider knowledge and skills. Technology, such as the use of high-fidelity human simulation and asynchronous learning, are shaping and changing the future of EMS education.

Key Terms

academy

accreditation

ARC Advanced First Aid

asynchronous learning

certifying examination

clinical behaviors and
   judgments

Commission on Accreditation
   of Allied Health Education
   Programs (CAAHEP)

Committee on Accreditation of
   Emergency Medical Services
   Professions (CoAEMSP)

competency

contact hours

continuing education

Continuing Education
   Coordinating Board for EMS
   (CECBEMS)

continuing education units
   (CEU)

distance education

distance learning

distributed learning

technology-enhanced learning

educators

essentials

high-fidelity human simulation

instructional guidelines

learning management systems

licensure

national certification

National EMS and Education
   Blueprint

National EMS Core Content

National EMS Education
   Standards

National EMS Scope of Practice

National Registry of EMTs

national standard curriculum

practice analysis

program director

protocol

provider levels

recertification

reciprocity

refresher training

regulators

relicensure

self-study

simulation

site visit

skills

standards or guidelines

student outcomes

technical training centers

terminal objectives

Review Questions

1. What are the major parts of the *EMS Education Agenda for the Future*?
2. What was the purpose of a national standard curriculum?
3. Which document serves as a guide for curriculum development?
4. Which organization provides a means for EMTs and paramedics to obtain reciprocity between states?
5. List six settings for EMS education and training.
6. Define asynchronous learning.
7. How is skills competency ensured once a prehospital provider is initially certified?
8. Briefly describe the CAAHEP accreditation process.

Additional Resources

Laerdal. (2000). Available at www.laerdal.com/html/annepop/html

National Academy of Sciences, National Research Council. (1966). *Accidental death and disability: The neglected disease of modern society.* Washington, DC: Author.

National Academy of Sciences, National Research Council. (1969). *Training of ambulance personnel and others responsible for emergency care of the sick and injured at the scene and during transport.* Washington, DC: National Academy Press.

National Highway Traffic Safety Administration. (2000). *Emergency medical services education agenda for the future: A systems approach.* Washington, DC: U.S. Government Printing Office.

National Registry of Emergency Medical Technicians. (1993). *National emergency medical services education and practice blueprint.* Columbus, OH: Author.

Picken, S. E. (1923). *The American National Red Cross: Its origins, purpose, and service.* New York: The Century Co.

5

Transportation

Objectives

Upon completion of this chapter, the reader should be able to:

- Identify the various types of EMS service providers.

- Define and differentiate between fixed-post staffing and event-driven staffing.

- State the role of a chase vehicle in providing ALS response.

- Identify BLS staffing and ALS staffing configurations.

- Describe the purpose and role of interfacility transport.

- State the role of the federal star of life ambulance specifications in ambulance development.

- Differentiate between the types of ambulance design.

- State the advantages and disadvantages of air medical transport.

- Identify alternative means for transport of patients.

- Identify alternative forms of prehospital transport.

The Transportation Attribute

Fundamental to any emergency medical system is the need for efficient conveyance of the patient to definitive care. Some form of specialized vehicle staffed with trained prehospital providers is the basic component of emergency medical services (EMS) transportation. This is most often accomplished using an ambulance. To fully understand the transportation attribute, it is necessary to look at it in three ways: who provides the service, how it is delivered, and how the EMS unit is staffed.

Service Providers

Who provides EMS varies greatly across the country and depends on the needs of a specific community. Although EMS is thought of as an important public service, it is not always provided as a governmental function. The relationship of EMS with other emergency service providers also varies from jurisdiction to jurisdiction. In most cases, however, systems have evolved to best suit the needs of the community. Various approaches to the delivery of EMS are presented here.

Fire Service

Perhaps the most traditional provider of EMS transportation is the fire service (**Figure 5-1**). Many fire departments took on the responsibility for ambulance service to provide support to their own personnel on the fire scene or as a public service when other providers ceased providing service. In many rural communities, the fire service was the natural choice because it already had a structure in place to deliver emergency services. In the early days of advanced life support (ALS) development, pioneering physicians such as Nagel in Miami and Cobb in Seattle saw the fire service as the ideal delivery system. The fire department already had trained personnel, strategically located stations, and response vehicles.

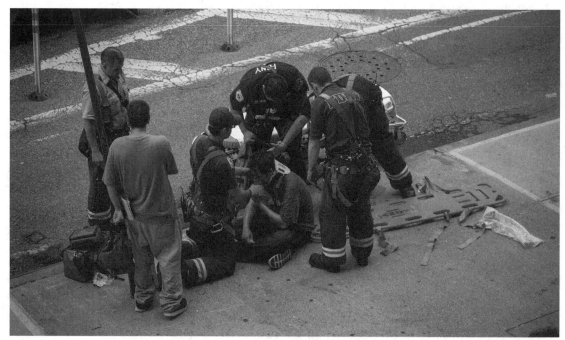

© Richard Levine/Alamy.

Figure 5-1 The fire service is a major provider of EMS in the United States.

In the latter part of the 20th century, the role and expectation of the American fire service changed. Budget issues, coupled with declining fire incidents, forced many communities to look at the role of the local fire service. Expanding the role of the fire departments beyond their routine work was seen as a means to increase efficiency. Today, the fire service is involved not only in EMS but also in hazardous materials response, urban search and rescue, and disaster and domestic terrorism response.

The fire service's embracing of EMS has not always been positive. As the role of the fire service began to change and the integration of EMS brought new training, personnel, and response patterns, some departments were reluctant to accept what has been called the "stepchild of the fire service." Demand for EMS exceeds the need for fire suppression. Stations with EMS units experienced increased alarms that disrupted traditional station routines. Personnel assigned to EMS units were often hired as EMTs and paramedics without fire training, thus leading to union membership issues, changes in labor standards, supervision conflicts, and promotion concerns. In some systems, engine company personnel were required to obtain EMS training as well as to respond with an engine or truck company on critical EMS calls. Individuals who had joined the fire department to fight fires soon found themselves spending most of their shifts responding to EMS calls. Over time, however, the fire service accepted EMS as one of its prime missions. Major fire service organizations, such as the International Association of Fire Chiefs (IAFC) and the International Association of Fire Fighters (IAFF), the predominant fire service union, have active EMS sections that support and encourage EMS in the fire service.

Commercial Service

Since the early inception of ambulance service, for-profit or commercial providers have played a vital role as a source of transportation. Just as most communities have a fire department, they most likely have a funeral home as well. Although one may not like to consider the similarities, a hearse has much in common with an ambulance, especially the early Cadillac ambulances. These were ambulances built on luxury-car chassis by Cadillac, Oldsmobile, and Buick. With a hearse, funeral directors could easily remove the rollers while retaining the hardware for a coffin, which was replaced by a stretcher. A removable "red light" was stuck on the roof and the hearse became an ambulance. Equipment and training were minimal at best. Through this transformation, the funeral director was able to expand his or her services and revenue while providing a needed public service. In areas of high demand, some funeral directors actually established separate ambulance divisions.

The need to provide nonemergency or **interfacility transport** service has been the impetus behind the founding of many commercial ambulance companies. In urban areas where 9-1-1 service is provided by the fire department, commercial operators handle the interfacility transports. In suburban and rural areas, the fire department or rescue squad may also provide interfacility transport. However, as the demand for 9-1-1 service increases and the availability of volunteers decreases, some services are forced to turn over this aspect of their operation to commercial providers. Often the need for an interfacility transport arises on short notice. This makes the task of finding a volunteer crew more difficult and also ties up the crew and vehicle for an extended period of time. Thus, many commercial operators are expanding their service areas.

Transport of patients by ambulance can be lucrative given the fact that such transports are billable to insurance companies as well as to Medicare and Medicaid. Operators can also charge for expendable items, oxygen, mileage, and night differentials in addition to the basic cost of the transport. Commercial operators often compete for exclusive contracts with hospitals, extended-care facilities, and managed care organizations. Increasingly, commercial services are becoming involved in **pathway management**. This is the management of how a patient enters into the healthcare system. For instance, there are several options for the patient who falls and injures his or her leg and cannot walk. The traditional action would be to dial 9-1-1 and request an ambulance. If the injury is not too serious, the patient could be transported to the hospital emergency department by a private automobile. With pathway management, the injured patient would call the dedicated telephone number of a managed care organization. A healthcare professional would question the patient and advise the best course of action. If an ambulance is needed and the situation is not life-threatening, a commercial ambulance service would be dispatched. This service would be one that has a contract with the managed care organization to provide transport at an agreed-upon rate that is less than the 9-1-1 service rate. The organization would transport the patient to a hospital or an urgent care facility that is also part of its plan. This also results in lower costs to the managed care organization. Such flexibility is not possible utilizing traditional 9-1-1 ambulance service.

In an effort to reduce cost, some municipalities and jurisdictions have abandoned public ambulance service in favor of commercial service. Commercial operators bid on a governmental contract to provide 9-1-1 service. The contract often contains a **performance clause** that specifies the required **response time** and **response coverage**. Failure to meet these requirements will result in fines and possible loss of the contract. Because delivery of 9-1-1 service can be expensive, the commercial operator will often negotiate a clause in the contract giving the operator exclusive rights to nonemergency and interfacility transports within the service area. The ambulance operator may also receive a **subsidy** from the local government to make up the difference between actual cost and insurance reimbursement schedules.

As the demand for commercial ambulance service increased in the 1980s and 1990s, the industry underwent a major change. Small "mom-and-pop" ambulance services were bought out by large consolidators. These acquisitions reduced local competition and increased the ability of large commercial operators to compete with public service EMS systems. National consolidators also provided "one-stop shopping" for managed care organizations interested in pathway management and interfacility transports at service locations across the country.

In addition to providing efficiency and economy of scale, commercial operators were not constrained by **fixed-post** locations and staffing patterns common with public service EMS systems, especially the fire service. This increased flexibility led to the development of **event-driven** posting strategies. This concept will be discussed in more detail later in this chapter. The interests of the commercial ambulance industry are served by the American Ambulance Association.

Third Service

The third service approach to EMS delivery involves the creation of a separate public safety service to deliver EMS. The term "third service" is derived from EMS being added to the traditional municipal services of police and fire. In a third service system, EMS is delivered by uniformed personnel who have their own vehicles, command structure, and in some cases their own stations. More often, EMS vehicles and personnel are posted to existing fire stations because they have the necessary facilities. However, the EMS personnel are not part of the fire department. Some municipalities have aligned their third service with the police department rather than with the fire department.

The third service concept solves many of the conflicts associated with the integration of personnel and services into a fire department. Often, the personnel and services do not fit the department's traditional structure and mission. However, such a system adds additional expense by duplicating much of the infrastructure already present in the fire service.

Public Safety Agency

Jurisdictions have traditionally provided fire and police protection for their residents. With the addition of EMS, a jurisdiction now has to provide three services at the taxpayer's expense. A concept that has developed in a few jurisdictions is to combine all of the public safety functions into one department of public safety that provides fire, police, and EMS services within a single organizational structure. Public safety stations may serve as a fire station, an EMS station, and a police station all in one. Jurisdictions that fully embrace this concept have public safety officers who are trained to provide all three levels of service.

As an example, if a fire alarm is received, a minimum crew responds to the scene with the fire engine. Officers on police patrol respond along with EMS personnel to complete the crew and provide command. In a medical emergency, a police car may respond to the scene with a police officer-paramedic who can upgrade the ambulance to ALS. In other jurisdictions, there may be a single public safety agency that employs police, fire, and EMS personnel, but each service is a separate division within the agency.

The main advantage of the public service concept is that it utilizes personnel to their maximum efficiency. A crucial disadvantage is that it requires personnel to maintain proficiency in diverse areas. There is also the potential for resource conflicts between the different services in the agency. **Figures 5-2** and **5-3** show the structure of these systems.

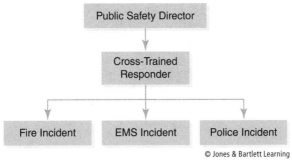

© Jones & Bartlett Learning

Figure 5-2 Consolidated public safety organization.

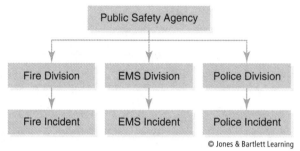

© Jones & Bartlett Learning

Figure 5-3 Public safety agency.

Police or Sheriff-Based Service

Just as the fire service has been used to provide EMS service to a community, so too have police departments or sheriffs' offices (**Figure 5-4**), although this is not a common model of EMS delivery. EMS services using a sheriff's office appear in some of the western areas of the United States.

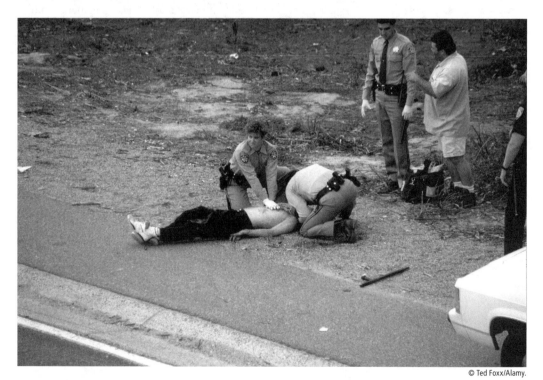

© Ted Foxx/Alamy.

Figure 5-4 Law enforcement EMS.

Hospital-Based Service

Hospitals have a long tradition of providing ambulance service. This was a natural extension of the hospital's role in the community. Today, few hospitals provide ambulance service. Changes in hospital ownership, business practices, and federal regulations have limited the practice of hospital-based EMS systems. Those still functioning most often provide ALS, interfacility, or specialized transport service.

As ALS was developing, various delivery models were tried. Early on, hospital-based providers were used to move ALS into the field setting. Doctors and nurses were placed on ambulances to provide ALS. In smaller communities, an ambulance would respond to the hospital and pick up a nurse before responding to the scene of a cardiac emergency. In those systems that chose not to exclusively utilize paramedics, hospitals developed **chase vehicle** systems, which use a nurse and paramedic combination. A hospital-based vehicle responds with a team of a nurse and a paramedic to upgrade a basic life support (BLS) ambulance. Based on local medical protocols, the nurse may be able to provide specialized interventions not normally permitted of paramedics. Having initiated the treatment of the patient in the field, the hospital-based crew is able to continue this care in the emergency department. When not responding to calls, the nurse and the paramedic assist in the emergency department as additional staff.

Through regulation and competition, the services provided by hospitals in a geographical area may vary and be regulated to prevent duplication of specialized services and thus to control cost. The business of health care has also resulted in a dramatic increase in the consolidation or networking of hospitals. A common configuration is to have a large, urban tertiary-care hospital take over or partner with local community hospitals in the area. Patients needing specialized care not available in the local hospitals are treated at the central tertiary-care facility. This change in the delivery of health care has resulted in the increased need for transport of patients between facilities.

To facilitate the transfer of patients, some hospitals have established specialized transport services, as shown in **Figure 5-5**. These services may include ground or air transport. Specialized vehicles, some as large as motor homes, are equipped to support patients during the transfer. Crew configuration varies, but at a minimum includes a critical care registered nurse (CCRN), a critical care transport paramedic, and a driver. For extremely critical patients, a physician and other specialist accompany the crew. To avoid the cost and management of a fleet of vehicles and personnel, some hospitals have contracted with commercial operators to provide transport service infrastructure.

First Responder

The term "first responder" refers to the rapid response of trained personnel to the scene to provide life-sustaining care until the arrival of definitive care and transport. Although not technically a transport service, first responder service is an integral part of the EMS system in many areas. An example of such a service would be a fire engine crew responding to a medical emergency to provide immediate care, such as airway management, oxygen, and vital sign assessment. Even in areas where the fire department

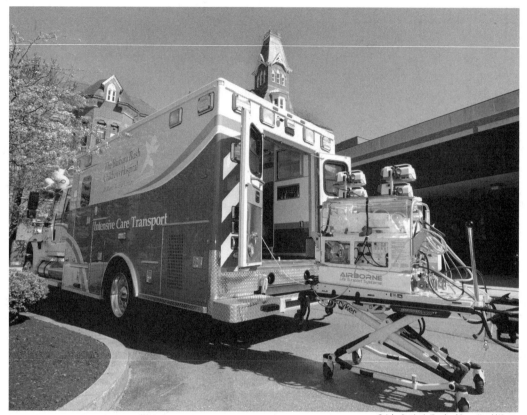

© John Patriquin/Portland Press Herald/Getty.

Figure 5-5 Specialized transport vehicle.

provides EMS service, it is not unusual for the closest emergency unit to be dispatched. In busy systems, the first responder unit can provide care until a transport unit arrives. Some jurisdictions have been creative in designating first responder units by utilizing police, public works personnel, and highway maintenance crews.

Public Utility Model

The public utility model for delivery of EMS utilizes a governing strategy similar to that used to provide basic utility services, such as electricity and gas. An EMS authority is established with the responsibility for providing EMS through contracts with a commercial provider. To ensure continuity of service, the authority usually owns the EMS vehicles and equipment. By owning the system's equipment, the likelihood of the commercial contractor defaulting is limited. The authority also establishes performance standards for monitoring the commercial contractor.

Integrated System

Given the different configurations for EMS systems, it is possible to develop other systems that combine aspects of two or more existing ones. An example of an integrated system would be a commercial ambulance operator providing BLS level transport and the fire department providing ALS upgrade service. In such a system, the fire department responds with paramedics who provide ALS. The paramedic then accompanies the patient to the hospital in the commercial operator's BLS ambulance. A similar system would be ALS provided by a hospital with transport by the fire department or commercial operator. There are even systems that have two different entities providing BLS transport and ALS transport. Integrated systems allow localities to custom design EMS systems to best meet a community's unique needs.

Delivery Systems

Just as there are variations in who delivers EMS, there are also variations in how EMS is delivered. Variables include how to determine the number and type of ambulances available to respond.

Fixed-Post Staffing

The traditional approach to the delivery of EMS has been for the provider, whether commercial or public safety, to respond from a fixed station to the incident scene. When a call is received, the dispatch center determines the closest available unit. Regardless of the demand for EMS service, the same number of units would be in service at any given time.

Fixed-post staffing systems develop for one of two reasons. In the case of a commercial provider, the operator has one central location, usually the company's headquarters, from which ambulances operate. This is where personnel report for work, restock units, bring units for maintenance, and return at the end of a shift. Some commercial operators covering large areas may have satellite centers that serve a similar function.

In the case of fire department EMS, ambulances are placed in the fire stations. For small communities, this may be a central location. In others, the fire department may have multiple stations. Interestingly, in many older urban centers the location of fire stations was determined by how far the horses that pulled steamer engines could run. Yet today, the location of these same stations determines the placement of EMS units.

Most fixed-post systems do not take into consideration the changes in the demand for EMS service that occur over the course of a day or according to the day of the week. On average, the demand for EMS service decreases during the late evening and early morning hours and rises during the day, especially around dawn and rush hour periods. Demand patterns also change between workdays and weekends. In a fixed-post system, the number of units in service remains constant, thus some units are used more than others depending on the time of day and day of the week. For example, a unit located in a downtown urban area would be busiest during normal working hours. However, this same unit would be underutilized at night and on weekends. Fixed-post systems may temporarily transfer units to cover open areas, but this is done on an ad hoc basis.

Although the fixed-post system attempts to provide uniform coverage for a given area, the system does not necessarily do so in the most efficient manner. Maximum utilization of units and personnel is not usually obtained by such a system.

Event-Driven Staffing

In contrast to fixed-post staffing, event-driven resource deployment matches an EMS system's resources to predicted demand using data on historical patterns. All high-performance EMS systems—that is, EMS systems that produce clinical quality care, response time reliability, customer satisfaction, and economic efficiency—simultaneously deploy event-driven resources. These techniques were first developed by Jack Stout, an EMS economist and consultant, in the late 1970s and early 1980s and were initially tested in the EMS systems of Tulsa, Oklahoma, and Kansas City, Missouri. They are referred to as "advanced system status management." **System status management** is "the process of preparing the system to produce the best possible response to the next EMS call" (Stout, 1983).

The Center for Economic and Management Research at Oklahoma University found that demand for EMS was similar to the demand for electricity from the electric utility industry (Stout, 1985). Demand for EMS fluctuates by the hour of the day and the day of the week, just as the demand for electric power varies. There is more demand for EMS on Saturday night at 10:00 p.m. than on Monday morning at 4:00 a.m. The center found that the geographic distribution of calls also varied by the hour of the day and the day of the week.

In recognition of these findings, high-performance providers use **peak load staffing**, which means they add units when demand is high and reduce units when demand is low. Therefore, these systems do not use typical fixed-shift patterns. Instead, they use a variety of shifts, including 8-, 9-, 10-, 11-, 12-, 14-, and 16-hour shifts. These shifts also start at various times throughout the day so that the supply of units closely matches the demand for those units.

EMS demand also shows a geographic pattern. As people move through the day, so does the demand for EMS. High-performance services study these geographic patterns and position their vehicles accordingly (**Figure 5-6**). They create **posting plans** for each hour of each day. These services use a process developed by Jack Stout in which maps showing the distribution of calls for each hour of each day are analyzed to determine the optimal location for their units. They start the analysis by determining where they would post one ambulance if there were only one unit available to the entire system, and then where they would post two units if that were all that were available, and so on. After one hour is done, the next hour is analyzed until posting plans for all 168 hours (one week) have been developed. This analysis is a great deal of work even when facilitated by computer-aided dispatch (CAD) software.

High-performance providers maintain ambulance fleets that are 120–130% in excess of the maximum number of units that might be scheduled at the peak hour of coverage. The **peak hour** is the hour in

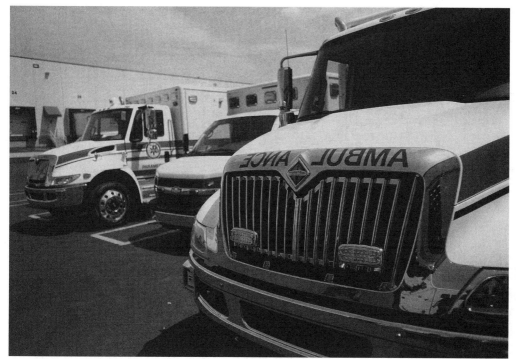

©Ty Wright/Bloomberg/Getty.

Figure 5-6 Ambulances at a posting site.

which the most ambulances are scheduled to be on duty at one time. These providers also hire vehicle service technicians whose primary function is to "**make ready**"; that is, they wash and stock ambulances and make them ready for the crew to go in service. The crew verifies the status of critical equipment and then advises the control center of their availability for service. Crews are dispatched to calls and to post locations throughout the day in response to the demand for service at that particular time and day.

Many high-performance systems are also full-service systems; therefore, the ambulance crews handle both emergency and nonemergency requests for service. As crews are assigned to calls, the remaining ambulances are repositioned so that the system is always configured to best respond to the next life-threatening emergency.

At the end of their shift, the crew returns the ambulance to the fleet facility, where the vehicle is washed and restocked. Vehicles are taken and returned throughout the day, and it is only in rare circumstances that a vehicle will be immediately given to another crew. All units are frontline units and are fully equipped. Crews are not always assigned to the same ambulance on successive shifts, but all the ambulances are identically configured. When there is a need for additional units, they can be quickly added to the system. The extra capacity also makes it possible to schedule routine and preventive maintenance of vehicles without reducing the number of ambulances available in the system.

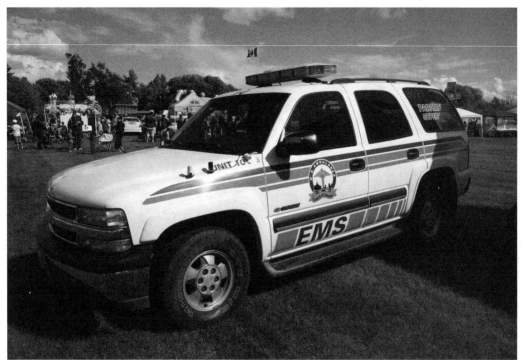

© Radharc Images/Alamy.

Figure 5-7 Chase vehicle.

ALS Intercept

The **ALS intercept** or chase vehicle delivery system combines fixed-post and event-driven systems. Chase vehicles, also known as "fly cars" or "chase cars," are most often used to provide ALS service (**Figure 5-7**). A non-transport vehicle staffed with ALS providers and equipment responds from a central location to upgrade a BLS transport unit. The chase vehicle can either respond to the scene or rendezvous with the ambulance en route to the hospital. Some systems staff the chase vehicle with two ALS providers and double equipment to allow the unit to return to service after transferring a provider and equipment to the transport unit.

The main advantage of a chase vehicle is that specialized services such as ALS can be provided to a large area with minimal staffing and equipment. One disadvantage is longer response times for ALS if the unit must cover a large geographical area. In some parts of the United States, police officers provide ALS chase vehicle service using specially equipped police cars.

Interfacility Transport

Although emergency or 9-1-1 transport accounts for a large part of ambulance transports, ambulance services also provide for the transfer of patients between medical facilities. These transports may be routine or nonemergency calls for such services as moving a patient from a hospital to a nursing home or even from the hospital to home, or from a nursing facility to a treatment facility and back. Such calls are usually scheduled in advance and require little or no medical intervention by the transport crew. Some services provide "wheelchair vans" specifically to transport wheelchair-bound patients, and others may provide transport only for ambulatory patients, similar to a taxi service.

With the consolidation and partnering of hospitals into networks as well as the availability of specialty services such as stroke and trauma centers, a means is needed to quickly and efficiently move patients to these facilities from primary care hospitals. The transfer of such patients is regulated by the Emergency Medical Treatment and Active Labor Act (EMTALA), also known as "COBRA." This act required that a certain level of patient care be maintained during transport of the patient, thus often requiring specialized transport personnel and equipment. To provide this level of care, training programs have been established for nurses and paramedics to become certified as critical care transport technicians. Ambulance vehicles are also modified or designed to accommodate advanced patient monitoring and life-support equipment.

Staffing Configuration

Just as there are variations in delivery systems, there are also variations in EMS unit staffing. A minimum of two individuals is needed for a transport vehicle: one to drive and the other to provide patient care. This may seem logical, but before the modern era of EMS, some services responded only with a driver who loaded the patient in the ambulance on a "one-man cot" before speeding off to the hospital. This led to the term "ambulance driver" being used to refer to anyone who rode on an ambulance. The reader is cautioned that staffing configuration varies greatly among jurisdictions. The following examples represent the most common configurations.

BLS Staffing

The staffing pattern for BLS units revolves around an EMT providing patient care on the scene and en route to the hospital. Thus it is possible to have only one crew member trained in patient care. Although not an optimal arrangement, especially when two-person skills are required, this configuration reduces crew cost and provides greater availability of drivers. The availability of someone to drive the ambulance may be a critical issue in some volunteer organizations. It is also possible to use as drivers other public safety personnel, such as first responders and firefighters.

The more common BLS crew configuration, as shown in **Figure 5-8**, is EMT/EMT. This crew involves two trained personnel to provide patient care on the scene. Additionally, the crew members can take turns driving and providing patient care. In the event of a multipatient situation, both crew members can provide initial patient stabilization. For critical patients, it is possible for both providers to assist with patient care during transport, with a first responder or firefighter enlisted to drive.

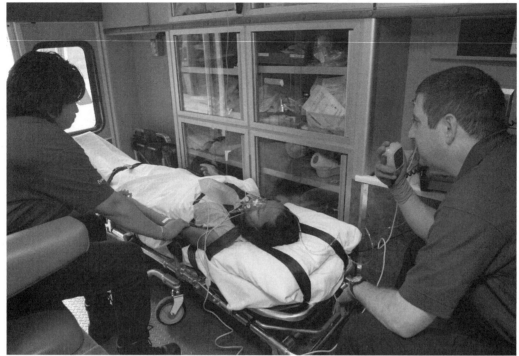

© Jones & Bartlett Learning. Courtesy of MIEMSS.

Figure 5-8 EMT crew en route to the hospital.

ALS Staffing

ALS staffing is more variable than BLS staffing given that there are two levels of ALS provider: AEMT and paramedic. ALS staffed crews can include a variety of combinations such as:

- AEMT/AEMT
- AEMT/EMT
- AEMT/other
- Paramedic/paramedic
- Paramedic/nurse
- Paramedic/AEMT
- Paramedic/EMT
- Paramedic/other

ALS staffing depends on the nature of the EMS system and the type of incident a unit responds to. In a single-tier system, an ALS unit will respond to both ALS and BLS calls. In a two-tier system, the ALS ambulance will respond only to ALS calls; thus, having two paramedics on board may be an advantage. Having a non-paramedic as the driver limits that individual to always driving and not practicing patient care skills. In rare instances, a driver with limited or no medical training may accompany a paramedic. Such an arrangement limits a unit's flexibility and places the total burden of patient care on the paramedic.

Most EMS systems have arrangements (either internal to the system or using external services, such as the fire department or police) to provide additional staffing to assist the on-scene crew. An example would be responding with two ALS units to a cardiac arrest. This additional staffing can assist with lifting and moving patients as well as with carrying ALS equipment and assisting with CPR. Services that provide on-scene quality assurance and scene command have supervisory personnel who are assigned to field response. These field supervisors—an additional source of on-scene staffing—respond to major medical and trauma calls to assist and guide responding personnel.

To increase the utilization of fire suppression units and staff, some fire departments assign a paramedic to an engine or ladder company. The vehicle is equipped as an ALS upgrade vehicle. Similar to the chase car concept, the **paramedic engine company** responds to an incident and provides a paramedic and equipment. The engine company can remain in service as a fire suppression unit while the paramedic accompanies the patient in the transport unit. In the event of a fire call, the engine company would respond similarly to a regular engine company and the paramedic would function as a member of the crew. This configuration has the advantage of providing enhanced EMS response along with maintaining fire suppression capability. Likewise, the addition of a paramedic to the crew enhances unit staffing. Expensive fire trucks and crews are more fully utilized.

Mobile Health Care

As managed care organizations search for new ways to provide lower-cost health services, taking services to the patient seems a less expensive alternative than having the patient come to the hospital or clinic. This has led to the concept of mobile health care, which not only responds to less critical acute situations but also provides continuing care for chronic medical problems, as well as wellness and prevention activities. Given that EMS systems already have trained personnel and vehicles available, EMS is seen as the best source for this type of service. As Medicare Shared Savings Programs develop under the Affordable Care Act and contract with Accountable Care Organizations (ACOs), the role of EMS and specifically that of the paramedic will expand. This expansion has already led to the community paramedic concept. (See chapter 10.)

EMS Vehicles

Having trained personnel respond to the scene of a medical or trauma emergency would not be effective if there were no means to transport the patient to definitive care. Thus a dedicated transport vehicle—an ambulance—is needed.

Ambulances have progressed from special chariots in ancient times to horse-drawn carriages during the Napoleonic period to motorized vehicles in the 20th century.

In 1969, the National Research Council, National Academy of Sciences, published *Medical Requirements for Ambulance Design and Equipment* (NAS, 1969). From these general recommendations, the National Highway Traffic Safety Administration developed the Ambulance Design Criteria (NHTSA, 1973). This document presented specific engineering criteria for ambulance design and construction. These specifications were adopted by the federal government and were required for any ambulance vehicle purchased with federal funds. The General Services Administration specification for ambulances was known as **KKK-A-1822**, followed by a sequential letter indicating version (KKK-A-1822F was current as of publication). Ambulances designed to specification are called **star-of-life ambulances** because originally they were the only vehicles allowed to display the federally registered "star-of-life" emblem. In 1997, the trademark held by the NHTSA for the star of life expired; thus, the designation of star-of-life ambulance has become more of a tradition than a regulatory compliance.

The purpose of the KKK specifications was to:

describe ambulances which are authorized to display the "Star of Life" symbol. It establishes minimum specifications, test parameters, and essential criteria for ambulance design, performance, equipment, appearance, and to provide a practical degree of standardization. The object is to provide ambulances that are nationally recognized, properly constructed, easily maintained, and, when professionally staffed and provisioned, will function reliably in prehospital or other mobile emergency medical service. (General Services Administration, 1994)

The most significant aspect of the KKK standards is the designation of four types of ambulance designs (as shown in **Figure 5-9**). Each design has a configuration "A" for ALS and a configuration "B" for BLS. Thus, you may have a type IIB ambulance that is a van chassis designed for BLS transport.

Type I

The **type I ambulance** is designed as a "conventional, cab-chassis with modular ambulance body" (General Services Administration, 1994). Essentially, a type I is a pickup truck with an ambulance module in place of the truck bed. This unit is designed so that the ambulance module can be removed and placed on a new chassis as needed. Most type I ambulances do not have a means to go from the cab to the ambulance module, an arrangement known as a "walk-through."

Advantages of the type I include a more robust chassis and easy access to the engine compartment. Disadvantages are a harder ride, a greater height from street to floor in the patient compartment, and lack of a walk-through.

Type II

The **type II ambulance** is a van converted into an ambulance. The KKK specification is "standard van, forward control, integral cab-body ambulance" (General Services Administration, 1994). A standard commercial van is converted to provide more headroom by adding a raised roof. A divider panel equipped with a walk-through is installed to separate the cab from the patient compartment.

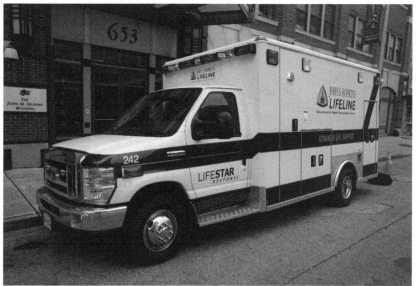

© Jones & Bartlett Learning. Courtesy of MIEMSS.

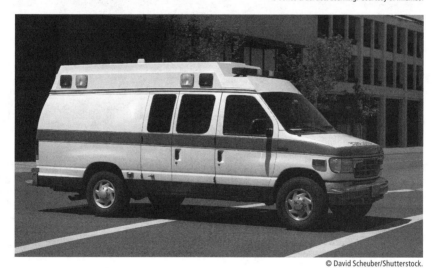

© David Scheuber/Shutterstock.

Figure 5-9 Types of ambulances: (A) Type I ambulance, (B) Type II ambulance, (C) Type III ambulance, and (D) Medium Duty ambulance.

The main advantage of a type II ambulance is cost. Of the three ambulance types, the type II is the least costly to produce. This makes it economical for BLS transport services that do not need a large patient compartment. The van is also more maneuverable. The main disadvantage is interior space. Because space is so limited, it is difficult to configure a type II ambulance for ALS, even though type II ambulances are used for ALS. The van generally does not last as long as type I and type III ambulances, which have heavier chassis construction.

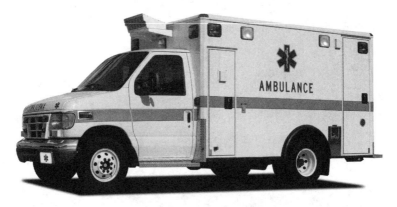

© Rob Wilson/Shutterstock.

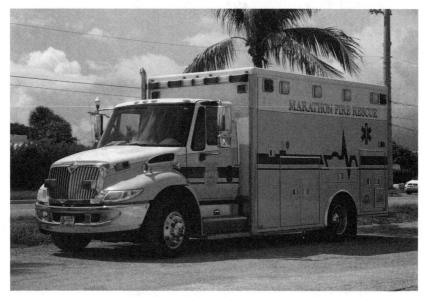

© Radharc Images/Alamy.

Figure 5-9 *(Continued)*

Type III

The type III ambulance combines the attributes of the type I and type II ambulances. It is the most common ambulance configuration in use today. A "specialty van, forward control and control integrated cab-body or combination containerized modular ambulance" (General Services Administration, 1994) describes the type III ambulance, which has a van-style chassis with a mounted modular ambulance body, similar to the type I configuration. The van chassis may be integral or connected directly to the modular body, or it may be separate from the body. A walk-through is almost always provided.

Advantages of the type III include a heavier chassis than the type II, a walk-through, and increased maneuverability. Disadvantages include poor access to the engine compartment and greater wear on chassis components.

Medium Duty

Some type I ambulances are built on larger 1-and-¼-ton chassis. These heavy-duty units are referred to as **medium-duty ambulances** by some manufacturers. These ambulances are currently not specifically addressed in the KKK standards. The larger chassis provides heavier brake and power-train components as well as the ability to mount larger patient compartment modules. Disadvantages of the medium-duty unit include decreased maneuverability with increased size and greater height from street level to patient compartment floor. Because this makes loading the ambulance stretcher difficult and unsafe, most medium-duty units are equipped with air shocks that deflate on the scene to lower the back of the unit.

The KKK Standards expired in October 2013 and have been replaced by the National Fire Protection Agency (NFPA) 1917 "Standard for Automotive Ambulances." The **NFPA 1917** is an industry-developed consensus standard. Using the standard format of the NFPA standards process, a technical committee consisting of ambulance manufacturers, providers, regulators, and safety researchers develop a draft standard that is then voted on and accepted by the NFPA general membership. Standards are routinely revised every five years. This process and the use of NFPA standards is well established in the fire service and brings the design and specifications of ambulances into line with standards for other emergency services vehicles. The standard also removes the federal government from the role of standard-setter for the ambulance industry.

Air Medical Transport

Although the vast majority of patients are transported for definitive care by traditional ground ambulances, there are times when more rapid transport or transport over long distances requires other forms of transportation. Such transports are most often handled by **air medical transport** units. Air medical transport utilizes rotor-wing (helicopter) (**Figure 5-10**) or fixed-wing (airplane) aircraft.

Advantages of air medical transport include:

- High speed;
- Greater response area;
- Not hindered by vehicle traffic;
- Access to remote areas (rotor wing); and
- Adequate patient compartment (fixed wing).

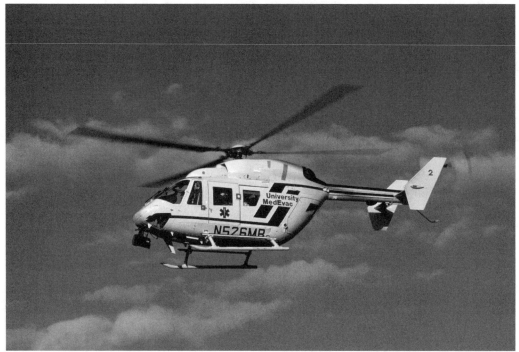

© John Greim/LightRocket/Getty.

Figure 5-10 EMS helicopter.

Disadvantages include:

- High cost;
- Weather limits;
- Increased training demand;
- Increased danger to patient and crew;
- Greater operational demand and control;
- Greater logistic coordination (fixed wing); and
- Requirement for landing strip (fixed wing).

Air medical transport can be used for on-scene response and transport or for interhospital transfers of critical patients. Crew configuration depends on the aircraft type and mission. The majority of helicopters are staffed with a paramedic and flight nurse. Fixed-wing aircraft, which are used for long distance transfers, often carry a physician or critical care registered nurse. Training of flight paramedics and nurses is based on the *Guidelines for Air Medical Crew Education* developed by the Association of Air Medical Services (AAMS), which builds on knowledge and skills obtained in paramedic and nursing education programs.

Regulation of air medical transport involves flight operations and medical control. Flight operations in the United States are under the jurisdiction of the Federal Aviation Administration (FAA). The FAA regulates aircraft airworthiness and flight crew certification as well as operational parameters. The Commission on Accreditation of Medical Transport Systems (CAMTS) provides voluntary accreditation for air medical services. Patient transfer regulations, such as COBRA, also apply to the transfer of patients by air.

Alternative Transport Modes

Although the ground ambulance and, to a lesser extent, the air ambulance are synonymous with EMS transport, geographic or system parameters may require the use of less traditional means to transport patients. Examples of such modes include watercraft and specialized land vehicles. Water-bound or water-related areas may use watercraft to facilitate patient access and transport. In areas of special terrain or extreme weather conditions, specialized land vehicles, such as tracked vehicles, sleds, and all-wheel drive, as well as units with high-output heating or air conditioning, may be used. One such example is the patient transport sled used by the National Ski Patrol. In the law enforcement community, there is also the need for specialized medical response vehicles to extricate victims from hostile situations as well as to protect responders.

One approach tried by some services has been to combine the functionality of response vehicles. An example of such a vehicle that has been around for some time is the rescue ambulance. This most often is a large and heavy-duty ambulance equipped with basic rescue equipment, such as a hydraulic rescue tool. Another approach to a combined vehicle that was tried but did not prove useful was a fire engine with a patient transport compartment. The idea behind this unit was to make the most efficient use of an engine company and its personnel. However, the cost and vehicle wear of transporting patients did not prove efficient or cost effective. The patient compartment was also very small and the ride comfort was not comparable with that of an ambulance.

Ambulance Equipment

Regardless of the type of ambulance configuration an EMS service uses, the vehicle alone would be of limited value if it were not properly equipped. Since 1961, the Committee on Trauma of the American College of Surgeons has produced a list of essential equipment for ambulances. Starting in 1988, the American College of Emergency Physicians produced a similar list. In 2000, the two lists were combined.

Ambulance equipment can be grouped into two broad categories: equipment for basic-level providers and equipment for advanced-level providers (ACEP and ACS, 2000).

Basic-level-provider essential equipment includes the following:

- *Ventilation and airway equipment.* Equipment for clearing and maintaining a patient's airway. Examples include suction apparatus, pocket mask, and bag-valve mask.
- *Monitoring and defibrillation devices.* Includes cardiac monitor-defibrillator or automatic external defibrillator (AED).
- *Immobilization devices.* Equipment for splinting bones confirmed as or thought to be broken.

Examples include cervical collars, splints, and backboards.

- *Bandages.* Equipment for control of bleeding and care of soft-tissue injuries. Examples include burn pack, gauze sponge, and roller gauze.
- *Communication equipment.* Equipment for two-way communications between provider, dispatch center, and medical direction.
- *Obstetrical delivery equipment.* Equipment for management of childbirth.
- *Miscellaneous.* Equipment used for patient assessment and patient transfer. Examples include stethoscope, blood pressure cuff, and ambulance stretcher.
- *Infection control equipment.* Equipment used for bodily-substance isolation. Examples include latex-free equipment.
- *Injury prevention equipment.* Safety equipment, including seat belts, helmets, eye protection, and fire extinguisher, for crew and passengers.

Advanced-level-provider essential equipment includes the following:

- *Vascular access equipment.* Equipment for initiation and maintenance of intravenous lines.
- *Airway and ventilation equipment.* Equipment for advanced management of the airway. Includes equipment for endotracheal intubation.
- *Cardiac equipment.* Portable cardiac monitor-defibrillator-pacer.
- *Other advanced equipment.* Includes nebulizer, glucometer, and pulse oximeter.
- *Medications.* Medications required for ALS.
- *Optional advanced equipment.* Automated monitoring equipment and specialized equipment for ALS procedures.

WRAP UP

Summary

An EMS system would not be able to function if it did not provide a means for the transport of patients for definitive care. How transport is provided, and by whom, varies widely. Traditionally, public safety agencies such as the fire department have been the usual providers of EMS service. In other areas, commercial operators provide transportation, often using an event-driven deployment system as opposed to the fixed-post staffing common to public safety agencies.

The vehicles used for EMS transportation have changed greatly over time. Through standardization developed by the federal government, ambulance vehicles are now built to a set standard based on one of three basic designs. For special, rapid transport, air medical transport using rotor-wing or fixed-wing aircraft has proven effective.

Key Terms

air medical transport

ALS intercept

chase vehicle

event-driven resource
    deployment

fixed-post staffing

interfacility transport

Guidelines for Air Medical
    Crew Education

KKK-A-1822

make ready

medium-duty ambulance

mobile health care

NFPA 1917

pathway management

peak hour

peak load staffing

performance clause

posting plans

public utility model

response coverage

response time

star-of-life ambulance

"star-of-life" emblem

subsidy

third service

type I ambulance

type II ambulance

type III ambulance

Review Questions

1. Differentiate between a public safety EMS provider and a commercial EMS service.
2. What is meant by an integrated EMS service?
3. Discuss the advantages of event-driven staffing versus fixed-post staffing.
4. List the various types of ALS staffing.
5. Why were ambulances built to KKK-A-1822 referred to as star-of-life ambulances?
6. State a situation when air medical transport by rotor-wing aircraft would be appropriate.
7. What is interfacility transport?

Additional Resources

American College of Emergency Physicians & American College of Surgeons. (2000). *Equipment for ambulances*. Dallas, TX: Author.

General Services Administration. (1994). *Federal specification for the star-of-life ambulance KKK-A-1822D* (GSA Publication AMBU-0001). General Services Administration: Washington, DC.

National Academy of Science. (1969). *Medical requirements for ambulance design and equipment*. Washington, DC: Author.

National Highway Traffic Safety Administration (1973). *Ambulance design criteria*. Committee on Ambulance Design Criteria and National Research Council: Washington, DC.

Stout, J. (1983). System status management: The strategy of ambulance placement. *Journal of Emergency Medical Services*, 8(9), 22–32.

Stout, J. (1985). Public utility model revisited: Part 1-origins. *Journal of Emergency Medical Services*, 10(2), 55.

6

Medical Oversight

Objectives

Upon completion of this chapter, the reader should be able to:

- State the role of medical oversight in EMS.

- Differentiate between medical control and medical oversight.

- Review the history of medical oversight in EMS.

- State the importance of regulation and legislation related to medical oversight.

- Describe models of medical oversight.

- Describe the relationship of medical oversight to advanced practice EMS.

- Differentiate between indirect and direct medical oversight.

- State the primary roles of an EMS system medical director.

- State the relationship between the EMS system medical director and the EMS provider.

- Identify a national position paper related to medical oversight.

- Differentiate between a protocol and a standing order.

Historical Background

For many years, the terms **medical direction** or **medical command** were used to describe physician involvement in emergency medical services (EMS). The physician who took responsibility for the practice of medicine by prehospital providers was the medical director. Such terminology implied a rigid hierarchy of control with the physician at the top and the EMT at the bottom. As EMS systems developed and became more sophisticated, and physicians became more comfortable with their role in EMS, the concept of **medical oversight** replaced the rigidity of medical control. Oversight implies more of a quality of care approach to medical direction than only physician authorization for providers to function. This approach is more proactive and ongoing than reactive and prescriptive.

Since these early formative years, medical oversight has also grown in scope to encompass all components of the EMS system. Medical oversight now starts with public-access defibrillation programs and continues through the highest levels of care. All EMS providers now have some connection to the medical director. Emergency medical dispatch protocols are now under medical oversight and include prearrival instructions for patient care by untrained lay persons. Emergency medical responders (EMRs) are now allowed to use an automatic external defibrillator (AED), which is a piece of medical equipment that requires special training and oversight. Emergency medical technicians (EMTs) can assist patients in taking the patients' own prescribed medications as well as by administering multiple medications approved by the medical director. Advanced EMTs and paramedics have the strongest connection to the medical director due to the variety of advanced life support (ALS) skills they utilize. The bottom line is that it is now nearly impossible to have an effective EMS system without medical oversight.

The history of medical direction and oversight parallels that of EMS system development. An early example of medical direction is the advice given to Napoleon by his physicians about evacuating injured soldiers. Later, during the American Civil War, physicians coordinated the treatment of battlefield casualties. World War II saw the introduction of trained "physician extenders" in the form of corpsmen.

In the 1960s and 1970s, the medical literature reported new advances in the resuscitation of sudden-cardiac-death victims. Recognizing time as an important aspect of these interventions, pioneering EMS physicians attempted to introduce techniques such as CPR, artificial ventilation, and defibrillation to the prehospital environment, all of which have become essential techniques and required training for all EMS providers. In 1969, Dr. Eugene Nagel began to train members of the Miami Fire Department to provide ALS. As part of the training for these early paramedics, and to show support for nonphysician delivery of ALS, Dr. Nagel allowed students to intubate and ventilate him. This was perhaps the ultimate testament of physician advocacy!

Physician support for ALS in the field was not limited to urban areas. In the rural county of Haywood in the Great Smokies area of North Carolina, Dr. Ralph Feichter worked with the local rescue squad to develop an all-volunteer ALS team. Through support from the local medical society and hospital, Dr. Feichter trained 40 volunteers in advanced cardiac life support in the late 1960s.

The first medical directors were recruited as part-time volunteer advisors, sharing their time between their EMS work and a career elsewhere in medicine. Momentum was developing to establish respect for the emergency medical physician's expertise in prehospital care. In parallel, legislation was sought to recognize the prehospital provider as a limited practitioner of medicine under physician oversight. By 1974, many states, local jurisdictions, and local medical societies were recognized by law as mandating medical direction for ALS providers. Although the earliest providers were very much interested in providing medical direction, the proliferation of ALS programs brought about by the availability of federal funding and the relative shortfall of available volunteer physicians led to a period of underemphasis of medical direction in EMS.

Through the 1980s, in some urban and suburban areas, a "modern director" emerged, possessing special credentials and a more clearly defined role. These professionals, many of them with academic ties and teaching experience in emergency medicine, were able to apply clinical knowledge to EMS systems. The American College of Emergency Physicians (ACEP) embraced the EMS cause by publishing a position paper in 1989 titled *The Principles of EMS Systems* (Roush, 1989). This paper called for active participation and involvement of physicians in all aspects of EMS, including design, implementation, evaluation, and system revision. General requirements for the physician in the role of medical director were also outlined. Further recognition of the activities of physicians in EMS as a unique vocation worthy of its own status led to the creation of the National Association of EMS Physicians (NAEMSP), which became the leading physician society for prehospital emergency care. Recognizing the lack of a national standard or job description outlining the specific activities of a physician director, in 1998 the NAEMSP published a position paper containing a job description and checklist against which systems could compare their medical direction. This position paper highlighted the various duties by classifying them under many of the subsystems inherent in EMS (**Table 6-1**). The position paper also defined essential and desirable qualifications of directors and made a statement advocating appropriate support for directors by jurisdictions or agencies (**Table 6-2**).

Table 6-1 Role of the Medical Director

- Dispatch
- Clinical Care, Including Continuous Quality Improvement (CQI)
- Physician Clinical Roles
- EMS Education
- Administrative Duties, Liaison Roles, Finance, and Legislation
- Public and Occupational Health Arena
- System Evaluation
- EMS Research

Table 6-2 Qualifications of the Medical Director

Essential Qualifications
- Licensed to practice medicine or osteopathy
- Familiar with local and regional EMS activity

Desirable Qualifications
- Board certification or board preparedness in emergency medicine
- Active clinical practice of emergency medicine
- Completion of an EMS fellowship

Acceptable Qualifications
- Board certification or board preparedness in a clinical specialty

The physician's role is seen as collaborative. An EMS system medical director is an advocate for the patient and public health as well as for the EMS system and the EMS provider. Physician involvement in EMS is not limited to medical practice issues but extends to all aspects of EMS. An effective EMS physician will be involved in processes before, during, and after the emergency incident.

Medical oversight has also been recognized as important for all levels of EMS providers. Traditionally, physician involvement was limited to providers delivering ALS. Now, with EMTs authorized to assist patients with medications and perform more advanced techniques, such as IV initiation and advanced airway control, along with EMRs being able to use AEDs, the need for medical oversight is critical at all levels.

The design of future EMS systems to include advanced practice paramedics relies on both medical oversight and a close relationship with physicians. In the future, paramedics may serve as extensions of entire healthcare systems or hospitals that include not only emergency medicine but preventative and long term **population based health care**.

Models of Medical Oversight

With the advent of the modern EMS physician, as described by NAEMSP, the term "medical oversight" became preferable. Over the years, the definition of medical oversight has been refined. It has become a system of physician-directed quality assurance providing accountability for medical care in the prehospital setting. It involves the implementation and supervision of the medical aspects of an EMS system— by a physician—designed to deliver emergency care in the prehospital setting. Oversight is now often provided by a combination of the medical director and an EMS coordinator (often a paramedic) or other designee, to assist in the growing amount of duties placed on the system. Future systems might include a relationship with primary care physicians, hospitalists, and the entire hospital as the focus shifts to prevention and lowering readmissions.

Through medical oversight, the physician is primarily able to affect a system of care rather than merely the individual patient being served. The physician involved targets the quality of care being routinely delivered and acts as a consultant for the medical aspects of delivery, which may involve each subsystem of EMS. The physician's understanding of the epidemiology of prehospital emergencies and the scientific basis for interventions drives the system's decision making. Often this may be seen in the addition or subtraction of new techniques or equipment at the provider level that may be the result of changing medical research, which the physician regularly consults and performs. Medical direction provides and creates a line of medical accountability from patient through physician extender to physician. There are two aspects of medical oversight: indirect and direct.

Indirect Medical Oversight

Indirect, off-line, or system medical oversight implies physician input that is administrative, involving all facets, but remote from the patient encounter itself. By far, the most relevant and comprehensive tasks for medical directors occur by indirect oversight. The basis for day-to-day care rests with the system medical director. Clearly, in the United States, the fact that physicians are not needed in the ambulance for the typical patient encounter has been established and accepted. Rather, medical consultation is needed to help develop and refine a system of care that is in place for any potential patient. As such, the medical director's role may vary, based on a system's structure.

Medical directors are now involved at all levels, including federal, state, and local, and sometimes even at the company level. NAEMSP and ACEP now promote the use of state medical directors in regular, full-time positions to provide system oversight, though this is often not the case. At the minimum, the medical director serves as the legal means for a system and providers to function. The involvement of such directors is often limited to just signing forms, testing, and approving personnel. Some jurisdictions have primary oversight by a committee, with the medical director serving as a physician advisor. In others, the medical director is a primary part-time or full-time position, with a contract or job description that supports local duties and authority and that gives management status to the position. In this set-up, the director might be the sole ultimate authority, working with other leaders to make decisions that maintain or implement changes in the system. Finally, the director might be in a cabinet position that is directly accountable to a mayor or county executive, as would be the director of public health. In each model, there are specific areas of EMS where off-line medical direction has a place and a key role.

In some areas, medical oversight has become such a large task that multiple medical directors or a planning council oversees EMS for a city or region. These offices are often staffed by an **EMS coordinator** to provide day-to-day support in the name of the physician for off-line issues such as training and quality improvement. EMS coordinators can be paramedics, registered nurses, physician assistants, or a variety of other healthcare professionals, but they usually have direct experience and exposure to the EMS system and can serve as the "eyes and ears" of the medical director on a daily basis.

System Design

The physician medical director brings a unique perspective to EMS system design. The physician can analyze the medical needs of a population, the available resources, the levels of providers, the geographic area, and hospital resources. The physician can then suggest design characteristics of a system that prioritizes calls and provides prearrival instructions, dispatches the most appropriate care, intervenes in a beneficial manner, and transports the client to the closest appropriate facility. This analysis may lead to system characteristics such as priority medical dispatch, tiered assignments, police or fire AED first response, and specialty referral policies.

In addition to the system care delivered by advanced providers, the creation of AEMT and emergency medical dispatch has added new practitioners and skills to the basic arena. Both the framers of the *EMS Agenda for the Future* (NHTSA, 1996) and the creators of national dispatch systems have advocated for strong medical direction. When the design of a system calls for these levels, state agencies place the responsibility of supervision of all levels of care on physicians. Physicians have had a growing impact on initial dispatch due to the refinement of prearrival instructions, such as how to provide CPR or deliver a baby, along with the ability of dispatchers to determine the use of lights and sirens for response.

Protocols

Many in the EMS community consider protocol development to be the most important off-line component of medical oversight. **Protocols** are preauthorized sets of instructions that guide patient care. Protocols often use a decision tree that flows from patient assessment to patient management. These flowcharts are called **algorithms**. A protocol consists of a series of algorithms for each of the medical and trauma situations a provider will encounter in the field. For example:

- Nontraumatic shock
- Cardiac arrest—nontraumatic (**Figure 6-1**)
- Trouble breathing
- Suspected myocardial infarction
- Limb amputation
- Allergic reaction

Depending on the level of medical supervision and communication capacity, system protocols may contain points at which the field provider must contact medical control for further treatment actions (**Figure 6-2**). This most often occurs in situations involving critical interventions or with conditions that are hard to differentiate in the field. The requirement for providers to contact medical direction varies by area and depends on the level of trust that the medical director has in the competency of the providers and the overall educational level of the providers. Current trends are to educate providers to a higher level and to allow them additional latitude in deciding the correct action through standing orders or protocols. As protocols expand, so must quality assurance and quality improvement efforts, as discussed later in this chapter.

Protocols are drafted to give the various levels of providers an appropriate amount of autonomy in intervening on a patient's behalf without immediate physician consultation. By definition, the protocols represent that part of EMS that truly parallels the practice of medicine. In addition, the medical director's input into the planning, implementation, and revision of these documents is a key reason for the EMS physician's existence. Despite the need for medical expertise, diplomacy and humility dictate that the protocol development process involves the EMS coordinator, managers, nurses, emergency department physicians, prehospital providers, and other interested professionals.

Protocol development and revision may be driven by the physician, providers, or changes in medical science. With the wide acceptance of **evidence-based medicine (EBM)**, existing protocols have been called into question and new ones are needed. Additionally, research into population-based health care and readmissions may lead to protocols that change based on a patient's recent treatment within a hospital. Protocols should be regularly revised to reflect changing research and consensus standards. Some protocols, such as cardiac-arrest resuscitation, may directly reflect consensus standards, such as the American Heart Association's CPR and ACLS guidelines, which are updated every five years. Protocol changes may require further education of providers, changes in equipment, and quality assurance—all duties of medical oversight.

CARDIAC EMERGENCIES: CARDIAC ARREST

1. Initiate General Patient Care.

2. Presentation
   Patient must be unconscious, apneic, and pulseless.

 EARLY DEFIBRILLATION IS A PRIORITY IN WITNESSED ARREST. FOR PATIENTS IN UNWITNESSED ARREST 5 CYCLES OF CPR SHOULD BE COMPLETED PRIOR TO DEFIBRILLATION.

 3. Treatment
   a) Perform CPR.

   b) Utilize AED as appropriate.

   c) Transport
      (1) If no shock indicated, transport immediately.
      (2) If shock indicated, defibrillate and transport ASAP.

   d) Identify rhythm and treat according to appropriate algorithm.

   e) Perform CPR.

   f) Utilize AED as appropriate.

 DO NOT USE AED FOR PATIENTS WHO ARE LESS THAN 1 YEAR OF AGE. USE ONLY PEDIATRIC AED FOR PATIENTS 1 TO 8 YEARS OF AGE.

   g) Transport
      (1) If no shock indicated, transport immediately.
      (2) If shock indicated, defibrillate and transport ASAP.

   h) Identify rhythm and treat according to appropriate algorithm.

Figure 6-1 ALS protocol algorithm.

**CARDIAC EMERGENCIES: HYPERKALEMIA
(RENAL DIALYSIS/FAILURE OR CRUSH SYNDROME) (NEW '10)**

1. Initiate General Patient Care.

2. Presentation
   Certain conditions may produce an elevated serum potassium level that can cause hemodynamic complications.

3. Treatment
   a) Patients must meet the following criteria:

      (1) Suspected hyperkalemia patient **(NEW '10)**
          (a) Renal dialysis/failure with poor or non-functioning kidneys or
          (b) Crush syndrome or patients with functional kidneys by history
          AND
      (2) Hemodynamically unstable renal dialysis patients or patients suspected of having an elevated potassium with bradycardia and wide QRS complexes.

   b) Place patient in position of comfort.

   c) Assess and treat for shock, if indicated.

   d) Constantly monitor airway and reassess vital signs every 5 minutes.

   e) Initiate IV LR KVO.

   f) Initiate Bradycardia protocol.

   g) Consider calcium chloride 0.5-1 grams slow IVP over 3-5 minutes. Maximum dose 1 gram or 10 mL.

   h) Consider sodium bicarbonate 50 mEq IV over 5 minutes. **(NEW '10)**

   i) Consider/ administer albuterol (high dose) via nebulizer 20 mg (if available) **(NEW '10)**

 FLUSH IV WITH 5 ML OF LACTATED RINGER'S BETWEEN CALCIUM AND SODIUM BICARBONATE ADMINISTRATION **(NEW '10)**

   j) Crush syndrome or patients with functional kidneys by history
      Consider/ administer sodium bicarbonate 50 mEq SLOW IV over 5 minutes and then initiate drip of sodium bicarbonate 100 mEq in 1000 mL to run over 30-60 minutes. (Reserve for patient suspected of crush syndrome or patients with functional kidneys by history.) **(NEW '10)**

Reprinted with permission of the Maryland Institute of Emergency Medical Services Systems.

Figure 6-2 ALS protocol algorithm requiring medical consultation.

CARDIAC EMERGENCIES: HYPERKALEMIA (Continued)

k) Place patient in position of comfort.

l) Assess and treat for shock, if indicated.

m) Constantly monitor airway and reassess vital signs every 5 minutes.

n) Initiate IV LR KVO.

o) Initiate Bradycardia protocol.

p) Administer calcium chloride 20 mg/kg (0.2 mL/kg) slow IVP/IO (50 mg/min)
   Maximum dose 1 gram or 10 mL.

q) Consider/administer albuterol via nebulizer
   (1) For patients 2 years of age or greater, administer albuterol 2.5 mg
   (2) For patients less than 2 years of age, administer albuterol 1.25 mg. **(NEW '10)**

 FLUSH IV WITH 5 ML OF LACTATED RINGER'S BETWEEN CALCIUM AND BICARBONATE ADMINISTRATION. **(NEW '10)**

r) Crush syndrome or patients with functional kidneys by history
   Consider/administer sodium bicarbonate 1 mEq/kg IV over five minutes. Maximum dose 50 mEq. (Reserve for patient suspected of Crush syndrome or patients with functional kidneys by history.) **(NEW '10)**

4. Continue General Patient Care.

Figure 6-2 *(Continued)*

Another term that is often used synonymously with protocol is **standing order**. In some systems, a standing order refers to the ability of providers to initiate treatment on their own without direct medical control: The standing order is part of the system protocol. Others define a standing order as direct orders issued to a provider to deal with a specific patient situation. For example, a paramedic may request, through direct medical control, a drug order to give Valium to a seizure patient in the event that the patient begins seizing. The physician's order to do so would be a standing order. However, the use of Valium in this situation is allowed under system protocol. Standing orders support protocols.

Education

Emergency medical service education is a cornerstone of prospective off-line medical direction. **Prospective** refers to physician involvement while a process or activity is happening before the emergency call, often through education and system development efforts. The role of the medical director in EMS education includes academic instruction, curriculum review, setting standards for class performance, evaluation, and student counseling. In most systems, the physician must rely on qualified nonphysician EMS educators to train providers. These EMS educators are often trained and approved by the medical directors to provide education on their behalf. Perhaps the ideal compromise is the physician who makes targeted appearances in the classroom, cadaver lab, megacode recertification, and drills, or in situations in which new information in medicine would be best disseminated by a physician. Whenever possible, EMS students should complete a clinical rotation with the medical director in the emergency department (ED).

Quality Systems

In the 1950s, one of the fathers of **quality improvement** (QI), W.E. Deming (1986), brought his message to a limited number of American industries and to Japan, where he facilitated a dramatic turn-around in the quality of industrial processes and goals. By the 1980s, a renewal of interest in quality, management skills, and ultimate output brought Deming's efforts back to U.S. industries. He laid out his 14 points for the success of Western management, which included positive goals for training: communications, morale, and the elimination of traditional barriers such as workforce fear, arbitrary standards, and meaningless slogans.

Joseph Juran (1989) was a synergistic force in the area of quality management with the development of a trilogy that describes a perpetual effort to maintain quality while looking for opportunities for improvement. In quality planning, one defines who the customers (recipients of products or services) are and what their needs are, determines the products that will serve those needs, and identifies the key processes and methods of operation that will generate those products. In quality control, the processes are monitored to ensure that they maintain the appropriate output of quality products. In quality improvement, the waste or inefficiency of the process is identified as an opportunity for beneficial change. This change is implemented in the process, and a new, better zone of quality control is established.

Avedis Donabedian (1980–1985) was one of the pioneers of quality systems with respect to health care. His well-known model focuses on three elements that are key to the delivery of services: structure, process, and outcome. The structure obviously determines the framework in which care can take place. The process implies the care itself and the method of its delivery. The outcome refers to the effects of the care and the subsequent health status of patients.

All three of these concepts and their authors have relevance to EMS medical oversight. The EMS physician can advocate for education, good morale, communication free of fear, and provision of constructive feedback, consistent with Deming's principles. The director can identify patients as customers and focus on the systemwide response to needs as endorsed by Juran. The structure can parallel system design and equipment, the process can relate to resources and protocols for all levels of provider and how they are educated, and the outcome can be determined through data-collection mechanisms best sanctioned by a physician.

Quality of care is the ultimate goal of any healthcare service. Many medical directors feel that their primary role is to be the ultimate authority on quality. This emphasis on quality has led to the change in terminology from "medical direction" to "medical oversight." Oversight infers a **continuous quality improvement (CQI)** approach to physician involvement in EMS systems. Integrated healthcare systems use data from EMS not only to improve care but also to connect patient outcomes in the hospital to prehospital treatments. Together, the physician and the EMS system can have dramatic impacts on long-term outcomes.

Providers who see the medical director infrequently may view with concern and suspicion requests for information about care. Traditional quality assurance (QA) focuses on evaluating individual cases in which problems have arisen and may lead to affixing blame to providers. An EMS system and medical director who uses CQI shifts the focus away from blaming the individual provider and toward studying and improving the system's process. CQI also uses a scientific process to collect and study data along with evidence-based medicine in order to make decisions, as opposed to the traditional system of decision-making with subjective opinions. The outcome may be determined through data-collection mechanisms that are best sanctioned by physicians. The result of the medical director's commitment to CQI is an evaluation method that looks at and corrects system problems first, promotes positive feedback using objective data, and uses reeducation to bring about cultural changes rather than encouraging individual negative feedback.

Growing EMS systems now often have a quality improvement or assurance program within the organization itself, along with that provided by the medical director. This tiered approach allows the agency the EMS provider works or volunteers for to have a direct impact on quality improvement; they can often handle "smaller" issues without the direct involvement of the medical director. Unfortunately, in systems in which providers have contact with the medical director only when there is a "big" issue, providers may feel even more distant from the director, causing further fear and suspicion.

In a system of CQI, there is still a place for retrospective review of care. **Retrospective** refers to the process of looking at or studying something after it has occurred, such as reviewing completed incident reports. Quality improvement takes place alongside QA and trends are identified that call for future reeducation. CQI responds differently to these trends. This method is described as solving more than 80% of quality concerns and may be handled by the in-house quality assurance officer or EMS coordinator rather than by the physician himself or herself. Only in very unusual cases, in which educational feedback and remediation have failed, is disciplinary action the best next course. In implementing a quality management system, the physician's biggest challenge will be to find the data-collection mechanism that captures long-term outcome parameters, which is often not available through the records of prehospital systems.

Quality improvement and assurance is rapidly changing, with expanding protocols for advanced providers, new skills for basic providers, and the integration of evidence-based medicine. EMS providers now have to commit to developing their expertise with the assistance of the medical director to improve patient care. Providers and physicians will have to work collaboratively to ensure that the workplace environment supports and challenges the providers to improve their expertise through a combination of experience, classroom training, and call reviews if EMS is going to continue to grow as a profession.

Direct Medical Oversight

Direct or online medical oversight implies real-time physician involvement in a patient encounter with EMS providers. This model entails communication by radio or telephone directed at obtaining advice in patient treatment. In some cases, physicians on scene personally provide supervision. Online medical direction is provided in several ways. First, it is most commonly described as an established consultation after the assessment of a patient and initiation of care until reaching a decision point that requires physician input. In this model, contact is delegated, either through medical legislation or directly by the system director, to other physicians who are on duty or available at the receiving hospital. Within such a system, several possibilities exist. The provider may call or radio into an approved ED physician at the receiving facility. The online contact may be directed to a physician at a regional base station that serves more than one receiving facility. In some locales, such as the city of Pittsburgh, the on-duty EMS physician may carry a portable radio and provide consultation regardless of location while on duty. Finally, the medical director may monitor system operations and provide online directions to providers by radio or phone in special situations. In some locations, for instance California, specially trained allied health professionals provide online medical command. Nurses or paramedics answer consultations and consult with physicians for difficult or special cases.

In a less common scenario, direct medical oversight is accomplished by a physician on scene. In this model, the medical director is most commonly involved. Some directors make a regular effort to ride in the field to monitor the process of care, as a mentorship program, to develop sensitivity to the provider's work, or to provide supervision. Physicians within the medical oversight system might work on scene at mass casualty incidents or other critical incidents where time is of the essence and multiple providers are involved. Some systems provide "fly cars" or emergency response vehicles for members of the medical oversight team to provide help on scene. Additionally, physicians may become involved in on-scene patient care when procedures outside the scope of EMS are needed, such as surgical amputations.

A physician who is not part of the EMS system may also be on scene. Such bystander physicians include office physicians or a physician who stops to render aid. The authority of a bystander physician to provide direct medical control varies. If a physician wishes to provide medical direction, he or she will often be required to accompany the patient to the receiving facility and provide appropriate identification. The medical oversight system should state the appropriate way to handle physicians on scene; it may be advisable to have the on-scene physician who is not involved in the EMS system speak directly to the medical director for clarification. In any case, the EMS provider should ensure that a physician on scene provides appropriate documentation of his or her credentials before accepting direct medical direction from the physician.

Although the advantage of online medical direction seems obvious to the casual observer, there remains true debate on the value of routine physician consultation. Indeed, not only does the medical literature point to a lack of positive impact on patient care, but also some studies have suggested that routine online direction is counterproductive.

However, consultation should be available for specific, critical patient presentations or when providers desire assistance. Achieving a balance between online and off-line medical direction can be difficult and will reflect the level of service provided and the service area. What may work in one system may not work in another, and medical directors are allowed to make changes to suit their local conditions.

Regulation and Legislation

Because ALS-level care requires the practicing of medicine without a license, most states have recognized the unique status of the paramedic. However, no state currently authorizes paramedics to function without medical oversight.

Thus, the medical director's medical license extends to the prehospital provider. The prehospital provider is practicing medicine under the medical director's license. Because of this, the medical director is responsible for the actions of the providers and incurs any liability associated with this relationship. It is this extension of licensure that is most often used to support the role of the medical director in all aspects of an EMS system. The legal role of the physician in the provision of ALS is not always as clearly defined as that of the paramedic. Consequently, the physician's authority varies and is often open to interpretation.

In the early years of EMS, the development of EMS systems, especially the provision of ALS, was highly dependent on support from the local medical society. Often, a local physician would become an advocate for EMS and champion its cause with the medical society and hospital. Some early EMS systems sought physician support and advocacy to institute ALS, whereas others were influenced by physicians to develop ALS. The willingness of a physician to place his or her license on the line was often the only form of official medical control and sanction for paramedics to perform ALS.

As ALS systems proliferated, the need for formal recognition of ALS providers and medical control was recognized. In 1970, California passed the **Wedworth-Townsend Paramedic Act**, which legally recognized paramedics. This act served as a model for similar nationwide legislation. Maryland's early EMS laws governing cardiac rescue technicians, the state's first type of ALS provider, mandated medical supervision starting in 1973. Other states followed this trend over time, although some states did not incorporate medical-direction laws until after 1991. The nature of medical direction specified by state laws and regulation varies and is often open to interpretation and regular revision.

Considered necessary for the delivery of ALS, medical direction has now been introduced for BLS services. This change was brought about by changes in the *EMS Scope of Practice* for the EMR, EMT, and Advanced EMT. States have had to change their EMS laws and regulations to expand the coverage of medical direction. Some states, such as California and New Jersey, require a designated medical director for each EMS service. In Maryland, providers can be state certified as EMTs only if they are affiliated with an agency that has established medical direction. In Connecticut, EMS providers can work or volunteer only as part of the EMS system; their certification at all levels is only good when under medical direction and as part of the EMS system.

WRAP UP

Summary

Physicians play an important role in prehospital care. Since the advent of advanced life support, prehospital care has come to be accepted as the practice of medicine by physician extenders. Thus, physicians must supervise the delivery of care. The nature of this supervision, which is now recognized as a quality assurance issue, has become known as medical oversight rather than the original approach of medical direction. In most states and jurisdictions, the role of the medical director is legally defined. The director is involved in system design, education, protocols, and quality management.

Key Terms

algorithms

continuous quality improvement (CQI)

direct or online medical oversight

EMS coordinator

evidence-based medicine (EBM)

indirect, off-line, or system medical oversight

medical command

medical direction

medical oversight

population based health care

prospective analysis

protocols

quality improvement (QI)

retrospective

standing order

Wedworth-Townsend Paramedic Act

Review Questions

1. Define medical oversight.
2. State the role of CQI in system medical direction.
3. Differentiate between direct and indirect medical control.
4. Differentiate between prospective and retrospective medical oversight.
5. Briefly defend the need for the medical oversight of BLS providers.
6. Compare the structure of your local medical oversight system with that of other systems.

Additional Resources

Deming, W. E. (1986). *Out of the crisis.* Massachusetts Institute of Technology.

Donabedian, A. (1980–1985). *Exploration in quality assessment and monitoring* (3 vols). Health Administration Press.

Juran, J. M. (1989). *Juran on leadership for quality.* Free Press.

National Highway Traffic Safety Administration. (1996). *Emergency medical services: Agenda for the future.* Washington, DC: Author.

Roush, W. R. (Ed.). (1989). *Principles of EMS systems.* Dallas, TX: American College of Emergency Physicians.

7

Public Access and Communications

Objectives

Upon completion of this chapter, the reader should be able to:

- Identify the universal access number in the United States, its development, and its use.

- State the role and function of a public safety answering point.

- State the role of nonemergency access numbers, such as 3-1-1.

- List the two major components of pathway management.

- State the importance of public education in the efficient operation of a 9-1-1 system.

- State the importance of communications in an EMS system.

- Identify the communications phases of an EMS incident.

- Differentiate between system and medical communications.

- List the roles of the EMS telecommunicator.

- State the importance of prearrival instructions.

- Define and state the importance of the FirstNet concept.

Public Access

A community could have the most sophisticated emergency medical services (EMS) system staffed with highly trained paramedics responding in modern ambulances, but if the public does not have a simple and effective means of activating the system, it is worthless. The American Heart Association, in the chain of survival, has recognized the importance of public access in EMS response. The chain links early access, early CPR, early defibrillation, and early advanced cardiac care together in a chain of survival for the victim of out-of-hospital acute coronary syndromes (AHA, 2005). Public access is equally important in noncardiac-related events, such as trauma and severe respiratory distress. Because emergency medical systems exist to serve the public, access to the system is as important as the system components themselves. **Public access** is more than just having the capability to call 9-1-1. Public access involves the ability of an EMS system to appropriately respond to a caller's needs regardless of the caller's socioeconomic status, age, or perceived need. An effective EMS system has the ability to provide differing levels of response depending on the caller's needs. Thus, an appropriate response might not be the dispatch of a traditional ambulance, but referral to another agency or response network.

EMS systems have traditionally functioned independently of other community health resources, both public and private. However, the integration of healthcare systems within a community and the effects of managed care have changed the role of EMS. As a focal point for entry into the healthcare system, they must be responsive not only to the patient's needs, but also to the needs and concerns of the total community healthcare system.

9-1-1

When one thinks of public access, the **universal access number** 9-1-1 most often comes to mind. The number 9-1-1 is available to almost 93% of the U.S. population (www.nena.org). Before 1968, however, a person needing emergency assistance "dialed" either a seven-digit number or "0" for the operator. In those areas of the country not covered by 9-1-1, a caller must still use a seven-digit number for assistance.

The development of 9-1-1 was encouraged by EMS and fire services. In 1957, the first suggestion for a universal access number came from the National Association of Fire Chiefs. The need for such a number to provide quick access to law enforcement emergencies was recognized in 1967 by the President's Commission on Law Enforcement and Administration of Justice. Responding to these concerns, the Federal Communications Commission (FCC) approached American Telephone and Telegraph (AT&T) in 1967 to see if such a number was possible. In 1968, AT&T introduced 9-1-1 as the universal emergency access number. Note that prior to the early 1970s, telephone service in the United States was solely provided by the Bell Telephone System, part of AT&T. Thus, action by AT&T was nationwide and covered all public phone systems in the United States. To further the development of 9-1-1, the U.S. Congress passed legislation supporting the nationwide implementation of 9-1-1, and in 1973 the White House Office of Telecommunications issued a national policy statement on the advantages of 9-1-1. The first 9-1-1 call was made on February 16, 1968, in Haleyville, Alabama. Advantages of the digits 9-1-1 include the following:

- The number is easily "dialed," especially for rotary dial phones that were common in the 1960s.
- The number is easy to remember.
- The number is unique, having never been assigned as an area code or a service code.
- Nationwide, people need to remember only one number (9-1-1).
- Having one number reduces problems related to contacting the proper emergency agency.
- Pay or restricted phones allow 9-1-1 calls to be made for free.

9-1-1 Operation

The main purpose of the number 9-1-1 is to connect a caller with an emergency to a **public safety answering point (PSAP)**. Once connected to a PSAP, the caller can be routed to the proper emergency services dispatching agency. Depending on the sophistication of the local PSAP, the person answering the 9-1-1 call may also be the emergency dispatcher. However, the ideal situation is for the PSAP to be staffed with call takers whose primary responsibility is to answer and forward 9-1-1 calls to the proper agency.

In addition to providing easy access to emergency services, 9-1-1 also provides basic information important for call dispatching. Such information includes the caller's telephone number and location. The first 9-1-1 system, known as basic 9-1-1, provided limited information about the caller. With the introduction of a digital database of phone numbers, a more sophisticated 9-1-1 was possible. **Enhanced 9-1-1** provides automatic number identification (ANI) and automatic location information (ALI). When a person calls 9-1-1, ANI identifies the calling number and ALI provides the street address of the caller. Enhanced 9-1-1 also has automated call routing that ensures that an emergency call is directed to the proper PSAP. This feature is important because telephone service areas usually do not follow city or county boundaries. A growing area of concern related to accessing 9-1-1 by telephone is the introduction of new phone services that do not use traditional phone service technology. Voice over Internet Protocol (VoIP) is one such example of technology that presents unique challenges for 9-1-1 service. To address such changes, the U.S. Congress passed the New and Emerging Number Technologies 911 Improvement Act of 2008. The National Emergency Number Association (NENA) has created technical specification NENA i3, which details how to move an Enhanced 9-1-1 system to an Internet protocol-based emergency communications system. Such a system will allow the networking and integration of PSAPs during an emergency or a disaster situation.

Two services intergrated with 9-1-1 are **geographic information systems (GIS)** and **global positioning system (GPS)** technology. Integration allows better location-finding of incidents as well as specific routing of emergency responders to the scene. GIS present different layers of information about local response areas and infrastructure from many different perspectives. This sophistication allows for improved resource deployment with an emphasis on risk avoidance. For instance, GIS facilitate mapping and comparing incident demand and type with local demographics. GPS technology is now present in many everyday devices, from cars to cellular phones, allowing for the more precise determination of incident locations. This is especially important in remote rural areas where traditional address information, such as house numbers and street signs, is not readily available or accessible. An example of such an application is the "OnStar Alarm System" available in some automobiles. The driver or passenger needs only to push a button to summon medical or police assistance. Sensors in the car relay the vehicle's position via GPS to a central monitoring station that contacts the appropriate PSAP. These systems are also capable of detecting a vehicle crash and initiating a call without input from the vehicle's passengers.

An expanding technology that has had a profound effect on 9-1-1 notification and locating is the cellular telephone. The FCC requires that all cellular phones nationwide, even those without a service contract, be capable of connecting to a 9-1-1 system. Because cellular telephones do not operate from a fixed location, dialing 9-1-1 creates challenges related to determining caller location. Like phone service areas, cells may not follow jurisdictional boundaries, or a caller may move between cells while on the line. Unless a caller is familiar with an area, it may be difficult to pinpoint the location of an incident. To eliminate this problem, various public safety groups persuaded the FCC to require all digital cellular phones manufactured after 2001 to have either GPS capability or some other means of identifying the caller's location. Thus, when a cellular 9-1-1 call is received, the PSAP has the latitude and longitude of the phone making the call. This technology is known as Wireless Enhanced 9-1-1.

Another change emerging in 9-1-1 notification is the use of text messaging. As more people rely almost entirely on text messaging for communication, it was only a matter of time before texting would be used to contact the PSAP. This has led to the FCC allowing demonstration projects at select PSAPs around the country to receive emergency text messages. Initial results have been positive and it is anticipated that all PSAPs will eventually be able to receive requests for emergency response via text messaging.

There have been a few reports of people requesting emergency assistance via social media. However, this is not a practical approach, as it requires a friend or follower to receive the post and make the actual 9-1-1 notification. It is also not possible for a PSAP to monitor everyone's social media. This use of social media should be discouraged unless social media is the only available means of communication in an emergency.

Public Safety Answering Point

The PSAP, shown in **Figure 7-1**, also sometimes called a public safety access point, is an integral part of public access. PSAPs have evolved over the years from a single dispatcher who answered the phone as well as determined the running assignment and dispatched the call to multilayer, multifunction central communication centers. Once a telecommunicator or call taker determines the nature of the caller's emergency, information needed to dispatch the proper emergency service is transferred to that service's **dispatch center**. Depending on the incident, the call taker may remain on the line, transfer the caller, or hang up. If the call is a medical emergency, the caller will be transferred to an emergency medical dispatcher, who will provide prearrival instructions. Simultaneously, the service dispatcher will alert and direct the necessary units to the incident scene.

Although the staffing and complexity of a PSAP will vary, all PSAPs serve as a focal point for public access to emergency services. By being a centralized point of contact, the PSAP is able to obtain necessary information and direct the caller to the proper response agency. If a PSAP were not part of the public access system, callers would need to know which service they needed when dialing 9-1-1. Prior to the establishment of PSAPs, the 9-1-1 operator would answer "police,

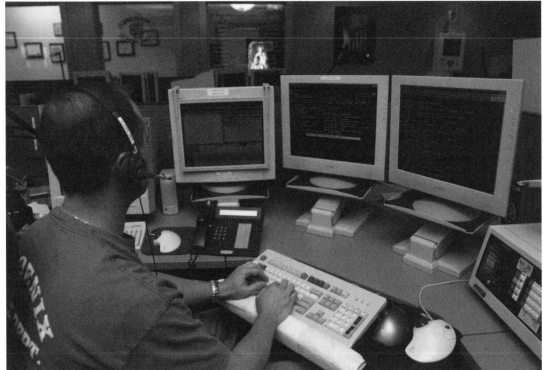

© Jones & Bartlett Learning. Courtesy of MIEMSS.

Figure 7-1 A 9-1-1 center.

fire, ambulance." Callers would have to pick which one they needed and then be transferred. Now, the PSAP telecommunicator will answer "911, what is your emergency?" and direct the call appropriately.

Call Processing

When people call 9-1-1, all they know is whether the phone is answered in time and the proper emergency services unit arrive on scene to help. Although this process may seem simple, it involves a number of interrelated steps, all of which must work together seamlessly to provide efficient access to emergency services.

Call Taking

When 9-1-1 is dialed, the caller is connected to the PSAP and to a person who answers the 9-1-1 line. Regardless of the ultimate responsibility and other duties of the person answering the call, at this point that person will function as a call taker. What happens next depends on the sophistication of the PSAP and the communications system.

In the simplest system, the call taker is the only person to handle the entire incident and may be the only person working at the PSAP. Once the information necessary for dispatching the call has been acquired from the caller and the 9-1-1 system, the caller is disconnected and the call taker assumes the role of a dispatcher.

In larger systems, the call taker may transfer the call to a dispatcher, who then determines the **response package** type and number of units needed to handle the call and alerts the indicated units. The caller may either remain on the line or be disconnected. If the caller remains on the line, he or she is either transferred to an **emergency medical dispatcher** or remains with the incident dispatcher; both will provide prearrival instructions.

In the most sophisticated PSAPs, the 9-1-1 call takers are a separate group of dispatchers who only answer 9-1-1 lines. They then transfer the calls to the respective agencies: police, fire, and EMS. The 9-1-1 answering center may not even be located in the same building or area as the service dispatch centers. This arrangement is common in most major metropolitan areas.

Dispatch Center

The dispatch center is responsible for receiving the 9-1-1 information, processing the call, and coordinating communications. The center may be service specific or it may handle dispatch for multiple services (e.g., fire and police). Because the dispatch center must constantly know the status of all response units in the service and select the most appropriate combination of units to handle a call, the centers utilize computer-aided dispatch, commonly called CAD. A CAD system is special software that tracks units' status and automatically recommends the proper response package for a given geographic location and incident type. Some CAD systems are capable of alerting units and sending location and incident information directly to the units electronically. Units may be equipped with **automatic tracking and status notification** that continually updates the CAD system via radio. The main advantage of a CAD system is speed and accuracy. Location information can be transferred directly to the CAD from an enhanced 9-1-1 (E-9-1-1) system. Location-specific information can also be stored, such as information about a handicapped person on premises or special hazards, and GIS data can also be tied in. The CAD always assembles the correct response package based on preprogrammed parameters and unit status and thus eliminates manual selection of units and proper response agencies. In addition to incident dispatch and coordination, the dispatch center may also serve as the notification agency for hospitals and other resources as well as the coordinating center for medical communications. The center also handles communications between the dispatch centers of the various emergency services and their units. For instance, if an EMS crew needs police assistance, the request would be forwarded to the police dispatch center via the EMS center.

Dispatch Life Support

Dispatch life support (DLS) is a term used to encompass emergency medical dispatch (EMD), **priority dispatching**, and prearrival instructions. More and more dispatch centers are using DLS as a means to provide increased services and better public access to EMS systems. The concepts of DLS have their roots in work done by Jeff Clawson, an emergency physician and fire department medical director from Salt Lake City, who began the concept of EMD in 1977. The importance of DLS was recognized by the National Association of EMS Physicians (www.naemsp.org) in 1989 with the publication of a position paper supporting emergency medical dispatching. The NAEMSP called for, among other things, recognition of the emergency medical dispatcher as an integral part of the EMS system. The paper also encouraged dispatch centers nationwide to adopt DLS.

If a dispatch center uses DLS, the 9-1-1 caller will not merely confirm the incident location and nature but also will be quickly interrogated using priority dispatch to determine the appropriate level of response (BLS versus ALS). Once the priority dispatch information has been obtained, the dispatcher can provide prearrival instructions. Depending on the complexity of the dispatch center, prearrival instructions may be provided by yet another telecommunicator. Most likely, the original dispatcher will remain on the line, and unit dispatch will be handled by another dispatcher. Transfer of information between the various dispatchers occurs via the CAD system. As new information is provided, or changes in the patient's condition are noted, the emergency medical dispatcher will pass this information on to the responding units. Arrival of EMS personnel at the patient's side ends the EMD phase of the incident.

Emergency Medical Dispatch (EMD)

EMD is the process of sending the right units to the right location with the right resources. It would be a waste to send an ambulance staffed with two paramedics to a call for a broken toe, but this cannot be avoided unless the dispatcher knows the true nature of the incident. EMD allows the dispatcher not only to function as a member of the EMS response team, but also to more efficiently manage system resources. This is accomplished through the use of priority dispatch.

Priority Dispatching

Priority dispatching is the process of using a scripted series of questions to interrogate the caller and determine the proper level of EMS system response. The emergency medical dispatcher asks a series of initial questions to clarify the nature and severity of the incident. After this quick interview, units are dispatched.

Prearrival Instructions

Prearrival instructions are a means to provide first aid instructions via phone. Instead of disconnecting the caller after the initial interrogation, the caller has the option of remaining on the line and receiving instructions on how to care for himself or herself or for the patient. The dispatcher follows a set sequence of questions and provides instructions based on the caller's answers. Instructions for complex activities, such as CPR and childbirth, can be given over the phone.

Nonemergency Access Numbers

As 9-1-1 became known as the most direct means to reach police and emergency services, people began using it as a general number for any type of governmental assistance. Callers have dialed 9-1-1 to ask directions, inquire about garbage pickup, complain about rodent control, or find the correct time. All of these inappropriate calls place a strain on the PSAP, especially in highly populated areas. Public education programs, such as "Make the Right Call," have helped to educate the public, but have not eliminated the problem. In major urban areas, the demand on the 9-1-1 service can become so severe that callers will receive a busy signal or recording when calling during peak times.

Looking for a way to reduce or eliminate inappropriate 9-1-1 calls, a number of cities have implemented **nonemergency access numbers**, of which the most common is 3-1-1. The first use of 3-1-1 occurred in 1996 in Baltimore, Maryland. The city developed a 3-1-1 system with support from the Department of Justice Office of Community Oriented Policing Services (COPS). The slogan "Where there is an urgency, but no emergency" was used to promote the number. After implementation of 3-1-1, Baltimore experienced a significant improvement in 9-1-1 system efficiency and responsiveness.

Because of the possibility of a real emergency being reported via 3-1-1, such services should be part of the PSAP operation. 3-1-1 systems should also have ANI and ALI capability to ensure proper handling of emergency calls. The number 3-1-1 must also be a local, non-toll call just like 9-1-1.

Pathway Management

Public access deals with the means by which a person enters into the EMS system. Entry into EMS is also a pathway for entry into the broader healthcare system. When people perceive that they have an emergency situation, they dial 9-1-1 for assistance. EMS is dispatched, and in most cases the person is transported to a hospital. After the event is over, the patient submits the bills to the insurance company for payment. In this situation, the insurance company has no control over the patient's decision to call 9-1-1, the EMS treatment provided, or the medical facility the patient is transported to. If the patient's perceived problem turns out not to be an emergency, the insurance company may deny the claim. If the insurance company or managed care organization (MCO) could control the patient's entry into the medical system, it could potentially reduce false calls or inappropriate use, thus saving money. The means by which MCOs have attempted to control access is through pathway management.

Pathway management is a process whereby an MCO subscriber calls a central number and speaks with a healthcare professional, usually a nurse. Using a set of algorithms, the call taker evaluates the caller's complaint and decides on the appropriate course of action. This may include calling 9-1-1 or a physician, seeing a physician, or self-treatment. Through the use of telephone triage, the MCO is able to control patient entry into the healthcare system and ensure that the patient accesses an appropriate level of care.

The concept of pathway management can also be applied to 9-1-1 service. By screening calls for EMS assistance, a call taker can reduce the number of inappropriate requests for EMS service, thus reducing EMS system demand. Some systems even go as far as calling a taxi to assist callers not in need of emergency services. To screen calls, 9-1-1 systems utilize field paramedics assigned to a call rotation in the dispatch center.

A comprehensive pathway management system operating through a PSAP must include two main components. The first is a means to triage emergency calls. This is accomplished through the use of

EMD, just discussed in this chapter. The second is nonemergency triage. This process involves medical interrogation of patients whose conditions do not require an EMS response. Nonemergency triage follows the same process as described earlier for MCO subscribers.

How best to provide these two services to the public remains controversial. Should they be handled through a public safety PSAP, or is nonemergency triage outside the scope of public safety? Would a combined public-private venture better serve the public? These questions will only be answered as the EMS community gains more experience with pathway management.

Public Education

To be effective as a means to serve the public, EMS must take steps to ensure that the public knows how and when to call 9-1-1. As entry into the healthcare system becomes more controlled through processes such as pathway management and preauthorization, it is critical for the general public to know how to get the help they need. One media campaign designed to educate the public about the appropriate use of 9-1-1 is the "Make the Right Call" program, sponsored by the National Highway Traffic Safety Administration. A newer version of the program, "Children Make the Right Call to EMS," is designed to educate children, especially those old enough to be left alone, about when to call EMS as well as to provide them safety prevention information.

Communications

An EMS system is made up of various components that must be able to effectively and efficiently work together. This coordination is accomplished through communications. Communication occurs at all levels of the system and takes various forms. Everything from a yearly briefing of constituent groups by a local EMS director, to the online medical consultation by an ambulance in the field, to the exchange of information by physicians in the emergency department is an example of EMS communications. However, this chapter focuses on the use of communications to coordinate the emergency response to a citizen's call for help and the system and medical communications associated with such a call.

Communications was one of the original 15 EMS system components and remains one of the 14 system attributes as defined in the *EMS Agenda for the Future*. The EMS Systems Act of 1973 called for a system of communications that addresses each of the following:

- Personnel, facilities, and equipment will be joined by a central communications system.
- Calls for EMS will be handled by a central communications center.
- Incoming calls will be medically screened.
- 9-1-1 will be utilized as the universal access number.
- The system will allow "direct communication connection and interconnections" with all parts of the EMS system and with other EMS systems.

"We can talk to astronauts on the moon, but an ambulance can't talk with a hospital ER" was a common statement during the early days of EMS. The statement acknowledged the availability of technology to improve EMS communications, but it also identified the poor condition, or lack, of operational EMS communications. Ambulances either did not have radios or would utilize citizen band (CB) channels and commercial frequencies that were often shared with other users. It was not uncommon for ambulances to just show up at the emergency room without any prior notification. A system for online medical direction did not exist. If EMS was going to advance, ambulances, paramedics, hospitals, and regional centers all needed the capability to connect to one another.

Role of Communications

As the "glue" that ties an EMS system together, communications serves a variety of roles in EMS. These include:

- Contact between persons needing help and dispatchers;
- Contact between dispatch and responding EMS providers;
- Contact between field providers and receiving hospitals;
- Contact between field providers and medical control; and
- Contact between field providers and other responders or units.

Effective EMS system communications provide for:

- System control and administration;
- Scene control and coordination; and
- Medical direction.

Perhaps the most important thing to remember regarding communications is that system personnel function as members of a team. The team can only function as efficiently as its communications. The typical EMS event can be broken down into a series of communication phases. These include the following:

- Occurrence
- Detection
- Notification
- Dispatch
- Prearrival instructions
- Response
- Scene communications
- Medical communications
- Transport
- Hospital arrival
- Return to service

Occurrence

Not all EMS events are as vivid as an auto crash. Some are very subtle and sensed only by the victim, such as a person who feels chest pain or has trouble breathing. Even then, not everyone will appreciate the significance of symptoms. For some, denial will influence their decision-making process and delay movement to the second phase, detection.

Detection

Someone must perceive that an event has taken place and recognize the need for EMS. An individual might see someone lying in a field. Is there a need for EMS, or is the person just sleeping? To be noticed, a person with chest pain needs to communicate, either verbally or through actions, that he or she is in distress. Others must be able to recognize the communication as a call for help.

Notification

Once the need for EMS has been established, the system must be called into action. This is most commonly accomplished by using the universal access number, 9-1-1. The victim or third party contacts the PSAP to request help. Once the nature of the call is understood by the call taker, proper units can be dispatched.

Dispatch

In order to help the victim, the proper services must be alerted to respond. Dispatch is the process of pulling together the proper response package and alerting units to respond. It also involves passing necessary response information—such as location, map coordinates, and nature of the call—to the responding providers.

Prearrival Instructions

After dispatching the call, some dispatch centers can provide assistance to the victim or caller by providing prearrival medical instructions. Using a set of standardized criteria, the dispatcher interrogates the caller and provides instructions on how to provide immediate, life-saving care. Prearrival instructions are given while responding units are en route to the scene.

Response

Having determined the nature of the call, the dispatcher selects the appropriate unit or units and alerts either the unit's station or the unit itself to respond. If more information about the incident is determined, it is passed on to responding units.

Scene Communications

Communications to and from the scene can be the most crucial of all incident communications. In addition to advising the dispatch center of arrival and departure from the scene, scene communications may include requests for additional resources, police assistance, updated call status, cancelling of responding units, and scene command and coordination.

Medical Communications

Once contact with the patient has been made, EMS personnel need to communicate with the receiving facility. If medical control orders are needed, personnel are put in contact with a medical command physician. Medical command is most often contacted via the medical radio system.

Transport

Once a transport destination has been determined, the EMS crew members need to advise the receiving hospital that they are en route. Notification can be made via the operational radio system or via a dedicated medical control radio system, depending on the EMS service's operating procedures.

Hospital Arrival

In addition to advising the dispatch center that the unit has arrived at the hospital, EMS personnel must also communicate their patient assessment and treatment to the emergency department staff. Even if the crew has notified the hospital via radio or phone, updated information and patient response to treatment needs to be conveyed. In some hospitals, this update is accomplished during a patient status report.

Return to Service

Once the unit is restocked and ready to handle another call, the dispatch center is notified that the unit is available for response. Depending on service procedures, the unit might not make any further contact with the dispatch center until alerted for another call. In fixed-base systems, the unit may advise when it has returned to its quarters.

Systems Communications Technology

Communications within an EMS system can be divided into two broad groups—**systems communications** and **medical communications**. Systems communications involves the communications necessary for operating and coordinating an EMS system. The main functions of systems communications are alerting and dispatching units and coordinating unit statuses. Medical communications are used to provide online **medical control** with a physician and to notify receiving facilities. Often, the two functions are integrated into one central communications system.

Systems Communications

The backbone of systems communications is the two-way radio. Radios have been used in fire and EMS vehicles since the 1930s. Technology developed in World War II made mobile radios more practical. War surplus and civil defense equipment also provided a source of radios for emergency vehicles. Development of the transistor in the 1950s made mobile communications equipment smaller and more reliable and also reduced the power needs of such units.

There are two basic components of a communications system. Messages are sent out to field units via a **central transmission system** that is capable of delivering a signal over the entire service area.

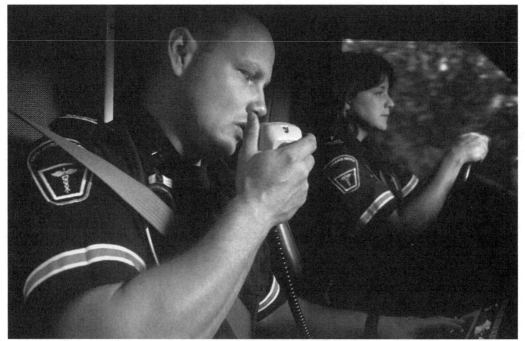

© Pat Lacroix/Getty.

Figure 7-2 The mobile radio unit is in the emergency response vehicle.

The second component of the radio system is the **mobile unit**. This is a radio unit, as shown in **Figure 7-2**, located in a vehicle. Powered by the vehicle's electrical system, the mobile unit allows contact with the dispatch center or with other mobile units. Vehicles and personnel may also be equipped with small **handheld radios** similar to a cellular phone that allow personnel to remain in contact with the dispatcher while away from their vehicle. Use of these portable units is not only convenient, but also provides increased safety for personnel, as they can quickly request help in an emergency or a threatening situation.

To speed up the communications process and to eliminate errors common to voice communications, radio systems are now incorporating direct computer-to-computer communications. Information received at the dispatch center is entered into the CAD computer, which integrates location information, unit status, and other factors to determine the optimal dispatch package to send to an incident. This information is transmitted directly from the center's CAD computer to field units and is displayed on a **mobile data terminal**. Two-way linkage also allows providers in the field to communicate, via the vehicle's computer, with the dispatch center or other sites for in-field information. In addition to call information, vehicle and crew status can also be transmitted. Linking mobile computers with vehicle GPS allows dispatch personnel to monitor vehicle movements in real time. GPS integration also provides mapping and travel route information directly to the vehicle crew. Continued evolution of the computer into the radio system results in direct links between prehospital providers and the dispatch center via computer, tablet, or smartphone-type devices. These devices integrate voice, data, and GPS functions in a single handheld or worn device.

Medical Communications

Paralleling the EMS communications system is medical communications. This can be a completely separate system or can be integrated into system communications. The medical communications system allows the prehospital provider to consult with medical control (**Figure 7-3**), pass patient information to a receiving facility, transmit biotelemetry (patient physiological parameters, such as an electrocardiogram (ECG)), and monitor the diversion status of facilities.

In the formative years of paramedic service, it was thought that paramedics would routinely transmit the patient's ECG to the base hospital for confirmation. Online medical consultation would also be

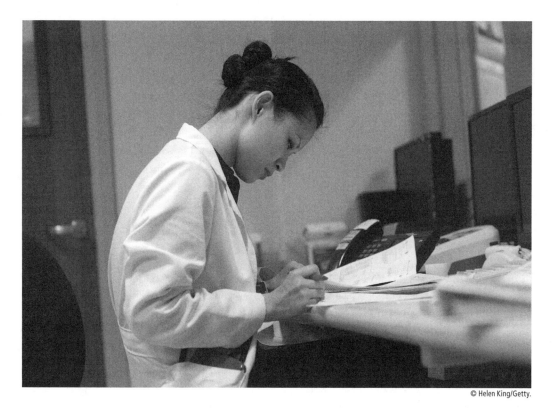

© Helen King/Getty.

Figure 7-3 Biotelemetry allows an ECG to be received by the hospital while the EMS crew is en route.

needed during the treatment of serious medical and trauma cases. To facilitate this increased communications' need, the FCC designed a set of frequencies in the ultra-high-frequency range (UHF) for exclusive nationwide use by EMS, known as the **national EMS radio system**, to which the FCC designated 10 pairs of frequencies. Two pairs of frequencies were for dispatch and system control and the other eight were designated medical channels for communications of patient information and biotelemetry. These same 10 frequency pairs are still in use today.

As paramedic practice became established, there came a decreased need for transmission of 3-lead ECGs to the base hospital for interpretation. Paramedics had proved their ability to accurately interpret ECGs in the field. Likewise, standing orders and protocols have allowed paramedics to treat most patients without having to obtain online medical direction. Thus, the use and nature of medical communications in many EMS systems changed. The system is now used more for notification and transfer of patient medical information than for online medical control.

Telemedicine

Although the transmission of simple ECGs from the field has decreased, new technologies are reversing this trend for more complex ECGs. Rapid and proper diagnosis of heart attacks is facilitated by the direct transmission of 12- or 15-lead ECGs to the hospital, usually using a facsimile system integrated into the cardiac monitor. Biomedical monitoring devices being developed by civilian and military researchers are providing increasing amounts of real-time patient data. Coupled with faster and more reliable communications networks, these devices can be used by field providers to directly send increasing amounts of information from the field to physicians and hospitals. Thus, a physician at a distant location can assess and treat a patient without even physically seeing or touching that patient. Trauma centers and emergency departments can be better prepared to quickly treat patients upon arrival based on medical data relayed directly from the field. This area of medical assessment and treatment is known as **telemedicine**. As computers and radios continue to be integrated, and miniaturization evolves, the future role of the prehospital provider may be more like that of a sensor technician.

National Emergency Response Communication System

The congressionally mandated First Responder Network Authority (FirstNet) is charged with developing an integrated nationwide system for first responder communications. The system is mandated to cover the entire continental United States, Hawaii, and Alaska, as well as U.S. territories. Using frequencies within the 700MHz radio spectrum, the system will integrate voice, video, and data for seamless communications among all first responders. An LTE system similar to that used by commercial cell service providers will provide the technological backbone for the system. Because commercial systems are more vulnerable to terrorism and natural disasters, the FirstNet system will use a dedicated infrastructure.

As with any program national in scope, politics and funding issues become a concern. It is questionable if the FirstNet system will even become a reality. Funding of $7 million was to be appropriated for the system but has not been made available and is assumed to be insufficient for a system of this scope. Because of such concerns, a number of states, including Maryland, Virginia, and California, have begun developing their own statewide systems.

WRAP UP

Summary

An EMS system is of no value if the public it serves cannot access it for service. Communications play a major role, not only by providing a means for public access, but as a critical element of the operational functioning of an EMS system. Centralized dispatch and coordinating centers accessible via 9-1-1 provide a convenient means for the public to request service and efficiently convey necessary vital information to receive a timely response of the appropriate resources. Staffed by trained and professional telecommunicators, these centers not only take caller information, but also provide additional services, such as prearrival instructions. The use of system and medical communications allows dispatchers, responders, and receiving facilities to coordinate the efficient care and transport of patients.

Key Terms

automatic tracking and status notification

central transmission system

dispatch center

dispatch life support (DLS)

Enhanced 9-1-1

geographic information systems (GIS)

global positioning system (GPS)

handheld radios

medical communications

medical control

medical interrogation

mobile data terminal

mobile unit

national EMS radio system

nonemergency access numbers

priority dispatching

public access

public safety answering point (PSAP)

response package

systems communications

telemedicine

universal access number

Review Questions

1. Define public access.
2. Why are the digits 9-1-1 used as the nationwide emergency access number?
3. What is a PSAP?
4. Why were nonemergency access numbers developed?
5. Why is public education an important part of public access?
6. Effective EMS communications provides for three functions. List them.
7. List, in order, the communication phases of an EMS incident.
8. Differentiate between system communications and medical communications.
9. What is telemedicine and what impact will it have on EMS?

8

Clinical Care and Hospital Emergency Medicine

Objectives

Upon completion of this chapter, the reader should be able to:

- State the importance of the receiving hospital as part of an EMS system and identify historical trends that have led to an increased utilization of the emergency department by the general population.

- Identify the recognition of emergency medicine as a medical specialty and as a positive factor in the improvement of emergency department care.

- Describe the basic organization of an emergency department and list common management positions within the emergency department.

- State the advantage of special emergency department areas, such as fast track and chest pain ERs.

- Differentiate between categorization and designation of medical facilities.

- Identify the clinical components of a trauma system.

- Identify the components of a trauma center and differentiate between the three levels of trauma center designation.

- List the major requirements of the Emergency Medical Treatment and Active Labor Law.

- Discuss the role of critical care transport.

- Discuss the expanded scope of practice for paramedics and community paramedicine.

Clinical Care

A community could be served by the best emergency medical services (EMS) system in the world, responding in the latest vehicles, and with the highest trained personnel, but that system would be essentially worthless if it could not transport patients for definitive care. For the average patient transported by EMS, definitive care is provided at the local hospital's emergency department (ED). Although modern EMS involves more than transportation, comprising the initial emergency medical care that would be provided in the ED, it is still a temporizing solution to a medical or trauma problem that most often requires resolution in a hospital.

Because EMS is a system of attributes that work together, the hospital is an integral component of a total community EMS system. The importance of clinical care was recognized both by Boyd in the original 15 components of an EMS system and as one of the 14 system attributes in the *EMS Agenda for the Future*. In addition to serving as the terminus for prehospital EMS, the ED is also a major supplier of medical care for the general public. In 2012, it was estimated that 19.5% of adults were seen at least once in EDs across the country (CDC, 2012). Although EDs have been used as a substitute for primary care, the number of adults visiting EDs at least once has gone down from 20.2% in 2000. For patients unable or unwilling to use their **primary care physician** or for those who do not have one, the ED is seen as a community "doctor's office" with a wide scope of quality services.

The current structure and function of the modern ED has evolved from a simple accident ward for charity patients or accident victims to a sophisticated medical care unit capable of handling the entire spectrum of medical and trauma emergencies. As a result of this evolution, the practice of emergency medicine (EM) has developed into a recognized medical specialty with five subspecialties: hospice and palliative care, medical toxicology, pediatric emergency medicine, sports medicine, and undersea and hyperbaric medicine. The American Board of Emergency Medicine now recognizes EMS as a medical subspecialty.

History of Emergency Medicine

In 1979, the American Board of Emergency Medicine (ABEM) was recognized by the American Board of Medical Specialties and the American Medical Association. This made emergency medicine the 23rd recognized **medical specialty**. This approval led to the development of residency programs in EM and certification of physicians as Fellows of the American College of Emergency Physicians (FACEP). Prior to this time, ED physicians were trained in a number of specialties, such as surgery, internal medicine, general practice, anesthesiology, and cardiology. The term "emergency room" was appropriate in the 1950s and 1960s, as many hospitals had a single room with one gurney and an outside door to serve as the place where emergency patients were admitted for definitive care. Some hospitals required house staff to cover shifts in the ED as part of their overall hospital duties, regardless of the physician's expertise or interest. EDs were occasionally staffed only by interns.

The demand for hospital emergency care grew rapidly after World War II, when a number of socioeconomic factors caused a significant shift in the way Americans sought medical care. A major force behind this change was the demise of the "house call" by private physicians. It was common practice for the local general practice physician to visit the sick at their home. Likewise, in cases of injury, the patient was either rushed to the physician's office or the physician was summoned to the scene. Only in the more populated urban areas where people lived close to a hospital were patients taken directly to that hospital for care. The second factor that changed the practice of medicine was the increased mobility of the general public. The availability of affordable transportation meant that more people were able to travel. The development of the "suburbs" required people to commute to work every day. This mobility resulted in increased auto crashes and demographic changes. People were less connected with the family physician than they had been in the past. The hospital ED replaced the local physician as the source of emergency and after-hours medical care.

In addition to the social changes of the postwar period, the practice of medicine was also changing. The experiences of physicians during World War II, coupled with advances in battlefield medical evacuation during the Korean War, were leading to the investigation and development of new approaches to emergency and trauma medicine. The advantages of rapid transport of the trauma victim, even by helicopter, were now being recognized.

As a result of increased national attention on EMS, EM began to develop along two parallel routes. The quality of medical care in emergency departments was improved as the importance and value of the ED was recognized by hospitals and medical staffs. At the same time, research into shock and trauma was leading to the development of a systems approach to the treatment of the severe trauma victim. The concept of a trauma system based on a trauma center was emerging. As these two paths continued to develop and, in some circumstances, intersect, the specialty of EM and the concept of the modern emergency department emerged. During the same period, advances were being made in critical care medicine. Anesthesiologists developed the new specialty of intensive care medicine from the care provided to patients during surgery and in the recovery room. These advances in critical and resuscitative medicine practices were easily adapted to the developing field of EM.

Scope of Emergency Medicine

Patients with a wide and varied spectrum of medical and trauma conditions are taken to EDs. This variety requires a medical staff with a broad preparation in all areas of medicine. The organizations representing emergency medicine—the American College of Emergency Physicians, American Board of Emergency Medicine, and the Society for Academic Emergency Medicine (SAEM)—have jointly developed a Core Content for EM (see **Table 8-1**). As stated in the Core Content's preamble:

> *The Core Content's purpose and function are threefold: It represents the breadth of emergency medicine practice. For the American Board of Emergency Medicine, it outlines the content at risk for examination in emergency medicine. Finally, it serves as a guide in the development of graduate and continuing medical education programs for those involved in the practice of emergency medicine. Because emergency medicine is changing rapidly, the Core Content, now called the Model of Clinical Practice, requires periodic revision.*

The Emergency Department

Hospital emergency departments serve as a direct point of contact with the public. They have been called the "front door" of the hospital. Nationally, approximately 55% of hospital admissions occur through the ED. Additionally, the ED serves as the primary care center for a significant portion of the population.

Hospitals have provided some form of emergency room or accident room almost since their inception. In the mid-17th century, physicians from the Hotel Dieu of Paris, France, held sessions on Wednesdays and Saturdays to assist the poor. Early emergency rooms were simply rooms in which a private physician would greet patients presenting with urgent conditions. In larger teaching hospitals,

Table 8-1 Model of Clinical Practice of Emergency Medicine

SIGNS, SYMPTOMS, AND PRESENTATIONS

- Abdominal and Gastrointestinal Disorders
- Cardiovascular Disorders
- Cutaneous Disorders
- Endocrine, Metabolic, and Nutritional Disorders
- Environmental Disorders
- Head, Ear, Eye, Nose, and Throat Disorders
- Hematologic Disorders
- Immune System Disorders
- Systemic Infectious Disorders
- Musculoskeletal Disorders (Nontraumatic)
- Nervous System Disorders
- Obstetrics and Disorders of Pregnancy
- Psycho-behavioral Disorders
- Renal/Urogenital Disorders
- Thoracic-Respiratory Disorders
- Toxicological Disorders
- Traumatic Disorders
- Procedures/Skills
- Administrative Aspects of Emergency Medicine
- Communications and Interpersonal Skills
- Research
- Risk, Legal, and Regulatory Issues

Data from American Board of Emergency Medicine. (2007). (Model of the Clinical Practice of Emergency Medicine [Online]. Available: https://www.abem.org.)

interns or residents were assigned to see patients in the emergency room. These early endeavors have given way to the modern emergency department that is staffed 24 hours per day, 7 days per week by trained emergency medicine specialists (**Figure 8-1**).

Hospitals that are accredited by The Joint Commission (TJC) are required to provide at least one of four levels of emergency care (**Table 8-2**). The most basic, Level IV, provides only assessment and immediate stabilization. The typical ED is categorized as Level II (TJC, 1991).

As a department within the hospital, the ED is most often a stand-alone service or division within the administrative structure of the hospital. In some hospitals, however, the ED is part of the department of surgery. Most EDs are managed by an emergency department director or manager. Traditionally, this has been a physician who also served as the ED medical director. More recently, administrators with special training in emergency services management have either assumed the position of director

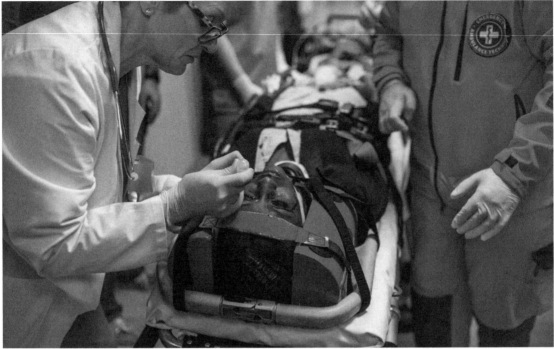

© Tashi-Delek/Getty.

Figure 8-1 Emergency department team of clinicians.

Table 8-2 Levels of Emergency Services

LEVEL I

A Level I emergency department/service offers comprehensive emergency care 24 hours a day, with at least one physician experienced in emergency care on duty in the emergency care area. There shall be in-hospital physician coverage for medical, surgical, orthopedic, obstetrical/gynecological, pediatric, and anesthesiology services by members of the medical staff or by senior level residents. Other specialty consultation shall be available within approximately 30 minutes. Initial consultation through two-way voice communication is acceptable. The hospital's scope of services shall include in-house capabilities for managing physical and related emotional problems on a definitive basis. The above requirements also apply to a comprehensive-level emergency department/service provided by a hospital offering care only to a limited group of patients, such as pediatric, obstetrical, ophthalmological, and orthopedic.

LEVEL II

A Level II emergency department/service offers emergency care 24 hours a day, with at least one physician experienced in emergency care on duty in the emergency care area, and with specialty consultation available within approximately 30 minutes by members of the medical staff or by senior level residents. Initial consultation through two-way voice communication is acceptable. The hospital's scope of services includes in-house capabilities for managing physical and related emotional problems, with provision for patient transfer to another organization when needed.

LEVEL III

A Level III emergency department/service offers emergency care 24 hours a day, with at least one physician available to the emergency care area within approximately 30 minutes through a medical staff call roster. Initial consultation through two-way voice communication is acceptable. Specialty consultation shall be available by request of the attending medical staff member or by transfer to a designated hospital where definitive care can be provided.

LEVEL IV

A Level IV emergency service offers reasonable care in determining whether an emergency exists, renders lifesaving first aid, and makes appropriate referral to the nearest organizations that are capable of providing needed services. The mechanism for providing physician coverage at all times shall be defined by the medical staff.

(Emergency Services Standards. Oakbrook Terrace, IL: Joint Commission on Accreditation of Healthcare Organizations, 1991.)

or have served as the department's administrative officer reporting to the ED director or ED medical director. The director usually reports to the hospital's chief operating officer.

The ED medical director is responsible for overseeing the clinical operation of the ED and the management of the medical staff. Hospitals, especially those that are not teaching hospitals, routinely contract out for ED medical staff services. Physician groups bid for contracts to provide physician coverage. Groups may include physicians' assistants and nurse practitioners as well as physicians. This practice reduces the administrative demand on the hospital to handle routine matters, such as staffing, hiring, and compensation.

In the early years of the ED, the head nurse performed many administrative and clinical duties, especially in EDs that did not have in-house or dedicated physician staffing. In the modern ED, the role of the head nurse has expanded to that of nurse manager or director. Nurse managers now have operational, personnel, and financial responsibilities. They oversee not only the nursing staff but also ED technicians, unit secretaries, and in some EDs, registration personnel. They report to the ED director as well as to the hospital's director or vice president of nursing. Unlike the ED physicians, the nursing and clerical staff are hospital employees.

Some EDs have created the position of EMS coordinator or liaison. The coordinator serves as the bridge between the hospital and the ED and the prehospital EMS community. This may be a full-time position or it may be assigned to a member of the nursing staff. The coordinator may also be responsible for providing training in prehospital EMS-related topics to the ED staff and prehospital providers. In addition to a training function, the coordinator ensures effective communication between EMS services and the hospital and assists with patient feedback information, quality improvement issues, medical direction and command, and ambulance restocking. The EMS coordinator may also be responsible for arranging ambulance transports and transfers to and from the ED or hospital at large.

Functions within the ED vary but can be categorized into the following basic activities:

- Triage
- Registration
- Nursing evaluation

- Physician evaluation
- Laboratory and radiology ordering
- Treatment
- Consultation
- Admission to the hospital
- Discharge from ED

Overcrowded Emergency Departments

Overcrowded emergency departments are a complex issue caused only in part by the increase in the number of patients seeking emergency care. The overcrowding issue became one of the primary reasons the Institute of Medicine (IOM) studied emergency care and released the 2006 three-volume report *The Future of Emergency Care*. ED overcrowding results in long waiting times for care and the boarding of patients in EDs who should be admitted to regular beds in the hospital. For ambulance services, it means patient parking (delayed patient offload times at the ED, up to one to two hours or longer) and ambulance diversion (when ambulances must take the patient to another hospital). In 2004, according to the American Hospital Association, close to 70% of urban hospitals diverted ambulance patients at least once during the year. Forty percent of urban hospitals reported daily overcrowding.

Hospital administrators have been trying to address this issue for two decades. Many patients come to the ED with nonemergent but urgent medical problems (see **Figure 8-2**). This chart illustrates the percentages of the different severity types that present to the ED. Semiurgent patients can safely be seen within an hour and nonurgent patients can wait up to 24 hours.

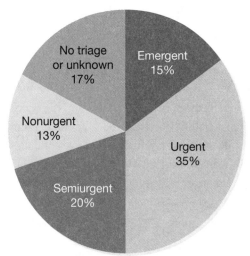

Data from Centers for Disease Control and Prevention, 2003.

Figure 8-2 Percentages of the different severity types that present to the emergency department.

Approaches to Relieving ED Overcrowding

One common approach to addressing the problem of ED overcrowding is the fast track ED. Walk-in patients arriving at the ED are quickly triaged. If their complaint is minor and not an emergency, they are sent to fast-track EDs where they are evaluated and treated. Fast tracks have their own dedicated staff and facilities. They often utilize physician extenders who lessen the burden on the ED medical staff. By having a separate facility, patients with minor conditions do not have to wait for a regular ED bed or tie up resources that may be needed for more urgent cases.

Occasionally, patients seen in the ED require a period of observation before being discharged. Because it is not practical to admit such patients to the regular hospital, they remain in the ED. If an ED does not have a dedicated observation area, such patients continue to tie up an ED bed and resources. As a result, some EDs have designated specific beds or even an area of the ED for observing patients. This makes it possible to keep patients in the hospital for up to 23 hours without having to admit them to a floor bed. Observation areas are also used for direct-admission patients not needing evaluation in the ED. A private physician can admit a patient to the hospital when a regular bed is not available. Such patients routinely enter the hospital through the ED and thus must remain in the ED area until a bed is available. During peak times, the presence of these patients may place a strain on the ED and limit its ability to deal with emergency patients. The observation area can also be used as a "staging area" for patients who have been evaluated and treated in the ED and are being admitted through the ED but for whom a bed is not yet available in the hospital.

Another strategy for hospital EDs that serve a large number of patients presenting with specific conditions or comprising a particular patient population is to open **specialty EDs**. Some hospitals open such units to increase their catchment area and thus increase revenue. Examples of specialty EDs include cardiac EDs, pediatric EDs, and psychiatric EDs. These specialty EDs are often similar to fast tracks for a specific patient group. Staffing includes medical specialists and nursing staff with special or advanced training as well as special resources and equipment.

Freestanding EDs

As hospital EDs become more crowded and the business of private physician services changes due to managed care, the availability of traditional primary care has also changed. Faced with an unexpected or a nonemergency medical condition, the patient has the choice of either waiting for an extended time in the hospital ED or seeing a private physician. As more and more physicians join HMOs and practice groups, the availability of the private physician becomes limited. To address this unmet need, freestanding urgent care clinics and true "freestanding EDs" have come into being, some of which are sponsored by hospitals as a means to reduce demand on the ED.

In some areas, hospital systems have built freestanding EDs that include CT Scanners, MRIs, and the ability to handle all emergencies that would not regularly result in an inpatient admission. These freestanding EDs may be an extension of a larger hospital and may share some of the same staff. Each state's regulations allow for different possibilities as well as whether EMS can transport to the location. EMS may also be an integral part of a freestanding ED because the need to transport patients for inpatient admission may be high. The result is that a freestanding ED may be a regular posting location for EMS units or destination in many areas.

The urgent care clinic is often open 24 hours per day, 7 days per week, or at least with early morning and late evening hours, to meet the needs of working clients. The centers are staffed with at least one physician and often a physician assistant, nurse practitioners, and nurses. Basic services, such as a clinical laboratory and radiology, may be available. Patients are usually seen on a walk-in basis, although some centers do make appointments for routine medical procedures and follow-up. Typical services include testing, treatment, or both for:

- Acute, non-life-threatening medical conditions;
- Asthma;
- Colds and flu;
- Pediatric ear infections;
- Wounds (including suturing);
- Minor fractures, sprains, and strains;
- Crisis intervention;
- Obstetrical conditions;
- STDs; and
- Allergies.

Although most EMS systems do not recognize all freestanding clinics as transport destinations, some systems allow prehospital providers to transport patients with minor complaints to freestanding clinics, thus lessening the burden on hospital EDs. This is especially true in rural areas with limited hospital services or long transport times. Urgent care clinics may also be found in remote or isolated areas, such as an island or mountain community that cannot support a community hospital. Clinics also operate at resort areas that have increased populations during certain times. Examples include clinics at ski and seashore resorts. Some major ski resorts operate clinics that are essentially hospitals without wards but that do have EDs as well as radiology, laboratory, and outpatient surgical services.

Yet, with all these efforts to improve the way our healthcare system manages unscheduled and emergency health care, the problem of overcrowded EDs persists. Some of the contributing factors include:

- The growth in the number of uninsured individuals who use EDs as their primary care;
- The unavailability of primary care physicians after regular working hours;
- Closures of hospitals, particularly in rural areas;
- An inadequate supply of hospital beds and nursing home beds, causing backups in the ED; and
- Reduced numbers of physician specialists willing to pay the increased medical malpractice premiums for providing care to emergency patients.

There is no solution in sight for these issues. Even so, the IOM report on emergency care recommended that the practice of ambulance diversion be ended.

Categorization and Designation

The Emergency Medical Services Systems Act of 1973 called for the regionalization of EMS and trauma care. The idea was to maximize the resources available in an area and to pool resources and patients at support centers to serve specific patient groups, such as spinal cord injury and burn patients. In order to bring about regionalization, it is necessary to first determine which resources exist in an area. This determination involves the process of **categorization**. Once all the facilities have been categorized, certain facilities can be designated for specific purposes. This is the process of **designation**.

Categorization is often thought of as being "horizontal" in its approach. For example, all of the EDs in a region would be asked to categorize their ability and resources related to emergency care, trauma care, and care of special patient groups. Only the capabilities of the ED would be assessed, not the total resources of the hospital. Although set criteria can be used, categorization is voluntary and based on the facility's own assessment. There is no independent verification. Also, categorization can change over time, as can the ED's ability to meet a previously assessed level. Categorization is nonbinding on prehospital providers. For example, merely because a hospital may categorize itself as providing pediatric ED services, prehospital providers are not required to transport all pediatric patients to that particular hospital. Although the basic reason for categorization is to regionalize services, categorization does not limit the number of hospitals in an area that can provide the same or similar services. Categorization and designation impact the EMS system in that transport **destination protocols** must be developed to properly direct the patients to the hospitals that will provide the best possible care for their particular emergency.

Designation, on the other hand, is a more formal process than categorization. The process is usually codified in local or state law. Designation is vertical in that it involves the resources and capabilities of the entire hospital, not just the ED. Approval for designation involves independent verification against established standards and criteria. Once designated, a hospital must continue to meet the designation standards and reapply for designation on a regular basis. Because designation is legally binding and designed to regionalize EMS and trauma resources, prehospital providers are required to follow transport protocols intended to deliver patients to the facility that will provide the best possible care for a given injury or illness. The most common example of a designated facility is the regional Level I trauma center.

Trauma Care

One of the driving forces in the development of modern EMS was the recognition of automobile crash injuries as a significant source of death and disability. But most significant was the realization that a large portion of automobile trauma deaths could have been prevented if proper emergency care were provided. Trauma victims were arriving alive at local hospitals, only to die a few minutes or hours later. Research showed that similar victims transported to large urban academic medical centers often survived (Cowley, 1976). This fact, coupled with the military's experience with battlefield casualties, led to the concept of a dedicated hospital service for trauma victims. These early shock-trauma centers developed into the modern-day trauma center that is at the hub of a trauma system. Such centers are necessary because the only definitive intervention for the trauma patient is rapid surgical intervention. The clinical intervention efforts of prehospital providers and EDs are only temporizing. If a trauma patient is to survive the "golden hour," that patient must receive rapid surgical intervention.

Trauma research has shown that there are three periods in which trauma patients are likely to die. The first is at the time of the incident, when death results immediately from severe injury, such as brain-stem injury, spinal cord laceration, aortic rupture, or heart rupture. The next grouping consists of those patients who live through the traumatizing event but die within one to two hours. R. Adams Cowley, one of the pioneering researchers in shock and trauma, called this timeframe the "golden hour." It is these patients that the EMS and trauma system are designed to save. The patients who make up the final group are those who die weeks later due to sepsis or multiple organ failure.

The EMS Systems Act of 1973 called for the availability of critical care units within each EMS region or in an adjacent region. Trauma care centers were identified as one of the critical care units that should be available in each EMS region.

Trauma Care System

The **trauma care system** is really a subsystem of the total EMS system. A trauma care system cannot exist without support from the many other attributes of an EMS system. In its simplest form, a trauma care system consists of a designated trauma center at the hub, which receives serious trauma patients either directly from the field or from other hospitals within the region. Protocols exist for the transfer of patients from the field to the trauma center by prehospital personnel. A system also exists for the transfer of critical patients from other facilities to the trauma center. Such systems are usually supported by an established communications system.

At the most sophisticated level, the trauma care system consists of a number of interrelated components. The trauma victim is evaluated by prehospital providers, who, with medical direction, decide on the appropriate receiving facility. The patient may go to a local trauma center, a specialty referral center, or the central Level I trauma center. A series of local or regional trauma centers, often designated Level II centers, serve the needs of the trauma patient with severe single-system injury or moderate multisystem trauma. Severe trauma patients are sent to the area-wide Level I trauma center, most often associated with an academic medical institution. Admission to the Level I center may be directly from the incident site, via a local trauma center, or as a referral from a community hospital ED.

The *Trauma System Agenda for the Future* (NHTSA-OEMS) identified the following key components of trauma systems:

- Injury prevention;
- Prehospital care;
- Acute care facilities; and
- Posthospital care.

In addition to the fundamental operational components of the trauma system, the following key infrastructure elements must be in place to support any comprehensive trauma care system:

- Leadership;
- Professional resources;
- Education and advocacy;
- Information management;
- Finances;
- Research;
- Technology; and
- Disaster preparedness and response—conventional and unconventional.

The Trauma Center

A typical trauma center consists of the following components:

- Trauma resuscitation area (may be dedicated space in the ED);
- Dedicated operating room(s) (**Figure 8-3**);
- Intensive care unit(s);
- Postsurgical units; and
- Rehabilitation services.

Depending on the center's level, these components may be dedicated solely to the needs of the trauma center or shared on a priority basis with the hospital.

The Committee on Trauma of the American College of Surgeons has established three levels of trauma center designation. All of these levels involve formal designation of facilities by the authority that has jurisdiction. These levels of trauma center designation should not be confused with the four levels of emergency care recognized by the Joint Commission and discussed earlier in the chapter.

Level I. This is the highest level of trauma care. Level I centers are usually associated with major urban academic centers (medical schools and hospitals that admit more than 700 trauma patients per year). Facilities, staff, specialists, and intensive care beds are available on site 24 hours per day. In addition to trauma care, the Level I center engages in trauma medical education, trauma research, and trauma prevention.

Level II. This level of trauma center is often found in major suburban community hospitals or associated teaching (residency program) hospitals. The clinical level of trauma care should be the same as found in the Level I center. The dedicated facilities and availability of 24 hour per day on-site specialty services of the Level I center are not required or possible. However, specially trained trauma surgeons and associated medical staff are available on site or on call.

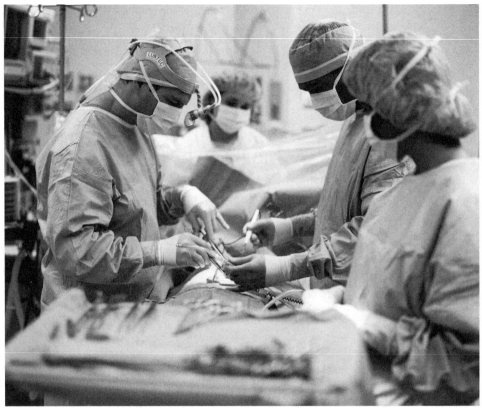

© Photos.com/Getty.

Figure 8-3 The trauma center has a dedicated operating room.

Level III. The Level III trauma center or facility is found in the neighborhood or community hospital. The primary role of the Level III center is to stabilize the trauma victim for transfer to a higher-level center. In such situations, the Level III center may be the only available trauma service. In this case, a means is provided for the local surgeon or emergency physician to consult with specialists at a Level I or II center. Depending on the availability of transport services, especially air medical transport, the extent of stabilization and treatment may vary. It is also possible that a team from a higher-level center will be transported to the Level III center to provide ongoing stabilization and transfer.

In addition to facilities, the Committee on Trauma has also established guidelines for the training of trauma care personnel, including surgeons, ED physicians, allied health personnel, and prehospital providers.

Specialty Referral Centers

Not all trauma patients experience severe multisystem trauma. Some patients suffer severe trauma to one particular body system, for instance, the auto crash victim who suffers blunt trauma to the spinal cord with loss of neurologic function. Such individuals may be transported to a trauma center but would be better served by a facility that specializes in spinal cord injury. The same would hold true for burn patients or for individuals who have experienced amputation with potential for reimplantation. Similarly, certain patient populations, most notably children, are better served in a facility with equipment and personnel geared to their needs. Examples of **specialty referral centers** include ones for:

- Spinal cord injuries;
- Head injuries;
- Burns;
- Eye trauma;
- Limb reimplantation;
- Pediatrics; and
- Hyperbaric services.

Trauma Registry

As trauma care systems developed, questions about their efficiency and efficacy were raised in light of the systems' high cost. Additionally, information about the patients seen in trauma centers and their injuries were of interest to public health and prevention researchers. What was needed was a means to uniformly collect patient data from all of the nation's trauma centers. This collection of data is known as a **trauma registry** and contains detailed information about moderate to severely injured patients admitted to a trauma center. It is cost-prohibitive to include information on all trauma patients. A trauma registry will include information on all trauma deaths, trauma patients transferred to another facility, patients cared for by a trauma system, and patients hospitalized for more than 48 hours and with specified discharge diagnoses.

Information entered into the trauma registry includes demographics, time intervals, type and severity of injury, physiological response to injury, treatment modalities, patient disposition, and discharge diagnosis. The process of reviewing a patient's medical records and entering them into the registry is called coding.

The purpose of a trauma registry is to provide a comprehensive database of trauma patients that can be queried by researchers and system administrators to assist with analysis and problem solving. It also provides baseline information for injury control and epidemiologic research. Additionally, the registry can assist with continuous quality improvement, resource utilization, and cost containment. By knowing the types of patients seen by a trauma system, local resources can be better managed and education can be tailored to the local case mix.

Because of the existence of various trauma registries nationwide, the American College of Surgeons has also developed the National Trauma Data Bank (NTDB). This subscription service is designed to collect data nationwide from the various commercial trauma registry programs. By combining data, a national repository of trauma data can be maintained. This will improve the scope of trauma and injury prevention research by providing data from a larger base population.

EMTALA Legislation

In the 1980s, the U.S. Congress passed legislation to bring deficit spending by the government under control. As a result of this action, changes were made to Medicare, including adoption of a prospective payment plan. Hospitals then saw an increasing number of uninsured or underinsured patients. To reduce their losses, private hospitals would immediately transfer patients to public or charity hospitals. The practice of transferring patients for economic as opposed to medical reasons became known as **patient dumping**. In extreme cases, ambulances found themselves driving from hospital to hospital with a patient nobody would accept. Other patients were transferred without initial stabilization and treatment, resulting in complications and even death. To put an end to patient dumping, Congress passed the Emergency Medical Treatment and Active Labor Act (EMTALA) of 1986 as part of the Consolidated Omnibus Budget Reconciliation Act (COBRA) (Public Law No. 99-272).

The purpose of EMTALA was to require hospitals receiving Medicare funding to provide initial assessment and stabilization to any individual presenting to an ED or to any woman in active labor. EMTALA also enacted strict guidelines for patient transfers. As the result of EMTALA and resultant economic losses from uncompensated care, some hospitals closed their EDs, obstetrical departments, or both.

The primary provisions of EMTALA are the following:

- Hospitals must provide an appropriate medical screening examination to determine if an emergency exists. This examination is the responsibility of the ED physician. The screening may include laboratory tests, radiological studies, and consultation as medically necessary.

- If a true emergency condition is found, the patient must be appropriately stabilized prior to discharge or transfer.

- A woman with contractions is considered unstable until the delivery of the child and placenta. Women undergoing complicated deliveries may be transferred if necessary.

- A patient may be transferred after evaluation if the physician feels such a transfer is medically necessary and the patient's condition is properly documented.

- Hospitals must maintain a list of on-call specialists who are available to evaluate the patient. If an on-call specialist is not available or fails to appear "in a reasonable period of time," the patient may be transferred.

- The hospital must agree to accept the patient, have a bed available for the patient, and have qualified staff and resources to care for the patient.

- An appropriate level of care must be maintained during the transfer. Requirements for transport must be specified by the referring physician.

- Hospitals not in compliance with the EMTALA regulations are subject to a fine and loss of Medicare reimbursement. Physicians can also receive sanctions that are not covered by malpractice insurance.

Of specific concern to EMS providers is the requirement for maintenance of care during transfer. Patient must be transported by personnel with the proper training and equipment. It would not be appropriate, for instance, for a patient with chest pains to be removed from a cardiac monitor and transferred by a basic life support (BLS) crew. It is not uncommon for a nurse to accompany some patients during transfer.

Critical Care Transport

There was a time when a person could go to just about any hospital and receive all the medical care needed. The attending physician and the hospital would just bill the person's insurance company. Today, this is not the case. With specialization, including new developments in medical equipment and procedures as well as new approaches to managing healthcare costs, patients may not be able to receive "full service" at a single hospital. To contain costs and to remain efficient, not all hospitals are able to afford every piece of major medical equipment and the staff to operate it. Hospitals now specialize in certain areas of care, such as cardiac care, stroke care, cancer treatment, and so on. Likewise, managed care organizations contract with specific hospitals for the most economic delivery of services. It is to the managed care organization's benefit for a member to go to a hospital or facility that offers a prearranged competitive rate. Because of all these changes and advances in medicine, it is not uncommon for patients to be moved from one hospital to another. In most cases, this transport occurs by ambulance.

The transfer of patients by ambulance can be as simple as a BLS crew moving a patient with a casted leg fracture or as sophisticated as the transfer of a patient from one intensive care unit to another intensive care unit. Transfers may require ambulances equipped with special medical devices and a specially trained staff of nurses and technicians. A typical critical care interfacility transfer crew consists of a critical care nurse and a paramedic. Depending on local medical protocols, advanced life support (ALS) units may transport stable patients without mechanical support such as respirators or balloon pumps.

As the demand for interfacility transports increases, there is a need to properly train paramedics and nurses to work in the critical care transport environment. For both the nurse and the paramedic, providing critical care life support in the back of an ambulance can be challenging at times. Because of this and the desire to increase the ability of paramedics to handle a wider scope of transports without the assistance of a nurse, special **critical care transport** training programs have been developed. The programs are offered either by the in-house nursing and medical staff of a medical institution that has (or contracts for) a critical care transport team or through an established EMS educational program such as the critical care transport course offered by the University of Maryland, Baltimore County (www.ehs.umbc.edu) and available nationwide. The critical care transport program is an intense 80-plus hours' program that introduces the paramedic or nurse to all aspects of critical care transport by both land and air. Topics covered in a typical critical care transport course include:

- The critical care environment;
- Breathing and airway management;
- Surgical airway management;

- Hemodynamic monitoring and management;
- Cardiac management;
- Pharmacological management;
- GI, GU, and renal management;
- Neurological management; and
- Transport considerations.

In 2003, with the implementation of the Medicare ambulance fee schedule, a new reimbursement level for specialty care transport was established. One of the requirements for this level is that the patient care provider be a registered nurse, respiratory therapist, physician assistant, or paramedic trained to a level beyond the normal paramedic in a program recognized by the particular state's EMS office. As the role of the paramedic in critical care transport becomes more defined and recognized in the ambulance fee schedule, state and regional EMS systems are developing protocols and amending the scope of practice to allow paramedics to assume an increasing level of responsibility during interfacility transports.

Expanded Scope of Practice and Services

Changes in healthcare delivery have also given rise to the idea that paramedics could do more for patients than just scene assessment, stabilization, treatment, and transport. It has been suggested that paramedics could be involved in population-based health care, including prevention and wellness programs and basic primary care. By adding additional knowledge and skills, the paramedic could help reduce healthcare costs by helping to prevent readmission, illness, and injury, as well as by providing care for minor medical and trauma conditions and diverting patients away from the high-cost emergency department. Patients with such complaints as a sprained finger or minor laceration would be evaluated on scene. Through physician consultation, the paramedic could transport the patient or provide initial treatment without transport and refer the patient to follow-up care. Paramedics could also provide routine health monitoring and immunizations (**Figure 8-4**).

Initial programs to expand paramedics' scope of practice have met with mixed but generally positive results, such as in Red River, New Mexico; Orange County, North Carolina; and Idaho. One key to success seems to be designing such programs to meet the needs of a defined population in a defined geographic area. Attempts to have paramedics provide services that have traditionally been within the scope of other healthcare providers, such as wound care and home health visits, have met with some resistance. Concerns related to the ability of EMS services to be compensated for expanded care have had and continue to have a chilling effect. Expanded scope continues to be discussed and investigated but remains an area of controversy. The Institute of Medicine's report on emergency care recommend that the Centers for Medicare and Medicaid Services (CMS) look at the issue of uncoupling Medicare payments from transport to allow for treatment without transport.

As health care shifts from a pay-for-volume model to a pay-for-performance model, additional focus is placed on keeping patients out of the hospital. Paramedics of the future may actually be community

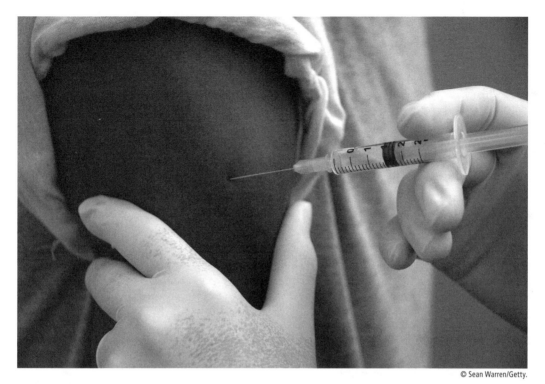

© Sean Warren/Getty.

Figure 8-4 Paramedics can also provide immunizations.

paramedics or part of a **Mobile Integrated Healthcare Practice (MIHP)**. In the MIHP type of model, the paramedic once again becomes an extension of the hospital, but now aims at preventing hospital readmissions. Programs have been developed across the country to utilize paramedics to prevent CHF readmission. Future research and healthcare finance changes will have a strong impact on whether or not community paramedics are a staple of the healthcare system.

WRAP UP

Summary

The development of modern clinical care has come a long way from unstaffed emergency wards to modern trauma centers supported by an established EMS system. The importance of time in the survival of the most critical trauma patients remains a primary reason for the establishment of trauma systems. In addition to trauma centers, emergency departments continue to provide the majority of clinical care to sick and injured patients, whether or not they are transported by EMS.

Key Terms

ambulance diversion
boarding
categorization
critical care transport
definitive care
designation
destination protocols

medical specialty
Mobile Integrated Healthcare
  Practice (MIHP)
overcrowded emergency
  departments
patient dumping
patient parking

primary care physician
specialty EDs
specialty referral centers
trauma care system
trauma registry

Review Questions

1. Discuss the development of the emergency department.
2. Describe how categorization and designation allow regionalization of EMS system hospital resources.
3. Identify the role(s) of a trauma registry.
4. Discuss the effectiveness of various initiatives to ease ED overcrowding.
5. Discuss how EMTALA regulations affect local EMS operations.
6. Discuss the role of critical care transport in interfacility patient transfers.
7. Discuss the role of the community paramedic or MIHP.

Additional Resources

American Board of Emergency Medicine. (2006). *Model of the clinical practice of emergency medicine* [Online]. Available: https://www.abem. org/public/_Rainbow/Documents/2007%20 EM%20Model.pdf

Cowley, R. A. (1976). The resuscitation and stabilization of major multiple trauma patients in a trauma center environment. *Clinical Medicine. 83*(14).

Joint Commission on Accreditation of Healthcare Organizations. (1991). *Emergency service standards.* JCAHO: Oakbrook Terrace, IL.

National Center for Health Statistics. (October, 2007). [Online]. Available: http://www.cdc. gov/nchs/products/pubs/pubd/hus/00tables. htm#Ambulatory Care.

Public Law No. 99-272, § 9121, 100 Stat. 82, 164. (1986). (Codified as amended at 42 USCA §§ 1395cc, 1395dd).

The Future of Emergency Care, Institute of Medicine. (2006).

9

System Finances

Objectives

Upon completion of this chapter, the reader should be able to:

- Identify the three types of organizations providing EMS.

- Describe the cost–income relationship for each of the three organizational types.

- Identify sources of income for each of the three organizational types.

- Describe basic accounting approaches used by each of the three organizational types.

- State the financial effects of reimbursement on ambulance services.

- Discuss the role of government in financially supporting EMS.

- Identify future issues in EMS funding.

System Finance

Healthcare costs in the United States now exceed $3 trillion every year and represent a cost of $9,523 per person. Despite efforts by the government and industry to control these costs, healthcare cost increases continue to substantially exceed the yearly rate of inflation as measured by the U.S. Consumer Price Index. Future projections of the demand and cost of health care show a significant increase based on two major factors: the aging of our population and the development of new and expensive medical technologies. **Third-party insurance** and individuals pay 60% of the fees paid for health care. **Medicare**, the federal health insurance for the elderly (shown in **Figure 9-2**), and **Medicaid**, the state- and federal-supported health insurance for people in poverty, make up most of the rest of healthcare fees paid. When it comes to emergency medical services (EMS), Medicare pays an even larger percentage due to the fact that the elderly use EMS more than any other demographic group.

No discussion of healthcare financing is complete without explaining the role of **bad debt**. Bad debt consists of fee-for-service charges that go unpaid for any reason. Part of bad debt is a result of governmental health insurance programs that pay below the fee rates. Healthcare providers must accept that

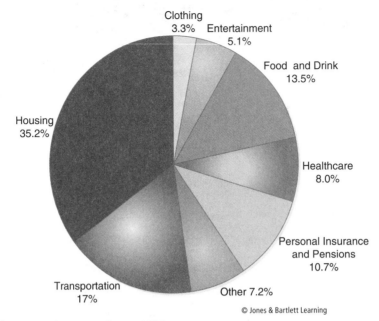

© Jones & Bartlett Learning

Figure 9-1 Personal consumption expenditures 1997.

level of payment and cannot attempt to collect from the individuals. Many people who have no insurance pay none or only some of what healthcare providers charge them for the service. This comprises the lion's share of bad debt. Healthcare providers attempt to **cost shift** to **commercial insurance** in order to make ends meet by charging commercial insurance more than any other payer. By the end of 2014, approximately 10% of U.S. citizens were uninsured despite the efforts of the Affordable Care Act.

There are other sources of revenue to support health care in the United States. Tax-based appropriations from local, state, and federal governments support the public healthcare system and much of the healthcare infrastructure, such as public hospitals and medical schools.

Nevertheless, EMS services, though they make up only a relatively small part of the total healthcare expenditures, face the same dilemma: increasing cost for personnel and equipment coupled with an increasing demand for services in an environment where government and industry are trying to control the costs. Because EMS services are a major entry point into the healthcare system, how these systems operate has taken on additional importance in attempts to control costs. EMS managers today must be concerned with the services they provide and must also understand the financial structure and constraints under which EMS systems operate.

System Organization

Every EMS system has a unique history and organization. The axiom "once you have seen one EMS system, you have seen one EMS system" holds true as it relates to system financing. Underlying any discussion of the financing of prehospital care and medical transportation is the business structure of

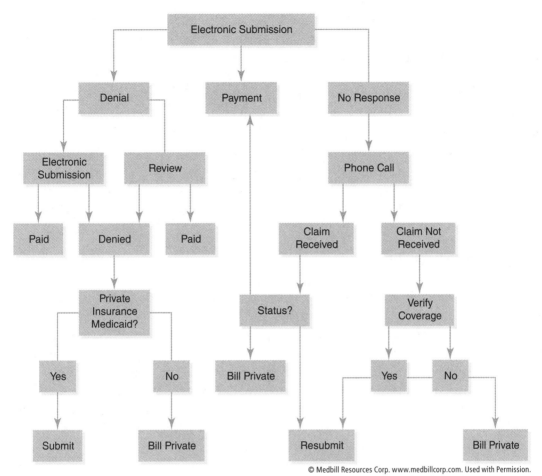

Figure 9-2 Example of the Medicare billing process.

the organization providing the service. The type of organization will, in large part, determine both the source of funds and how these funds are managed. Three major types of organizations provide services: nongovernmental organizations, governmental agencies, and volunteer organizations.

Nongovernmental Organizations

There are both for-profit companies and nonprofit companies in this category. They might be as small as a single ambulance "mom-and-pop" company or as large as the multistate companies that developed in the 1990s. For-profit businesses are organized by business owners or investors who expect to earn money on their investment of equity in the company. Therefore, there is an incentive for the company to operate so that revenues exceed expenses; a portion of the resulting profit is shared with the investors. A company that cannot generate a profit will not stay in business very long because investors will seek other opportunities for their investments.

Nonprofit companies are often owned by hospitals or are organized as services that are held accountable to community boards. The primary difference is that because the nonprofit company cannot make a profit, all its excess revenues are poured back into the organization or the community rather than going to the owners or investors.

For nongovernmental organizations, revenues are primarily based on **fee-for-service** charges to service customers (patients and their insurers) and depend on the volume and type of services provided. Prices charged for these services are constrained by competition from other companies as well as governmental reimbursement policies. The nongovernmental organizations strive to increase revenues while controlling costs; however, they are constrained in their cost-cutting by the necessity to maintain an acceptable quality or risk losing market share. Often, nongovernmental organizations serve a community based on a contract with performance requirements regarding response times and other critical **performance measures**.

Governmental Services

Governmental services, or agencies, are exempt from taxes and do not have owners or investors to share in the profits. They are authorized by legislatures, are operated by the executive branch of local governments, and depend on their legislatures to provide a yearly operating budget from tax revenues, which may be augmented by fees and grants. Increasingly, governmental services are looking to fee-for-service revenue to financially support their operating costs. The financial focus tends to be on accountability rather than efficiency, ensuring the legislature that the funds provided were spent properly in accordance with policies set by the government. Funds received in excess of need are usually returned to the government's **general fund** and may even result in action to reduce future appropriations by the legislature. This practice tends to encourage governmental agencies to expend all allocated funds each year and shifts the incentive for cost containment to the legislature.

Volunteer Companies

Volunteer companies are organized as independent nonprofit companies. Such businesses do not have investors and are organized under special provisions within the federal tax code to encourage the provision of services for social welfare. Such organizations are exempt from taxes, and donors can deduct donations made to the organization from their taxes. One of the major financial supports for volunteer organizations is the free labor provided by the volunteers, which significantly reduces the operating costs of the organization. Because they do not have to return money to investors, there typically is less incentive to increase revenue over costs. Any excess funds (profits) are retained within the company for future use. In order to ensure their future viability and maintain the confidence of lenders and donors, including the government, volunteer organizations must be concerned with efficiently providing services and responsibly handling their funds.

Nothing in the general descriptions of the three types of organizations should be interpreted to imply that one form is better suited to provide services than another. Examples of the best and the worst can be found in each of the organizational types.

Sources of Funds

In order to understand the funding of EMS, imagine yourself as the owner of a nongovernmental ambulance service, the chief officer of a governmental service, or the chief of a newly formed volunteer service. You have two major financial concerns. First, you must find the money to meet the start-up costs of housing and equipping the service, and then you need to be able to meet the ongoing operational costs.

Nongovernmental Organizations

If you run a nongovernmental for-profit organization, you will need to raise your start-up money in the private sector. You may invest your own savings in the business or bring in partners or other investors by selling shares of the company. In addition, you may turn to commercial banks to lend you a portion of the start-up cost. Once you are in operation, you will need to generate revenue through patient billing and contracts to meet your operational costs, compensate your investors, pay the interest on the bank loans, and generate funds for future development.

Because of the number of payment mechanisms and their complexity, billing for services has become a major component in the successful operation of EMS service (**Figure 9-2**). Between 7% and 10% of the workforce in an ambulance service is dedicated to the billing department. In some cases, you will bill the patient directly in what is termed fee for service. This is a simple business transaction in which you provide the service and the patient pays you directly out of pocket for the services provided. Your only problem is ensuring that the patient pays the bill.

Patients are most likely to have some sort of commercial health insurance or be involved in federally run medical programs that insure elderly, totally disabled, or poor individuals. These insurance programs, termed **third-party payers**, pay all or a portion of the billed charges, depending on the program. While the patient remains responsible for the bill (with the exception of Medicaid), you will need to assist in filing the paperwork necessary to support the insurance claim. Under some programs you will be paid directly by the insurance company, while in others the companies will pay the patient and you must collect from the patient. In the case of Medicare, your allowable charges will have been established in advance by the government, based on the ambulance fee schedule. Under most insurance programs, including Medicare, the patient is still directly responsible for a small portion of the bill called the co-pay, so you will still need to bill the patient directly or consider offering your own form of buyers' club through a subscription program. Under such a program, individuals pay a set annual fee to the ambulance service; if they need to use the ambulance service that year, all co-payments are waived.

Instead of billing the patient for services, you may enter into contracts with healthcare facilities and insurance programs to provide services to the patients in their program or you may agree to accept a reduced fee-for-service charge based on the expected volume of service or other operational considerations.

In order to ensure that necessary services are provided to all their constituents, state and local governments have established several programs to assist patients who cannot pay for services. The best known of these programs is the state-run Medicaid program, which uses federal and state funds to compensate healthcare providers for services to program enrollees who would otherwise be unable to pay for services. Under federal-government guidelines, states determine who will be covered and what services will be provided. The states also determine the rates of reimbursement that will be paid to providers.

These rates are usually significantly less than what would otherwise be billed. If a company bills Medicaid, it must accept the state reimbursement in full satisfaction of the claim and cannot bill the patient for the difference. Another mechanism that is used by local governments to ensure service is to provide a **subsidy** (to compensate a nongovernmental company for providing service to an area that would otherwise not be financially viable). The size of subsidies varies greatly depending on the performance expectations for the service, the percentage of uninsured patients, and other sources of bad debt. One should understand that on average Medicare pays six percent below the average cost of providing ambulance services, according to a report produced by the Government Accountability Office (GAO) in 2007, so the percentage of Medicare patients can impact the size of a needed subsidy.

Some local governments contract out their ambulance service system rather than directly provide the service. This method often uses a competitive-bid process to select a nongovernmental ambulance service to provide services in lieu of the governmental service. There are a few variations with this method. In some cases, the local government directly oversees the contract with the selected contractor. In other models, the local government establishes an independent oversight authority, which is responsible for securing a contractor and managing the contract. In some other models, the authority owns some or all of the assets of an ambulance service, including the vehicles, equipment, and facilities. The ambulance authority may also do the billing. The ambulance authority in turn contracts with the selected nongovernmental ambulance service to provide the staffing and run the day-to-day operations of the service. There have also been new models developed in which the governmental and nongovernmental ambulance services form partnerships and cooperative arrangements and the entities share service provision and revenues.

One significant aspect of governments contracting for services is the development of **performance-based contracts** that require the nongovernmental ambulance provider to meet specified performance standards. Most typically, these standards relate to response times to emergency requests for services, but may also include standards related to the clinical level of the crews, staffing configurations, and vehicle age, to name a few. Failure to meet these standards can result in financial penalties and even early termination of the contracts.

Governmental Services

As the director of a governmental EMS service, most of your start-up funding will come from the legislative body of your local jurisdiction. In addition, some grants from the state and federal governments as well as from private foundations may be available to purchase equipment and to assist in training. Grants are made by these organizations in order to encourage development and assist in improving services. Unlike business contracts, there is no specific product or service returned directly to the organization making the grant. Grants are usually made for a limited time period and are not meant to pay for ongoing operational costs.

As with start-up costs, most of the operational cost of the service will be provided by the legislature through an annual or biannual budget process. Some charitable giving may be generated by grateful patients and their families. These funds are kept separate and used for specific charitable projects that improve the service.

Increasingly, governmental services have turned to patient billing as a way of reducing the pressure on tax revenue. Usually, the local government does the billing and payments are returned to the general fund of the government. While some jurisdictions have handled the process well, in many cases there have been problems because taxpayers feel they are paying twice for the same service. As the billing process is complex, municipalities increasingly outsource this task to medical billing service companies.

Volunteer Organizations

To meet the start-up costs of a volunteer company, you will need to depend upon charitable giving, grants, and business loans. Charitable giving can take many forms, from responses to direct solicitations to participation in fund-raising events. Volunteer members can sponsor fund-raising activities, such as bingo or fairs, and use the proceeds tax free under the special provisions of the tax code for charitable organizations.

As a private business, volunteer organizations may also borrow money from commercial banks as long as they can show that their assets and expectations of future revenue will allow them to repay the debts. In order to meet ongoing operational costs, the volunteer company will rely on several methods, including charitable giving, governmental subsidies, patient billing, contracts, and subscription programs similar to those offered by nongovernmental businesses.

Charitable giving, the traditional method of fund-raising for volunteers, remains a most important source of funds, but these funds are proving inadequate to meet the costs associated with modern EMS systems. Consequently, volunteer units have had to rely more heavily on governmental funding in order to meet their obligations. Most local governments subsidize volunteer companies to some degree, but there are wide disparities in the amounts. In some areas, local governments will pay all or almost all of the organization's operational costs and consider it a bargain in that they do not have to provide a government service or contract with a nongovernmental provider. In other areas, local governments have been unwilling or unable to make more than a token contribution to the volunteers. State governments also assist in meeting the operational costs of volunteer units through grants to replace and upgrade equipment, to develop programs to train personnel and provide tuition assistance, and to offer tax breaks and other fringe benefits.

If a volunteer organization decides to bill patients for services, it faces all the complexities of the nongovernmental ambulance provider. Because of the time and the experience required to do the billing effectively, many volunteer organizations contract with billing services that specialize in ambulance billing. Volunteer organizations are very concerned with maintaining the goodwill of their donors and therefore tend not to pursue payments from individuals too aggressively and, in many cases, sponsor subscription programs to lessen the burden on individuals.

Table 9-1 is a recompilation of the various funding sources used by the different types of EMS organizations. No matter what type of EMS organization is providing the service, all must follow some

Table 9-1 Funding Sources for EMS Organizations			
	EMS Organization Type		
Funding Source	**Government Services**	**Volunteer**	**Nongovernmental**
Donations and Charitable Fund-raising Events	OO	M	OO
Grants	F	F	O
Governmental Subsidies	M	F	O
Contracts	OO	OO	M
Fee-for-Service	FO	F	M
Medicare	FO	F	M
Medicaid	FO	F	M
Subscription Programs	O	OO	OO
Business Loans	F	M	
Stock Investment	OM		
Direct Governmental Operational Funding	M		

M = Major Funding Source
F = Frequent Funding Source
O = Occasional Funding Source

form of accounting practice—but as you will see in the accounting section, these practices vary sharply, largely because of the varying sources of funds described in this section.

Financing Other EMS Components

While ambulance service is financed by a combination of fee-for-service and local tax-based governmental support, other components of the EMS system are supported by tax-based local, regional, state, and federal funds. Local government generally funds first response, 9-1-1, and communications systems. State EMS offices are funded through a number of mechanisms, from general funds to state excise taxes. 9-1-1 is also supported through excise taxes on telephone service. The regional communications systems, established in the 1970s with federal support originating with the Emergency Medical Services Systems Act of 1973, are antiquated, but there is no dedicated funding at the federal level to support EMS infrastructure.

There are many federal funding streams that provide some limited support to various components of local and state EMS systems. For example, the National Highway Traffic Safety Administration EMS Office provides funds to states to develop the National EMS Information System (NEMSIS). But, when it comes to disaster preparedness, since 2003 the various federal grant programs to states to support first responders have consistently provided a woefully inadequate four percent of the total funding for EMS (**Table 9-2**).

Table 9-2 First Responder Funding	05 Enacted	06 Enacted	07 Enacted	08 Enacted	09 Request	09 House	09 Senate
Basic State Formula Grants	1100	545	525	950	200	890	890
							Senate includes 50 million for REAL ID
Operation Stonegarden						60	0
LE/National Security			375	0	110	0	0
Terrorism Prevention Grants	400	396					
Firefighter Assistance Grants	650	540	547	560	300	570	560
SAFER	65	109	115	190		230	170
Emergency Management Performance Grants	180	183	200	300	200	315	300
Discretionary Grants	**1250**	**1143**	**1327**	**1929**	**1245**	**1870**	**1848**
Urban Area Grants	885	757	770	820	825	850	825
Port Security Grants	150	173	210	400	210	400	400
Rail and Transit Security Grants	150	148	175	400	175	400	400
Intercity (Over the Road) Bus Security Grants	10	10	12	11.5	12	12	12
Trucking Security Grants	5	5	12	16	8	8	8
Buffer Zone Protection Plan Grants	50	50	50	50	0	0	50
REAL ID Grants	0	40	0	50	0	50	0
Interoperable Communications Grants	0	0	0	50	0	50	Funded under State Grants
Metropolitan Medical Response System	30	30	33	41	0	50	33

Table 9-2 (Continued)

	05 Enacted	06 Enacted	07 Enacted	08 Enacted	09 Request	09 House	09 Senate
Technology Transfer Program (CEDAP)	50	50	50	25	0	0	10
Citizen Corp	15	20	15	15	15	15	15
Regional Catastrophic Preparedness Grants	0	0	0	35	0	0	35
Emergency Operation Centers Grants	0	0	0	15	0	35	10
Subtotal, First Responder Grants =>	*3740*	*3056*	*3089*	*3929*	*2055*	*3935*	*3768*
National Programs	**291**	**294**	**304**	**299**	**145**	**236**	**291**
National Domestic Preparedness Consortium	135	144	145	150.5	79	139	164 Includes Center for Domestic Preparedness
National Exercise Program	52	51	49	50	40	40	40
Technical Assistance	30	20	18	12	10	10	12
Demonstration Training Grants	30	30	30	28	0	0	25
Continuing Training Grants	25	25	31	31	0	31	31
Evaluations and Assessments	14	14	19	19	16	16	19
Rural Domestic Preparedness Consortium	5	10	12	8.8	0	0	0
Total, First Responder Funding =>	***4031***	***3350***	***3393***	***4228***	***2200***	***4171***	***4059***

Courtesy of Advocates for Emergency Medical Services, President Kurt Kruperman.

Accounting and Budgeting

Over the years, attempts have been made to compare the different types of prehospital EMS service providers based on their financial records. Such attempts have immediately run into problems, because accounting and budgeting practices logically differ according to the form of the organization. For comparison, the following is a brief description of the accounting and budgeting practices of each of the major prehospital care provider types.

Nongovernmental For-Profit Company

For-profit ambulance services keep their accounting records like other for-profit businesses, using the traditional report forms. The balance sheet records the assets, liabilities, and owner's equity at a point in time and the income statement reports the revenue and expenses for a given period. The business may be organized as a corporation, partnership, or sole proprietorship based on such factors as size, need for capital, and liability. Most larger firms will be organized as corporations, but they can differ from the large corporation that offers ownership shares to the public to the closely held corporation with limited shareholders. Regardless of the type of the for-profit organization, the financial goal is the same: increase revenue, reduce costs (including taxes when possible), and return a profit to the owners or investors.

The particular form of the business determines how reports are made to the Internal Revenue Service (IRS) and how profits and losses are apportioned for tax purposes. Firms that offer shares of ownership to the public are required to have a yearly audit by an outside accounting firm that attests to the company's compliance in following generally accepted accounting principles (GAAP).

In accordance with IRS guidelines, costs associated with the capitalization of assets, such as depreciation, are allowed as expenses before taxes are computed for for-profit businesses. Because taxes are not a concern for governmental and nonprofit providers, the same expenses may be disregarded by these organizations.

Budgeting in a for-profit business usually involves managers developing goals regarding the type and volume of services to be provided in terms of the expected return on investment. Each item on the balance sheet and income statement is projected forward based on past experience and anticipated cost and revenue. Progress is monitored during the budget year for variances, and corrections and adjustments are made to the projections.

Governmental Services

In contrast, governmental agencies rarely use the financial reports used by for-profit businesses, because they do not apply. Because governmental services do not pay taxes, they do not report to the IRS except to report salaries paid to their employees. Liabilities are usually limited to current purchases and there is no owner's equity to be considered. Instead, the most important financial activities are focused on developing and justifying the budget and measuring variances against approved appropriations. Rather than profit, the emphasis is on accountability, that is, were funds spent appropriately in accordance with established guidelines.

As stated earlier, the tendency is to ensure that all appropriated funds are spent because the "reward" for saving money may be a reduced budget in the future. It is the legislature that normally acts to limit expenditures through the budgeting process, although the state governor or local chief executive officer may intercede and curtail spending in economically stressed times. During normal times, agency budgets tend to grow incrementally as agency requests for additional funds are only partially pared down by the legislature. This usually provides a mechanism for auditing how the agency has expended its funds.

Nonprofit and Volunteer Organizations

Nonprofit organizations usually follow accounting practices somewhere between those followed by for-profit businesses and those followed by governmental agencies. The larger the organization, the more likely it is to follow for-profit procedures. Profit is not a primary goal, but the organization must track its revenue and expenses to ensure its ability to meet current and future needs. Consequently, income statements are frequently prepared. Although the organization is exempt from taxes, it is required to file a yearly report with the IRS concerning its activities and financial transactions, so it must maintain records for this purpose. Nonprofit organizations do not have investors to report to, or to share profits from the operation with, but typically they are accountable to a community board of directors or commissioners. However, they frequently incur long-term liabilities through loans and therefore may be required to keep financial records to demonstrate to lenders their ability to meet future payments on the debt.

Nonprofit organizations usually budget in a manner similar to for-profits, with an emphasis on meeting future demands for the services the organization provides. Nonprofit organizations are established with boards of directors or commissioners who are responsible for the organization's conduct and procedures. This can be a challenge if no board member can assume knowledgeable leadership for the safeguarding of funds. Nonprofit organizations depend on the continued goodwill of the community, donors, and supporters, so any evidence of fraud by management can be devastating. Unfortunately, this is not an unusual occurrence and many well-known organizations have had to deal with the consequences of a lack of financial oversight.

In accounting, form follows function, and each of the provider types discussed follows the procedures that are important for its operation. The result is that comparisons are difficult and often flawed or biased by individuals and groups with a particular agenda. An example of this difficulty is the GAO study of ambulance service providers released in 2007. While the GAO surveyed all provider types, it could not use the data received from governmental services with confidence due to the incomplete and sometimes unreliable cost accounting found in the survey responses.

Issues for the Future

Several issues related to EMS financing are problematic and in some cases controversial and will challenge the financial stability of EMS in the coming decade.

1. With the below-cost reimbursement by government payers it will likely become increasingly more difficult to continue to shift costs to commercial payers.
2. The lack of dedicated funding for EMS infrastructure will likely result in infrastructure-component failures.

3. The lack of adequate funding for EMS disaster preparedness will continue leaving communities with inadequate EMS capability to respond to disasters.

4. If the trend of declining volunteerism continues, rural EMS systems may fail or be forced to convert to using paid staff, significantly raising the cost of rural EMS without sufficient funding to support the increased costs.

5. Service payments for EMS are based on transports. Some systems are exploring clinical approaches to care that would reduce transports by providing more services on scene or referring patients to their primary care physicians. These approaches may reduce the cost of health care but will not be widely implemented as long as fee-for-service reimbursement is based solely on transports.

WRAP UP

Summary

The financing of EMS will continue to be a challenge for EMS managers. At present, a variety of providers are pursuing a number of funding sources. To manage EMS successfully will require managers to understand the financial functioning of their organization as well as the healthcare-financing environment.

Key Terms

bad debt	general fund	performance measures
commercial insurance	Medicaid	subsidy
cost shift	Medicare	third-party insurance
fee-for-service	performance-based contracts	third-party payers

Review Questions

1. Briefly describe the various funding streams for EMS systems.

2. Compare and contrast the three types of organizational groups providing EMS services.

3. Discuss the role of accountability in governmental EMS operations.

4. Discuss the sources of EMS bad debt.

5. Explain why fee for service is complicated.

10

Legislation and Regulation

Objectives

Upon completion of this chapter, the reader should be able to:

- Summarize Public Law No. 93-154.

- Differentiate between a law, a regulation, and a consensus standard.

- Summarize federal legislation related to EMS.

- Describe how funding is related to legislation.

- Differentiate between categorical funding and block grants.

- State the purpose of federal regulations related to EMS.

- Define lead agency at both the federal and state levels.

- State the role of the NHTSA in federal EMS.

- Identify the major components of a state-level EMS lead agency.

- List three areas common to state legislation.

Overview of Legislation and Regulation

To fully appreciate the role of **legislation** and **regulation** in emergency medical services (EMS), it is necessary for EMS personnel to have a basic understanding of the governmental process and how to be involved in and influence the legislative and regulatory processes. Laws are created by a legislative body, enforced by an executive, and interpreted by the courts. This three-legged approach is central to our democratic tricameral form of government, intended to create a balance of powers. Although most often evident at the federal level, this approach applies to state and local governments as well (**Figure 10-1**).

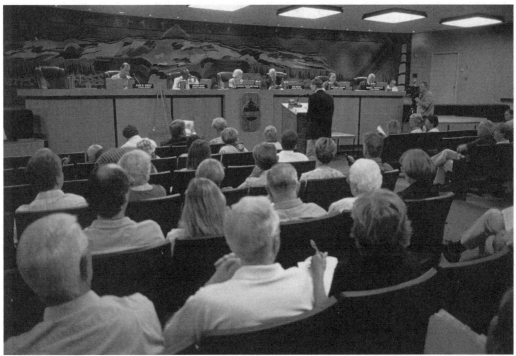

© David R. Frazier Photolibrary, Inc./Alamy.

FIGURE 10-1 City council meeting.

There are four sources of law: constitutional, statutory, common, and administrative. **Constitutional law** is derived from the U.S. and state constitutions. Examples of constitutional laws include those related to civil rights, privacy, and due process. Laws passed by a legislative body become **statutory laws**. These laws are found in a state's code of laws or on the local level as ordinances. When people think of breaking the law, they are usually referring to a statutory law. **Common law**, also known as case law, is derived, in most areas of the United States, from British common law. Common law differs from statutory law in that it is not derived from the actions of a legislature but from judicial precedent. The courts apply it, based on the social needs of the community; thus, the common law is less rigid and fixed than statutory law. An example of common law applied to EMS would be malpractice. What constitutes malpractice cannot be specifically defined; the standards must be established by judicial action.

The executive branch of government is charged primarily with enforcing laws. However, it may be given the authority to enact laws or regulations that are more specific or complex than those traditionally passed by a legislature. As an example, Congress has passed a law establishing the Occupational Safety and Health Administration (OSHA). It would be too time consuming and involved for Congress

Federal Regulation Process

Once a governmental agency has been given the authority to make a regulation, the agency must follow an established procedure involving publication of each step in the *Federal Register*. Agencies receive authority to make regulations by federal statute or executive order from the president. A governmental agency must publish a notice of proposed rulemaking in the *Federal Register*. This lets interested parties know that the agency is in the process of developing rules and regulations. Once the regulation is developed, the draft is published in the *Federal Register*. This step begins a public comment period of 30, 60, or 90 days. Information on how to make comments on the proposed rule as well as how to receive additional information is also published. At the close of the public comment period, the agency reviews the comments received and either approves the rule as proposed or makes changes as a result of the public comments. The notice of final rule-making ends the process with the publication of the final rule. The agency is required to provide responses to the received public comments regardless of whether the comments are incorporated into the final rule.

An interesting alternative path exists for rulemaking, known as negotiated rulemaking, in which stakeholders affected by the regulation and the responsible governmental agency negotiate the content of the proposed rule within parameters set by the agency. For example, in 1997, Congress passed the Balanced Budget Act of 1997 and called upon the Health Care Finance Administration (now the Centers for Medicare and Medicaid Services (CMS)) to establish a fee schedule for ambulance service using the negotiated rulemaking process. Representatives of the various EMS stakeholder groups, such as the American Ambulance Association, the International Association of Fire Chiefs, the American Hospital Association, and several others, met with CMS representatives for a year and hammered out a consensus on a draft rule that ultimately went into effect in 2002.

to pass all the regulations needed to ensure occupational safety and health. Therefore, it passes enabling legislation that allows OSHA to make such laws and rules. These laws and regulations are known as **administrative law**. The promulgation of such laws follows an established **rulemaking** process. As with other forms of law, failure to follow administrative law may result in fines, imprisonment, loss of professional status, or loss of legal status necessary to conduct business.

In addition to laws and regulations, EMS systems and providers are also affected by standards established by nongovernmental agencies. Professional associations and standard-setting organizations often develop standards and requirements (**Table 10-1**). Trade groups may establish standards for processes or products related to a particular occupation or service. These peer-developed standards are known as **consensus standards**. The process is similar to that used in the development of federal regulations. Usually, a committee of the organization develops a draft standard. The draft is circulated among the organization's members for input and comment. The committee responds to received comments and develops a revised draft. After an established period of time for review, the revised proposed standard is presented to the

TABLE 10-1 Trade, Professional, and Standard Development Organizations Providing Consensus Standards for EMS

- Ambulance Manufacturers Division of the National Truck Equipment Association
- American College of Emergency Physicians (ACEP)
- American College of Surgeons (ACS)
- Association of Air Medical Services (AAMS)
- American Society for Testing and Materials International (ASTM) Committee F-30
- Commission for the Accreditation of Ambulance Services (CAAS)
- Commission for the Accreditation of Air Medical Services (CAAMS)
- Committee on Accreditation of Emergency Medical Services Professions (CoAEMSP)
- National Association of EMS Physicians (NAEMSP)
- National Fire Protection Association (NFPA)

organization's full membership for approval. Compliance with the standard is usually voluntary or may be required for continued membership in the group that set the standard. Governments can pass regulations or laws that require conformity to these voluntary standards. An example of a consensus standard in EMS is the list developed by the American College of Surgeons of minimum essential equipment for ambulances. Although consensus standards do not carry the force of law, they may be used in court proceedings to establish a standard of care. Therefore, EMS systems and providers should be aware of applicable standards.

The Federal Legislative Role

Federal involvement in EMS developed through efforts to reduce death and injury from automobile crashes. As early as the 1920s, the U.S. Department of Commerce convened the National Conference on Street and Highway Safety, which led to the development of uniform traffic codes. However, traffic safety at this time was considered a state responsibility. The Federal-Aid Highway Act of 1956 called for the federal government to investigate means to improve highway safety.

It was not until the presidential election campaign of 1960 that a candidate, John F. Kennedy, observed that "traffic accidents constitute one of the greatest, perhaps the greatest, of the nation's public health problems" (Kennedy, 1960). Upon becoming president, Kennedy directed further investigation of traffic safety and accident prevention. Federal investigation identified areas of deficiency and also recognized that highway safety required a systems approach. One component of the system so identified was the human element.

In 1965, the President's Commission on Highway Safety published *Health, Medical Care, and Transportation of the Injured*. This report made recommendations similar to the National Academy of Science/National Research Council report *Accidental Death and Disability—The Neglected Disease of Modern Society*. Following the Kennedy administration's lead, President Lyndon Johnson proposed a Traffic Safety Act in his State of the Union Message of 1966. Congress responded by passing the Highway Safety Act of 1966 and the National Traffic and Motor Vehicle Safety Act of 1966. Passage of these bills established a defined federal role in EMS involving coordination and financing for states to develop highway safety programs. (See chapter 2 for more information.)

Legislation

The federal role in EMS is grounded in a series of legislative actions taken by the U.S. Congress (**Figure 10-2**). Significant federal legislation related to EMS includes:

- The Highway Safety Act of 1966, Public Law No. 89-564, established the Emergency Medical Services Program in the U.S. Department of Transportation. This act identified highway safety as a public health concern worthy of federal attention.
- The Emergency Medical Services Systems Act of 1973, Public Law No. 93-154 (appendix A), established a systems approach to the provision of EMS. The bill called for the establishment of comprehensive and integrated regional EMS systems. The 15 components of an EMS system were defined in the legislation as mandatory components of regional EMS systems. Funding

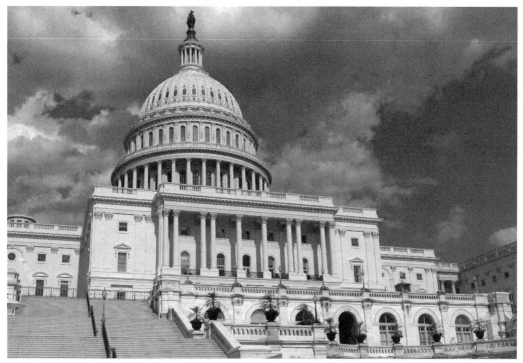

© Vacclav/Shutterstock, Inc.

FIGURE 10-2 The federal role in EMS is grounded in a series of legislative actions taken by the U.S. Congress.

was provided for planning, establishment, expansion, research, and training for EMS systems. This funding provided the start-up money for many statewide and regional EMS systems across the country.

- The EMSS Act Amendments of 1976, Public Law No. 94-573, and the EMSS Act Amendments of 1979, Public Law No. 96-142, provided funding for EMS project grants in feasibility studies and planning; burn treatment; trauma, burn, and poison demonstration projects; and additional funding for training.

- The Omnibus Budget Reconciliation Act of 1981 (OBRA), Public Law No. 97-35, marked the end of funding for EMS as established by the EMSS Act. Instead, funding was consolidated into preventive health and health services block grants (lump sums to be used for broad program areas) to the states. In addition to EMS, states had the option of funding programs in health incentives, urban rat control, hypertension, fluoridation, health education risk reduction, and home health care. Thus, the level and extent of federal funds going to EMS was now controlled by the states. This shift in funding patterns had a major and generally negative effect on EMS systems at the state level.

- The Trauma Care Systems Training and Development Act of 1990, Public Law No. 101-590, was an attempt by the original sponsors of the EMSS Act to revitalize federal involvement in EMS. The act was directed toward the development of coordinated trauma systems and improved EMS communications. After moving through various congressional committees, the act was finally passed in 1989. Funding included in the bill was appropriated for fiscal year 1990–91. The act established an office within the Health Resources and Services Agency (HRSA) of the U.S. Department of Health and Human Services (DHHS). This office was charged with developing model trauma systems and providing grants to state and local agencies to plan comprehensive trauma systems.

Funding

Federal funding for EMS began with the Highway Safety Act of 1966, which provided funding for development of EMS systems as a means to reduce highway fatalities. Section 402 of the act provided matching grants to the states for demonstration projects and studies. In 1972, the Health Services and Mental Health Administration of the U.S. Department of Health, Education, and Welfare (DHEW) was directed by the president to support the development of five EMS demonstration projects that were designed to develop comprehensive EMS systems. Contracts totaling $16 million were authorized. Passage of the EMSS Act in 1973 provided the most significant level of federal funding for EMS. The cost of the act was estimated to be $500 million. However, between 1974 and 1981, the federal government awarded grants under the act totaling $308,456,000 (Boyd, Edlich, & Micik, 1983).

States, regions, and local jurisdictions were able to use federal funding for the development of comprehensive EMS systems. The act limited funding to five years and required that at least 25% of each annual appropriation be given to rural areas. To ensure proper development of EMS systems, the act required recipients to utilize the 15 components of an EMS system as outlined in the act. In addition, local matching funding was required. Matching funding means that for each federal dollar provided, the state or region had to provide a dollar of its own funds. This approach ensured that the local recipients were involved and committed to the funded project.

Funding through the EMSS Act and amended versions is often referred to as 1200-funds money. This is derived from the various sections of the act:

- Sections 1202/1 and 1202/2: Feasibility studies and planning;
- Section 1203: Establishment and initial operation;
- Section 1204: Expansion and improvement;
- Section 1205: Research;
- Section 1221: Burn demonstration;
- Section 1221: Trauma, burn, and poison demonstration; and
- Sections 776 and 789: Training.

Federal funding for EMS continued under the EMSS Act until 1981. Changes in political philosophy that sought to reduce the role of the federal government, coupled with a desire to reduce the federal budget deficit, resulted in passage of the OBRA of 1981. This act changed the way the federal government provided funding to states. Primarily, the federal government controlled funding under the EMSS Act. Thus, states had less direct involvement in the development of EMS systems. The type of funding provided by the EMSS Act is known as **categorical funding**, funding provided to support specific programs or initiatives. The OBRA of 1981 changed funding to **block grants**, which provide lump sums of money to states to address broad programmatic or target areas. Under block grants, the state is given more authority to set priorities and commit funds than under categorical funding.

The OBRA of 1981 moved funding for EMS through the "1200 monies" (1200-funds) into the Preventive Health and Health Services block grant program of the DHHS (the successor to DHEW). The block grant program reduced the federal role in EMS, turning responsibility for funding local EMS over to the states. Today, still, 16 state EMS programs are funded through these block grant moneys. States were free to determine the level and use of funds provided for EMS. As a result of this change, initial funding for EMS under the block grants decreased in many states. This reduction was in part due to a lower level of funding by the federal government under the block grants. In the face of this shortfall, states used a variety of strategies to maintain funding levels. These included using funds remaining from categorical funding programs, transferring funds between block grants, and increasing the use of state funds. Because EMS programs had enjoyed a high level of federal support and control, some states were initially reluctant to assume this role.

As state support for EMS stabilized in the 1980s, significant changes occurred in many state EMS programs. Competition for funding resulted in state EMS lead agencies evolving from planning and development agencies with strong central control into offices supporting a regulatory and technical assistance role. This role change often came about as the result of staff and budget downsizing. In some states, however, alternative funding sources were developed (often tied to vehicle or license registration fees) to maintain funding of a comprehensive statewide EMS system.

Although direct federal funding for EMS was reduced, federal funds were still flowing to the states through highway safety funding administered by the National Highway Traffic Safety Administration (NHTSA). This funding source still continues today. Known as 402 funds, these block grants cover six primary areas: EMS, occupant restraints, speed enforcement, drug and alcohol enforcement, traffic records, and highway construction. Given that the states have control over how the block grant money is used, it is easy to see how EMS might not be considered a high priority.

Concerned over the effect of the DHHS block grants created by the OBRA of 1981, two of the original sponsors of the EMSS Act introduced the Trauma Care Systems Training and Development Act of 1990. This legislation authorized grants to states to develop trauma care systems, improve rural trauma systems, and establish a national Advisory Council on Trauma Care Systems. Funding to support 9-1-1 services was added in fiscal year 1993. Grants were also to be made available to trauma centers for uncompensated care resulting from drug-related violence and for residency programs in emergency medicine. Although $5 million was appropriated for the act, this amount was insufficient to meet grant demands, and funding for uncompensated care was never supported. The provisions of the act were terminated in 1995 and the Division of Trauma and Emergency Medical Systems within the Bureau of Health Resources Development of HRSA was closed. Since then, there has been no further federal legislative interest in EMS.

EMTALA

In addition to passing legislation to provide for the general welfare of the population and the associated funding to support such legislation, the federal government also passes legislation to address specific problems or citizen concerns. An example of such legislative action is what has come to be called the Emergency Medical Treatment and Active Labor Act (EMTALA). The EMTALA or antidumping laws require that the hospital provide initial stabilizing care to all patients regardless of their ability to pay. The law also establishes guidelines for the transfer of patients from one facility to another. (The law derives its name from section 9121 of the Consolidated Omnibus Budget Reconciliation Act of 1985 (COBRA), which contained the EMTALA legislation.) It is a common political practice for Congress to add unrelated amendments to legislative bills in hopes of getting the legislation approved.

EMTALA applies to every hospital that has an emergency department. The stimulus for the law came out of the practice by some hospitals of either refusing to treat uninsured patients or "**dumping**" them onto another facility. Of primary concern to EMS systems are the requirements for an authorized patient transfer. Services providing interfacility and critical care transports come under the scrutiny of the EMTALA statute. To provide for the enforcement of EMTALA, civil monetary penalties are specified in the statute for both the institution involved and the transferring physician. Depending on the size of the hospital, a fine of up to $50,000 per occurrence and loss of Medicare and Medicaid reimbursement can be imposed on both the hospital and the physician. EMTALA has helped ensure that all U.S. residents have access to emergency medical care; however, there is not a corresponding guarantee of payment. This has placed a tremendous financial strain on emergency health services that has yet to be addressed.

Federal Regulations

Federal regulations are laws promulgated by federal agencies and are contained in the **Code of Federal Regulations (CFR)**. The authority to create regulations is contained in legislation passed by Congress and signed by the president or through a presidential executive order. Regulations address specific areas too detailed or dynamic to be codified in a public law. Because of the complexity of some federal regulations, the administrative head of a governmental agency issues rulings that are similar to the interpretation of laws by the courts. They provide clarification and interpretation of complex or ambiguous provisions of laws or regulations.

It is beyond the scope of this text to list all of the federal regulations related to EMS. However, some representative sample federal regulations are presented here.

- 42 C.F.R. § 434.30—Contracts with Health Maintenance Organizations (HMOs) and Prepaid Health Plans (PHP5): Contract Requirements, Emergency Medical Services. This regulation defines the nature of contracts to provide emergency medical services with HMOs and PHPs that receive Medicare reimbursement. The regulation is administered by the CMS. CMS promulgates many regulations related to Medicare and Medicaid that apply indirectly to EMS because many EMS providers bill for service, especially for interfacility transports.

- 42 C.F.R.§ 489.24—Special Responsibility of Medicare Hospitals in Emergency Cases. This regulation defines the responsibilities of Medicare hospitals (a hospital that bills Medicare for patient services) under 42 U.S.C. § 1395 (EMTALA). This regulation also defines the requirements for Medicare hospitals under the law and sets fines and penalties for failure to comply with those requirements.

- 42 C.F.R. pt. 493—Laboratory Requirements. The Clinical Laboratory Improvement Amendments of 1988 (CLIA) were enacted to ensure that medical laboratory tests are properly performed. Enforced by CMS, this regulation applies to the performance of medical laboratory tests in an ambulance, specifically blood glucose testing. The regulations require ambulance services to apply for a waiver to perform glucose testing if they use devices approved for home use. If an ambulance service wishes to perform other medical tests, its ambulances must be licensed as medical laboratories.

- 29 C.F.R. pt. 803—Medical Device Reporting (MDR). A Food and Drug Administration (FDA) regulation, the MDR procedures require the reporting of any failure of biomedical equipment. If the cardiac monitor on an ambulance fails while in use, the incident must be properly reported to the FDA.

- 29 C.F.R. § 1910.1030—Blood-Borne Pathogens. A regulation of the OSHA, this section of the Code of Federal Regulations sets forth standards for the safe handling of blood and body fluids as well as requirements for personnel handling such materials.

Congressional EMS Caucus

At the end of the 110th Congress in 2008, a Congressional Emergency Medical Services Caucus was formed. **Congressional caucuses** organize members of Congress who have a particular interest in supporting a specific cause. The caucus helps its members be more effective in promoting and passing legislation on a specific topic—in this case, for EMS. The founding chairs of the EMS Caucus were Representative Ruppersberger of Maryland, Representative Boustany of Louisiana, and Representative Walz of Minnesota.

Federal Lead Agency

At present, no single federal agency is designated by law to serve as the lead agency for EMS in the United States. The NHTSA's EMS Office is the federal entity most closely filling this role. A lead agency was defined in the EMSS Act of 1973. The role of a federal lead EMS agency passed through various divisions and bureaus within DHEW and its successor, DHHS. The role changed as federal legislation related to EMS changed. With the end of categorical funding, a strong federal focus on EMS also ended. Today, the two federal agencies most involved in EMS within DHHS are CMS, through its administration of the Medicare and Medicaid programs, and the Bureau of Maternal and Child Health within the HRSA.

The federal agencies currently providing the most visible federal leadership in EMS are the NHTSA and the Maternal and Child Health Bureau. Through its Office of EMS, NHTSA provides technical assistance and program guidelines for EMS system development and review. The NHTSA Office of EMS has been responsible for developing the new education curriculum and standards for EMS. The NHTSA is also responsible for NEMSIS—the next generation of 9-1-1 technology—and guidance for the EMS response to pandemic influenza. It is NHTSA's philosophy that good EMS systems will ultimately improve survival from transportation-related incidents. The Maternal and Child Health Bureau has been instrumental in increasing awareness of the special EMS needs of children. Through a memorandum of understanding, these two federal agencies have agreed to combine efforts to promote EMS development nationwide. Additionally, in 2008, NHTSA established the National EMS Advisory Committee, a federal advisory committee that consists of 25 nonfederal experienced EMS leaders and provides expert consultation to the NHTSA administrator on matters of importance to the national EMS community.

A number of other federal agencies also impact EMS across the nation. The Department of Homeland Security (DHS) administers grants for first responder preparedness, although only four percent has been directed to EMS. The Federal Emergency Management Agency (FEMA) provides training for disaster response and other emergency topics through the U.S. Fire Administration (USFA). OSHA develops and enforces regulations related to worker safety. The blood-borne and respiratory protection regulations are two that are most relevant to EMS. The Government Services Administration (GSA) develops the specifications for ambulances that the federal government purchases. The Indian Health Services (IHS) operates EMS on many of the Indian reservations in the United States.

In 2005, when Congress reauthorized the Department of Transportation, Congress established the Federal Interagency Committee on Emergency Medical Services (FICEMS). Under the administrative management of the NHTSA EMS Office, FICEMS has representatives at the assistant secretary level from the various federal agencies that have EMS programs, including the NHTSA, DHS, DHHS, DOD, and FCC. Its purpose is to coordinate the federal agencies involved with EMS, provide a national EMS needs assessment, recommend new or expanded programs, streamline release of federal reports to EMS, and assist in setting priorities based on needs assessment. FICEMS must submit a report to Congress detailing its progress. At approximately the same time FICEMS was established, the Institute of Medicine (IOM) issued a report on emergency medicine. While one of its recommendations was the establishment of a lead federal EMS agency, the IOM did acknowledge that FICEMS was a step in the right direction. Through the coordination of the NHTSA Office of EMS, the activities of FICEMS and NEMSAC work in concert.

Field EMS Modernization and Innovation Act (2015)

In October 2002, the National Association of EMS Physicians (NAEMSP), the National Association of Emergency Medical Technicians (NAEMT), and the National Association of State EMS Officials (NASEMSO) formed a coalition dedicated to promoting, educating, and increasing the awareness among decision-makers in Washington on issues related to providers of EMS. The coalition was known as Advocates for EMS (AEMS) and contracted with a professional lobbying firm to coordinate its advocacy efforts. The coalition was expanded to include the National Association of EMS Educators (NAEMSE) as well as two at-large board positions representing corporate sponsors and individual members. In 2015, AEMS was dissolved as a coalition and its advocacy and lobbying efforts became the responsibility of NAEMSP.

Prior to the dissolution of AEMS, the coalition worked extensively with a broad constituency of EMS providers and supporters to formulate a legislative initiative to focus congressional attention on the needs of EMS at the operational level. This resulted in the 2011 introduction in the U.S. House of Representatives of the Field EMS Quality, Innovation and Cost-Effectiveness Improvement Act, H.R. 3144. The act sought to:

- Designate the DHHS as the primary federal agency for EMS and trauma through the establishment of the Office of EMS and Trauma within DHHS;
- Create three grant programs to improve EMS services:
  - Field EMS agency grants;
  - State grants; and
  - Education grants;
- Improve quality and accountability, primarily through increased emphasis on physician oversight and medical direction of EMS;
- Evaluate innovative delivery models, including alternative transport destinations;
- Enhance research through creation of a Field EMS Practice Center; and
- Provide funding for the bill by establishing a trust fund financed by voluntary contributions made by taxpayers on their federal tax form.

Since its introduction in 2011, the original legislation has evolved into the Field EMS Modernization and Innovation Act. This revised legislation, still known as the "Field EMS Bill," has the following goals as presented by the NAEMT:

- **Aligning Federal Leadership for Emergency Medical Services:** Clarifies DHHS as the lead federal agency for emergency medical care as recommended by the IOM (DHHS is already the lead for public health emergencies). A properly functioning emergency care system is a prerequisite for preparedness and response to major public health emergencies.

- **Promoting Innovation and Quality Through Field EMS Reimbursement:** Establishes the evaluation of field EMS alternative delivery models and a voluntary quality incentive program—with the goal of improving outcomes and lowering costs.

- **Modernizing Field EMS Capability:** Establishes grant opportunities for providers that demonstrate a need to improve preparedness response; enhances medical oversight through physician-led guidelines and identifies impediments to quality improvement; and recognizes field EMS as a health profession and establishes a grant program to ensure the availability, quality, and capability of field EMS practitioners, managers, medical directors, and educators.

- **Improving the Evidence Base of Care in the Field:** Requires the Secretary of DHSS to evaluate the extent to which research related to field EMS is conducted across DHHS and requires the Agency for Healthcare Research and Quality (AHRQ) to establish a Field EMS Evidence-Based Center of Excellence. www.naemt.org/advocacy/FieldEMSBill.aspx (accessed Oct. 30, 2015).

Patient Protection and Affordable Care Act

In March 2010, President Obama signed into law the Patient Protection and Affordable Care Act, known as the ACA. The ACA was designed not only to provide health care for millions of uninsured Americans but also to fundamentally change the nation's healthcare system. The ACA:

- Addressed issues related to Medicare and controlling Medicare costs;
- Provided health insurance for the uninsured;
- Implemented strategies to control healthcare costs;
- Emphasized quality and efficiency as means to reduce cost and improve care;
- Made changes to health insurance coverage, for example restrictions on covering patients with preexisting conditions; and
- Focused on prevention and wellness.

Perhaps the most important change brought about by the ACA was the way in which healthcare services would be paid for. The traditional method of paying for health care was the fee-for-service model wherein a healthcare provider performed a service and the patient was directly billed for the cost of that service. If the patient had insurance, the insurance company was billed instead, in a system known as third-party billing. If there was a difference between what the insurance company would cover and the actual cost, the patient was responsible for this co-pay. Ambulance services that bill for transport have used this system, referred to as reimbursement. It is important to note that reimbursement is based on the type and number of transports, with no consideration for the quality or efficiency of the service provided.

The ACA changes the way healthcare providers are reimbursed for services provided (including ambulance services). Instead of a simple fee-for-service model, the ACA would set reimbursement rates based on the quality of service provided. Providers would get paid more for keeping their patients healthy and out of the hospital. Accountable Care Organizations (ACO) would be formed, consisting of a wide range of healthcare providers who would work together to achieve increased quality and value of the care provided.

So how does the ACA affect the delivery of EMS and ambulance services? Implementation of the ACA is ongoing at the time of this writing and changes to EMS services are just beginning to be recognized. However, EMS and ambulance transport services will most likely be affected in the following areas:

- Transport EMS services will become part of an ACO, working with other healthcare providers to ensure quality and control cost.
- Reimbursement for transport will move from a fee-for-service model to a value-added model. EMS may even be compensated for not transporting some patients!
- The role of the EMS provider will change to place an emphasis on wellness and prevention as well as emergency and emergent care.
- New roles for EMS providers, such as the community paramedic, will develop.
- Quality of care will be closely monitored and directly tied to reimbursement level. An EMS system that provides consistently poor care will either not be reimbursed or will receive less than a service that has provided high-quality care.

The State Role

The EMSS Act of 1973 also had a profound effect on EMS at the state level. Not only did the act provide funds to the states through the 1200 grants, it also required the establishment of state lead agencies. Prior to the act, many states had statewide organizations and associations that fostered the interest of rescue squads and ambulance units in EMS. However, there was no office at the state level devoted to the coordination and delivery of EMS. Likewise, states often lacked legislation specific to EMS and EMS services.

Charged with improving EMS nationwide, the Division of Emergency Medical Services attempted to establish an identifiable lead agency within the health service of each state. In large metropolitan areas, local lead agencies were also developed. The same was true of more rural areas that came together to form regional EMS systems. A primary incentive for many states and regions to cooperate was the requirement of a lead agency to receive and manage 1200-funds.

Lead agencies sought to bring providers and consumers together to develop a systems approach to EMS delivery. The agencies provided coordination, technical expertise, and medical direction. They also administered the 1200-funds grants at the local level and provided fiscal oversight and management. Additionally, they were to work with professional groups, public and private agencies, and public safety agencies to coordinate and develop the delivery of EMS.

The original intention of the EMSS Act was to support the development of regional lead agencies as opposed to working with state-level health departments. It was thought that regional agencies would be more focused on EMS than specific state agencies. The regional approach also allowed areas with specific or common needs to work together. The regional and state agencies worked to establish legislation and regulation to accomplish their mission of EMS system coordination and control. In order to establish and develop an EMS system in a state, the lead agency needed the authority and regulatory ability to control system components. In many cases, the new roles given to personnel and system providers required state legislative changes or entirely new laws. For the first time, prehospital providers and ambulance services found themselves regulated and licensed by the state.

As federal funding for EMS changed in the 1980s, states suddenly found themselves with functional lead agencies required by law, but with little or no funding support. States had to either make up the lost funds or scale down the lead agency to fit available budget support.

In those states with strong support for EMS, alternative funding sources were developed. Because EMS was tied to highway safety, a few states developed programs that earmarked a portion of vehicle registration or driver's license renewal fees for EMS. Without federal 1200-funds' dollars to administer, the roles and responsibilities of the state EMS lead agency changed. The lead agency was seen more as a source of technical assistance to developed and functioning local EMS systems than as a central point for control and funding.

Components of a State Lead Agency

State-level EMS lead agencies in general have five major components: a state EMS director, a state EMS medical director, a governing board, training, and a licensing and regulatory function. The state EMS director serves as the chief operating officer of the state EMS agency and may be appointed by the governor, secretary of health, or public safety director. The director reports either to a state department secretary or to the state EMS governing board. In most states, the director is not a physician. The director is responsible for ensuring that EMS-related policy is developed and carried out as well as for enforcing laws and regulations passed by the legislature. The National Association of State EMS Officials (NASEMSO) represents the interests of state directors at the national level and provides a forum for networking among the directors. In those states with strong statewide control of EMS, there is an EMS medical director who is a physician responsible for coordinating statewide medical direction and quality assurance.

Following a requirement of the EMSS Act, many states maintain a statewide EMS governing or advisory council. The council brings together representatives of the many components of the EMS system. If the council has policy-making authority, it is the body that passes regulations and issues policy statements that are carried out by the state director and the lead agency. The council may work through the governor's office to propose legislation and request funding for EMS. If the council plays only an advisory role, it serves to provide guidance and initiative to the director. It may review the operation of the state lead agency and make recommendations, but it has no authority to craft policy or allocate funds. It may make recommendations to the governor or other authority concerning system operations and legislation. In order to carry out its mission, the state EMS council may work through regional and local EMS councils.

Another component of a state lead agency is a division or office responsible for training and education. This office is often combined with the certification function of the lead agency. The state training coordinator is responsible for ensuring that the training and certification of EMS providers follow applicable regulations and laws. The training function often sets the requirements for continuing medical education (CME) for EMS providers and, in some cases, develops curriculum for special training and education needs. State training coordinators have an organized section in NASEMSO.

There is a regulatory function that involves licensing of EMS providers, vehicles, and EMS services. In some cases, the lead agency may be responsible for designation of hospitals as specialty centers for certain categories of emergency patients, such as burn patients and stroke patients, as part of their regulatory capacity. In some states the lead agency has enforcement powers related to regulations, whereas in others it provides only technical assistance related to compliance with regulations.

State Legislation

Legislation related to EMS at the state level is as varied as the states themselves (**Figure 10-3**). Some states have very specific requirements, including licensing of ambulances, personnel, and medical facilities. Others provide only minimal state-level oversight. However, three areas of legislation common to all states include Good Samaritan laws, 9-1-1 service, and provider authorization.

"Good Samaritan" laws exist to provide legal protection relief to individuals who, of their own accord, stop and render aid at the scene of a medical or trauma emergency. In most cases, the person must do so without compensation and provide care consistent with his or her level of training. However, Good Samaritan laws only provide coverage from acts that do not constitute gross negligence.

The federal government fostered the development of 9-1-1 as the universal access number for emergency assistance nationwide. At the state level, legislation requires local telephone service providers to provide 9-1-1 service. Regulation of 9-1-1 is accomplished through a statewide "Numbers Board."

With the development of new levels of emergency care providers, the states were forced to change their medical practice acts, especially in regard to advanced life support (ALS) providers. States passed laws and regulations governing the scope of practice, requirements, education, licensing, and relicensing of prehospital providers. Regulation of prehospital providers is one of the key roles of the state EMS lead agency.

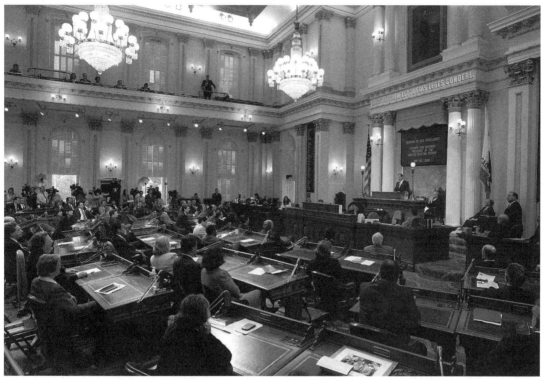

© Justin Sullivan/Getty.

FIGURE 10-3 State legislature in session.

Model State EMS Systems

In 2008, NASEMSO, along with technical assistance from NHTSA-OEMS and FICEMS, developed a template and tools to develop model EMS systems at the state level that includes a self-assessment tool, implementation tools, and model-state-enabling legislation. This process looks at the following 10 subsystems:

- Leadership and policy;
- Financial support;
- Human resources;
- Transportation;
- Facility regionalization;
- Public access and 9-1-1;
- Public information, education, and prevention;
- Clinical care and medical direction;

- Information and evaluation; and
- Disaster preparedness.

These assessments are designed to develop action steps for state EMS system improvements in the future.

Advocacy

It is not enough for EMS providers and administrators to know about EMS laws, regulations, and standards and how they are made. They also need to be aware of proposed legislation and regulation standards that may have a direct effect on them and their service. Political action is a necessary activity for EMS personnel, but it requires some degree of political savvy. Professional associations and trade groups often retain professional lobbyists to represent their interests to the government. At the local level, a well-planned appearance of an EMS leader and uniformed personnel at a town council meeting may be all that is needed to influence the political process.

A number of national EMS organizations formed a coalition in 2003 to raise awareness of EMS issues in the U.S. Congress and to advocate with a unified voice. Advocates for EMS (AEMS), formed by the National Association of EMS Physicians, the National Association of State EMS Officials, the National Association of EMTs, and the National Association of EMS Educators, have formed a number of national and other associations, and provider organizations have joined the coalition, including the American Ambulance Association, the National Volunteer Fire Council, the Emergency Nurses Association, the American College of Emergency Physicians, the National EMS Managers Association, and the Association of Air Medical Services, to name a few. AEMS has advocated for legislation and appropriations that support all components of EMS, regardless of provider type. AEMS has increased the profile of EMS in Congress and has been instrumental in securing funding for NEMSIS, EMS-C, and the creation of the Congressional EMS Caucus.

WRAP UP

Summary

Legislation and regulation are an integral part of EMS. At the federal level, legislation passed by Congress has had a profound effect on the national development of EMS. Legislation has served to authorize funding for states to develop EMS systems. In addition to public laws, various agencies within the federal government have regulatory authority over EMS-related activities.

At the state level, EMS lead agencies provide leadership through legislative mandates to coordinate and assist EMS systems. The lead agency accomplishes its mission under a state director guided by an advisory council. The agency's mission is supported by regulatory authority.

Legislative and regulatory initiatives of the future will be directed toward the integration of EMS into the overall healthcare system, especially as it relates to the reimbursement of EMS services through federally supported healthcare programs. Future regulation will seek to improve the quality of the workplace environment and provide for the safety of EMS providers.

Key Terms

administrative law

block grants

categorical funding

Code of Federal Regulations (CFR)

common law

Congressional caucuses

consensus standards

constitutional law

lead agency

legislation

patient dumping

regulation

rulemaking

statutory laws

Review Questions

1. List the four types of laws and describe each.
2. Explain how consensus standards affect the delivery of EMS.
3. Select one federal legislative act involving EMS and describe its effect on EMS systems development and funding.
4. Discuss the importance of the 1200-funds to the development of statewide EMS systems.
5. Discuss the status of a federal EMS lead agency.
6. List the major components of a state-level EMS lead agency.
7. List legislative or regulatory actions you would suggest that could improve the delivery or coordination of EMS.

Additional Resources

Boyd, D. R., Edlich, R. F., & Micik, S. H. (Eds). (1983). *Systems approach to emergency medical care*. Norwalk, CT: Appleton-Century-Crofts.

Kennedy, J. F. (1960). *Quotation from campaign speech*. In U.S. Department of Health, Education, and Welfare. (1968). *Report of the secretary's advisory committee on traffic safety*.

Washington, DC: U.S. Government Printing Office.

U.S. General Accounting Office. (1986). *Report to Congressional requesters: Health care: States assume leadership role in providing emergency medical services*. (GAO/HRD-86-132). Washington, DC: U.S. Government Printing Office.

11

Public Education and Injury Prevention

Objectives

Upon completion of this chapter, the reader should be able to:

- State the role of public education in EMS.

- List the stages of the public education process.

- Identify activities related to the three components of PIER.

- Describe the benefits of public education to the EMS organization, the patient and public, and EMS providers.

- Value the role of PSAs in public education.

- State the importance of technology in the delivery of public education.

- Identify the magnitude and components of the injury problem.

- Differentiate between intentional and unintentional injuries.

- Describe countermeasures against injury.

- Be familiar with the interpretation of Haddon's matrix.

- Identify the three E's of injury prevention.

- State the role of EMS in injury prevention.

Introduction

The provision of emergency medical services (EMS) is a public service. As such, EMS providers must effectively communicate with the public they serve. This communication can take many forms and serve various purposes. Members of the public are EMS customers; EMS has the responsibility to market the services provided to these customers and make sure they are informed about how to use these services. For instance, an EMS provider may want to inform residents about a new level of service being offered, or the importance of using 9-1-1 to call for assistance, or how to call an information line for nonemergency issues. A system may also utilize public education to gain community support (**Figure 11-1**). Many EMS services are tax funded, so maintaining public support is important because there are multiple organizations competing for the same funds.

Another, more contemporary form of public education in which EMS is becoming involved is population-based health, including wellness and injury prevention. Preventing illness and injury has not traditionally been seen as a concern of EMS. However, changes both in healthcare delivery and in attitudes within EMS have focused on this area. This idea will be discussed in more detail later in this chapter. However, public education is an integral part of any prevention strategy. To be effective at preventing illness and injury, members of the public must be well informed. The fire service has been effective at this through efforts such as fire prevention, but unfortunately EMS has been ineffective. As we move to a model of population-based health, prevention and education become the focus, just as fire prevention has changed the fire service. Many EMS organizations are already actively involved in some form of public education. This

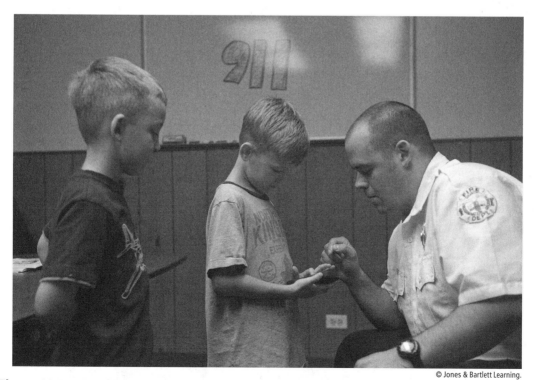

© Jones & Bartlett Learning.

Figure 11-1 Public education can help gain community support.

is especially true of volunteer organizations that rely on the public for direct financial support. Commercial and municipal organizations have started to become more engaged with promoting EMS as a profession to the public and improving its image. Following are some of the methods that promote EMS:

- Signs and billboards at the EMS offices or fire station
- Newspaper articles
- Direct mailings
- Door-to-door solicitation
- Blood pressure checks at shopping areas and malls
- Participation in community events
- Station open houses
- Visits to schools and daycare facilities
- Presentations to civic organizations
- Reports to governmental boards and councils
- Websites
- Social media

Forms of Public Education

As seen from the previous list, public education can take many forms. A common acronym to describe these activities is **PIER**—public information, education, and relations. PIER was developed by the National Highway Traffic Safety Administration (NHTSA, 1994) and the Federal Emergency Management Agency (FEMA) to assist EMS agencies in effectively interacting with the public.

Public information activities involve communicating to the public about an event or incident. It is "news." When a reporter arrives at an incident scene, information provided by EMS is public information. Public information may also include announcements of upcoming events, fundraisers, membership drives, awards presented to members, and so on. Public information is anything a service wants to tell the public about. Many services have a **public information officer (PIO)** who is responsible for public information activities and who serves as a focal point for the news media. Individual EMS providers are discouraged from speaking to the press unless under the guidance of a PIO due to the complexities involved in this process. Privacy issues, such as HIPAA restrictions, have dramatically limited the amount of information about patients that EMS providers can give to the public, but the press continues to be an ally for events and for publicity in general.

Changing the public's knowledge or skills is the goal of **public education** (**Figure 11-2**). It is the process of educating the public about an issue of importance to EMS. A community CPR class that is designed to teach the public the skill of CPR would be an example of public education and is often part of a public access defibrillator program.

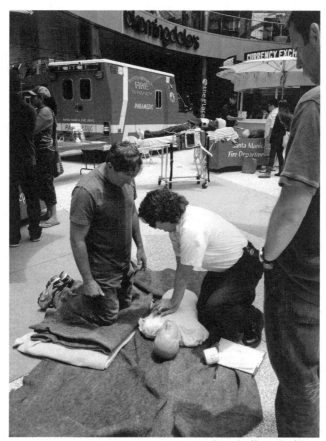

© Anna Bryukhanova/iStock/Getty.

Figure 11-2 Community CPR class is an example of public education.

Of the three components of PIER, **public relations** is probably the hardest to accomplish and the most overlooked. Public relations is the process of shaping public opinion. It is the activities an organization engages in to convey a particular image or to change the public's perception. For instance, if the local government is planning to cut taxes, the rescue squad may try to convince the public that this tax cut is bad because it will reduce funding for EMS. The squad will use public information and public education to garner support for its position. Maintaining a professional image at all times helps organizations, whether paid or volunteer, to show the public the pride they have in their service.

Public relations is something an EMS organization must be constantly concerned about. Everything an organization does is subject to public scrutiny. And how the public perceives something may not be the reality of a situation. Take, for instance, the simple act of a duty crew taking an ambulance to the local ice cream shop for a snack while on duty. Some members of the public may see this as unnecessary vehicle wear and tear or fuel usage. They do not see this as an incentive for personnel to be at the station and available for emergency response. It is important for EMS systems to constantly be aware of how their actions will be viewed and interpreted by the lay public. Appearance includes the way each provider acts, dresses, and provides service. EMS is a reflection of the individuals within the system, and everyone must do their part to advance the profession.

Benefits of Public Education

Engaging in public education and the broader PIER activities benefits not only the EMS system but also the people served by the system and the individual EMS provider. The benefits of PIER to EMS are listed in **Table 11-1**.

Public Education Process

Public education activities can take many forms. However, all such efforts involve the same basic steps. For public education to be effective, an EMS service must target programs for a specific community's need to thus reach the right people. But most importantly, all public education must provide a consistent message. It is important to constantly evaluate the effectiveness of every program and activity.

Delivery of a public education program begins with planning, which allows for the identification of program goals and objectives. It is important to consider a community's most critical need when planning public education activities. Planning also helps to identify the resources needed to carry out the

---

Table 11-1 Benefits of PIER to EMS

Benefits to EMS
- Increases efficient use of existing resources by educating the public to prevent or properly respond to emergencies
- Increases political exposure and support
- Increases public support for additional resources
- Increases service membership and retention of current members
- Improves morale through positive public and internal recognition

Benefits to the Patient and Society
- Reduces the number of deaths and disabilities by educating the public on self-care, first response, and bystander care
- Reduces costs (for both the patient and health care in general)
- Reduces emotional trauma
- Improves EMS response
- Increases community pride, which aids in recruiting new businesses and residents

Benefits to Providers
- Increases recognition and rewards for community service
- Increases job security and ability to move up in ranks
- Increases personal satisfaction
- Improves the working environment

Reproduced from National Highway Traffic Safety Administration and Federal Emergency Management Agency. (1994). EMS PIER Manual: Public Information, Education and Relations in Emergency Medical Services (FA-151). Washington, DC: U.S. Government Printing Office.

educational activity. How to measure success must also be identified during the planning process. Evaluation should be planned; it is not something that is done only after the activity has occurred.

As an example, an EMS service recognizes that bystanders are frequently removing young children involved in car crashes from car safety seats prior to the arrival of EMS. To address this problem, the EMS service plans a public education program. During the planning process, a working group would identify the specific problem to be addressed—in this case, removing children from car seats. Next, the group's members would set a goal for their educational effort. This should be obtainable and measurable. A realistic goal might be to reduce the number of children removed from car safety seats by 50% within 6 months. Now that a goal has been set, the working group decides on a strategy (or strategies), as presented in **Table 11-2**, to reach its goal. They also decide that they will measure attainment of the goal by reviewing EMS incident reports for six months after the initiation of public education activities.

The scope of a public education activity may be such that the EMS system alone cannot support it or that it must reach members of the public not routinely affected by EMS. This will require the development of partnerships and creative alliances to effectively deliver the proper message. Examples include working with civic organizations, church groups, special-needs populations, social clubs, or government agencies. The local news media should not be overlooked as a source of assistance. The media already has an established delivery system. Working with the media will help to develop a positive relationship that can lead to "more favorable press."

Table 11-2 Targeted PIER Strategies

EMS Organization Members
- Websites and social media
- Newsletters
- In-house communication pieces
- Recruitment materials
- Presentations
- Classes/courses
- Recognition programs
- Customer service training

Medical Community, First Responders, Nursing Homes, etc.
- Websites and social media
- Direct-mail brochures
- Print or public broadcasts
- EMS system access materials
- Articles in local and national trade magazines
- Press kits
- Newsletters
- Audiovisual lectures and presentations
- Mock-disaster exercises
- Support and assistance with other medical community programs
- Presentations

Table 11-2 *(Continued)*
Local Government and EMS Regulators
■ Newsletters
■ Press kits
■ Community service projects
■ Presentations
■ Brochures and reports
■ Information and professional EMS lobbyists
General Public
■ Community education programs and certifiable EMS training
■ Community involvement—health fairs and civic organizations
■ Public information through the media, websites and social media
■ Public safety campaigns

Reproduced from National Highway Traffic Safety Administration and Federal Emergency Management Agency. (1994). *EMS PIER Manual: Public Information, Education and Relations in Emergency Medical Services (FA-151)*. Washington, DC: U.S. Government Printing Office.

Using the child-safety-seat example, the EMS service realizes that it alone cannot get the message out to the general public. The working group meets with representatives of the local print media and radio stations. Together, they develop a public safety announcement (PSA) to be printed and aired over the next two months. The EMS service also uses websites and social media to provide real-time updates and information.

Evaluation of a public education activity must consider all aspects of the activity. Because an activity may be designed to change public behavior, immediate success cannot always be determined. For example, a three-month campaign educating the public about when to call EMS might not give immediate results. However, after reviewing and comparing a year's worth of run statistics, it might be seen that the number of inappropriate calls has declined. Evaluation should address issues of program planning, program monitoring, impact assessment, and resource utilization. In simpler terms, did the EMS system target the right population, reach that population, achieve its goal(s), and do so cost-effectively? Regardless of the success or failure of a program, it is important to share the results with other EMS systems, public safety organizations, and community groups. By exchanging information, EMS systems and community organizations can work together to more effectively educate the public.

Public Service Announcements

It is beyond the scope of this chapter to present and discuss all the methods available to reach the public. But one approach that is commonly associated with EMS is the **public service announcement (PSA)**. These are free spots on broadcast media or ads in print media. Broadcast stations are required to engage in some form of public service by the Federal Communications Commission (FCC). Stations often meet this requirement by providing free airtime to public safety and civic organizations. Stations often assist with the scripting and production of PSAs. State or national EMS organizations might make prerecorded PSAs available to local EMS services for broadcast in their area. A common example would be announcements supporting local EMS during National EMS Week. State EMS agencies may produce PSAs to support EMS in general statewide. Broadcast PSAs typically run in 10–15-second spots. For newspapers and magazines, professionally developed ad copy is available. Some copy can be altered to include the name of the local EMS agency.

Although not a true PSA, community calendars are sold by many civic organizations. Local residents can pay to have a birthday or anniversary listed. Meeting and fundraising dates are frequently included for public safety agencies free of charge, as are fire and safety messages. An example of this approach that has been especially helpful is PSAs reminding people to change the batteries in their smoke detectors.

Public Education and Technology

Changes in communications technology will affect the delivery of public education. Integration of the traditional telephone with cable television and the Internet has led to new possibilities for information exchange. Many EMS services have webpages or pages on social networking sites such as Facebook. Websites provide information on almost every topic of interest to the public. EMS systems must be aware of new opportunities to reach the public and have the resources to effectively communicate in new and emerging media. With the addition of streaming video, EMS agencies may be able to provide a multimedia presentation that packs a punch on the web. Many EMS agencies have started to use Facebook and Twitter to provide real-time updates and ongoing education.

Caution is needed in using technology and the Internet. The always-on and easily accessed nature of social media has led to both positive and negative changes. With almost every EMS provider having a smartphone, videos and photos of scenes can be very easily taken and quickly posted. All online postings should come from the public information officer or person in a similar position. EMS providers should be educated on what should and should not be posted. Many agencies have gone as far as to prevent all photo taking on scenes to prevent HIPAA violations. In particular, any photos or videos should be approved in advance, and EMS providers should be held accountable for their posts on Facebook or Twitter.

Injury Prevention

Injury is the single greatest killer of Americans between the ages of 1 and 44. Every year, nonfatal injuries cause one in three Americans to seek medical attention or render them unable to perform normal activities (National Research Council, 1985). The cost of injury in the United States is estimated to be over $460 billion annually, and more than 50 million traumatic injuries were medically treated in the United States during the year 2000 (Corso et al., 2006). This amount is more than twice the cost of cardiovascular disease and cancer combined (Campbell, 1998). Injury is the fifth leading cause of death and disability in all age groups and accounts for more **years of potential life lost (YPLL)** than any other health problem.

The modern view of injury began in the early to mid-1900s with the idea that some personal responsibility should be taken for injury. Motor vehicle crashes, house fires, drownings, assaults, and all the other ways in which injuries occur are not, as we used to think, accidents—random, uncontrollable acts of fate. They are understandable, predictable, and preventable. Injury, a public health problem, must be addressed by all healthcare personnel because it has consequences for the health of all Americans. Traffic injuries alone have produced more fatalities than all the wars in which the United States has fought, combined (National Committee for Injury Prevention and Control, 1989). Understanding what injuries are and how they can be prevented will provide a solid foundation for any outreach program.

The Injury Event

An **injury** is any unintentional or intentional damage to the body resulting from acute exposure to thermal, mechanical, electrical, chemical, or radiating energy or from the absence of such essentials as heat or oxygen (National Committee for Injury Prevention and Control, 1989). Examples of the various types of injury relating to energy are found in **Table 11-3**.

In this section, we will use an **epidemiological model** to discuss injuries and to examine the injury process. It is often helpful to view an injury from an epidemiological perspective, because injuries have elements similar to those of other diseases and include, as outlined in the **Haddon Matrix** (Haddon, 1963), a **host**, **agent**, **vector**, and **environment**. Injury events are also classified as occurring pre-event, event, and post-event. In addition, injuries can also be characterized by epidemic episodes, seasonal variation, long-term trends, and demographic distribution.

The host is the person injured. The actual agent of injury is energy, and the mechanism by which that energy is transferred is the vector. For example, an automobile can be a vector for physical energy

Table 11-3 Injuries Relating to Energy		
Energy Type	**Explanation**	**Example**
Thermal	Results from contact with source of heat or cold.	Burns, frostbite, heatstroke, hypothermia, etc.
Mechanical	Most common of all injury-causing energy types. Involves transfer of force (motion) between two moving objects.	Motor vehicle crashes, falls, penetrating injuries, etc.
Electrical	Involves the human body being subjected to an electrical field or current.	Lightning strike, contact with source of live electric current
Chemical	Involves the introduction of a chemical into the human body. Includes the ingestion of drugs.	Industrial incidents, HAZMAT spills, poisoning, overdose, chemical burns
Radiating	Exposure to radioactive isotopes that cause cellular mutation, illness, etc.	Nuclear incidents, industrial incidents, military actions

Table 11-4 Relationship Between the Injury, Host, Agent, Vector, and Environment				
Disease/Injury	**Host**	**Agent**	**Vector**	**Environment**
Fall	Human	Mechanical (kinetic) energy	Flight of stairs	Poorly lit stairwell with no handrails
Poisoning	Human	Chemical energy	Toxic substance	Chemicals in non-childproof containers
West Nile Virus	Human	Flaviviridae	Mosquito bite	Areas with mosquito carriers present

in a car crash, just as a faulty appliance can be a vector for electrical energy. In some cases, however, injury may also result from a lack of essential elements, such as oxygen or heat. The environment comprises the surroundings in which an injury occurs. The environment provides an opportunity for the agent to be transferred to the host. For example, the environment may be a poorly lit road on a rainy night that contributes to a car crash (Gordan, 1949; Gibson, 1961; Haddon, 1963). **Table 11-4** identifies the relationships between the injury, host, agent, vector, and environment. Note that the third example compares the components of the injury event to a classic infection.

Injury Types

Throughout history, injury has been a major cause of premature death. In modern America, injury takes a high toll on the lives of residents and is the leading killer of children, teenagers, and young adults.

Injuries are often classified by the behaviors and events that preceded them, as well as the intent of the people involved. The commonly used major subdivisions of injuries include **intentional** and **unintentional injuries**. Intentional injuries, those caused with an intent to harm oneself or others, include homicides, suicides, war, and assaults. Unintentional injuries, those caused without an intent to do harm, may include falls, motor vehicle crashes, and drowning. Although the events leading to intentional and unintentional injuries may be different, the mechanisms of injury and the injuries themselves are usually similar. For example, ingesting a toxic substance will always produce similar outcomes even though the spectrum of behavior can range from completely unintentional, as when a person is not aware of the presence or nature of a drug or its potential effect, to overtly suicidal self-poisoning.

There are a variety of potentially preventable injuries, including falls, drownings, poisonings, motor vehicle crashes, violence, and bicycle accidents. Understanding how these injuries can be prevented and how often they occur is essential knowledge for an EMS professional. Individual localities may have higher or lower incidences of injury, but national trends provide insight into how people are being injured or killed. Public education cannot stop until all preventable injuries are addressed.

Falls

Falls are the leading cause of injury deaths among people 65 years old or older, with traumatic brain injury accounting for 46% of fatal falls (CDC, 2009). Factors that contribute to falls include problems

Table 11-5 Top 10 Leading Causes of Death in the United States for 2006, by Age Group:[1] National Highway Traffic Safety Administration's National Center for Statistics and Analysis

Cause and Number of Deaths

Rank	Years of Life Lost[2]	Infants Under 1	Toddlers 1-3	Young Children 4-7	Children 8-15	Youth 16-20	Young Adults 21-24	Other Adults 25-34	Older Adults 65+	All Ages	35-44	45-64
1	Malignant Neoplasms 23%(8,913,260)	Perinatal Period 14,423	Congenital Anomalies 462	MV Traffic Crashes 449	MV Traffic Crashes 1,398	MV Traffic Crashes 5,685	MV Traffic Crashes 4,587	MV Traffic Crashes 7,047	Heart Disease 530,926	Heart Disease 652,091	Malignant Neoplasms 14,566	Malignant Neoplasms 149,645
2	Heart Disease 20%(7,876,528)	Congenital Anomalies 5,552	Accidental Drowning 437	Malignant Neoplasms 391	Malignant Neoplasms 835	Homicide 2,571	Homicide 2,717	Suicide 4,990	Malignant Neoplasms 388,322	Malignant Neoplasms 559,312	Heart Disease 12,668	Heart Disease 103,311
3	MV Traffic Crashes 5%(1,755,247)	Heart Disease 368	MV Traffic Crashes 370	Congenital Anomalies 205	Suicide 459	Suicide 1,905	Suicide 2,120	Homicide 4,752	Stroke 123,881	Stroke 143,579	Accidental Poisoning 6,729	Diabetes 16,992
4	Stroke 4%(1,579,544)	Homicide 306	Homicide 328	Exposure to Smoke/Fire 140	Homicide 440	Accidental Poisoning 896	Accidental Poisoning 1,553	Accidental Poisoning 4,386	Chronic Lwr. Resp. Dis. 112,716	Chronic Lwr. Resp. Dis. 130,933	Suicide 6,550	Chronic Lwr. Resp. Dis. 16,724
5	Chronic Lwr. Resp. Dis. 4%(1,575,270)	Septicemia 302	Malignant Neoplasms 279	Accidental Drowning 135	Congenital Anomalies 297	Malignant Neoplasms 764	Malignant Neoplasms 825	Malignant Neoplasms 3,601	Alzheimer's 70,858	Diabetes 75,119	MV Traffic Crashes 6,491	Stroke 16,409
6	Suicide 3%(1,155,478)	Influenza/Pneumonia 265	Exposure to Smoke/Fire 160	Homicide 126	Heart Disease 259	Heart Disease 425	Heart Disease 624	Heart Disease 3,249	Influenza/Pneumonia 55,453	Alzheimer's 71,599	HIV 4,363	Chronic Liver Disease 14,643
7	Perinatal Period 3%(1,130,784)	Nephritis/Nephrosis 159	Heart Disease 141	Heart Disease 73	Accidental Drowning 218	Accidental Drowning 353	Accidental Drowning 252	HIV 1,318	Diabetes 55,222	Influenza/Pneumonia 63,001	Homicide 3,109	Suicide 11,201
8	Diabetes 3%(1,107,065)	MV Traffic Crashes 140	MV Nontraffic Crashes[4] 113	MV Nontraffic Crashes[4] 52	Exposure to Smoke/Fire 137	Congenital Anomalies 257	Congenital Anomalies 201	Diabetes 617	Nephritis/Nephrosis 36,416	Nephritis/Nephrosis 43,901	Chronic Liver Disease 2,688	MV Traffic Crashes 10,466

Table 11-5 (Continued)

Rank	Infants Under 1	Years of Life Lost[2]	Toddlers 1-3	Young Children 4-7	Children 8-15	Youth 16-20	Young Adults 21-24	Other Adults 25-34	Older Adults 65+	All Ages	35-44	45-64
9	Stroke 126	Accidental Poisoning 2%(917,659)	Influenza/Pneumonia 100	Stroke 42	MV NonTraffic Crashes[4] 105	MV NonTraffic Crashes[4] 142	Accidental Falls 138	Stroke 546	Septicemia 26,243	MV Traffic Crashes **43,667**	Stroke 2,260	Accidental Poisoning 8,990
10	Malignant Neoplasms 75	Homicide 2%(855,969)	Septicemia 75	Influenza/Pneumonia 41	Influenza/Pneumonia 87	Accidental Firearms 109	Pregnancy/Childbirth 120	Congenital Anomalies 436	Hypertension Renal Dis. 21,265	Septicemia 34,136	Diabetes 2,045	Nephritis/Nephrosis 6,169
ALL[3]	28,440	100% (38,441,580)	4,034	2,484	6,354	16,048	16,672	41,925	1,788,189	1,759,423	84,785	458,831

The columns 8-15, 16-20, 21-24, 25-34, 65+ fall under the span **Cause and Number of Deaths**.

[1]When ranked by specific ages, motor vehicle crashes are the leading cause of death for each age 3 through 34.

[2]Number of years calculated based on remaining life expectancy (2005 data from CDC) at time of death; percentages calculated as a proportion of total years of life lost due to all causes of death.

[3]Not a total of top 10 causes of death.

[4]A motor vehicle nontraffic crash is any vehicle crash that occurs entirely in any place other than a public highway.

Note: The cause of death classification is based on the National Center for Statistics and Analysis (NCSA) Revised 68 Cause of Death Listing. This listing differs from the one used by the NCHS for its reports on leading causes of death by separating out unintentional injuries into separate causes of death, e.g., motor vehicle traffic crashes, accidental falls, motor vehicle nontraffic crashes, etc. Accordingly, the rank of some causes of death will differ from those reported by the NCHS. This difference will mostly be observed for minor causes of death in smaller age groupings.

Data from National Highway Traffic Safety Administration.

with gait and balance, neurological and musculoskeletal disabilities, psychoactive medication use, dementia, and visual impairment (Judge, Lindsey, & Underwood, 1993). Environmental hazards such as slippery surfaces, uneven floors, poor lighting, loose rugs, unstable furniture, and objects on floors may also play a role (Tineui, Speechley, & Ginter, 1988).

Falls from heights—which include falls from open windows, off roofs, from maintenance equipment, and so on—have also been a significant source of injury. In large cities, as well as communities with multiple-family dwellings, falls from open windows are a serious problem. Cities such as New York have taken steps through building and fire code modification to ensure that a child cannot open windows wide enough to conceivably fall through. Many occupational-related falls from heights have been prevented by regulations imposed by the Occupational Safety and Health Administration (OSHA). OSHA provides safety regulations for individuals working in hazardous environments. Its role in injury prevention has saved countless lives.

Drownings

There were 3582 fatal unintentional drownings in 2005, averaging 10 deaths per day (CDC, 2008a). Children aged 14 years old or younger accounted for one-fourth of these deaths; of all deaths among children ages one to four, 30% were from drowning. Males are four times more likely than females to die from drowning, and African Americans are 1.3 times more likely than Whites (CDC, 2008b). Drowning risk factors identified by the CDC include:

- Lack of barriers and supervision around water sources;
- Age (especially younger than five years old);
- Recreation in natural water settings such as lakes, rivers, and oceans;
- Improper boating, especially without the use of life jackets;
- Alcohol use (associated with half of adolescent and adult drowning fatalities and one in five boating-related fatalities); and
- Having a seizure disorder (drowning, most often in a bathtub, is the leading cause of unintentional death for persons with seizure disorders).

Poisonings

In 2005, there were 32,691 poisoning deaths in the United States, making poisoning the second leading cause of unintentional death behind motor vehicle crashes (CDC, 2008).

Poison control centers help millions of people each year and are extremely cost-effective, ensuring that poisonings are treated rapidly and correctly. In 2008, the average number of calls per day to all poison control centers was 6,825 (an average of one call each 12.7 seconds). Children younger than 3 years old were involved in 38.7% of exposures, and children younger than 6 years old accounted for half of all human exposures (AAPCC, 2008). According to the annual report of the American Association of Poison Control Centers (AAPCC), the leading causes of poisoning for all age groups were analgesics (13.3%), cosmetics or personal care products (9 percent), household cleaning products (8.6%), sedatives, hypnotics, or antipsychotics (6.6%), and foreign bodies or miscellaneous (5.2%) (Bronstein et al., 2009).

Violence

Violence is defined most broadly as the use of physical force with the intent to inflict injury or death upon oneself or another person. From a public health perspective, the fact that acts of violence may result in physical injury is the primary motivation for involvement. Violence or intentional injury manifests itself in many forms. From blunt to penetrating trauma, violence affects everyone, everywhere. One of public health's most significant contributions to violence prevention has been the use of a model of injury focusing on interactions among the host, the agent, and the environment. This model examines the importance of victim–offender relationships and provides a framework through which these relationships can be understood and analyzed (National Committee for Injury Prevention and Control, 1989).

Motor Vehicle Crashes

Motor vehicle crashes are the leading cause of injury-related deaths for Americans aged 1 to 34 years old. In 2008, 37,261 people died on the nation's roads and highways, and another 1.63 million suffered nonfatal injuries (NHTSA, 2009). However, the number of deaths on U.S. highways has been declining because of the tremendous efforts of many groups over the last 35 years, advances in the design of vehicles and roads, laws requiring and regulating the use of life-saving devices such as safety belts, and changes in societal attitudes toward destructive behaviors such as drinking and driving (CDC, 2000).

Bicycle Crashes

In 2007, 698 bicyclists were killed in crashes (NHTSA, 2009). Wearing a bicycle helmet reduces the risk of serious head injury in a crash by as much as 85% and the risk for brain injury by as much as 88% (Thompson, Rivera, & Thompson, 1989). In fact, if each rider wore a helmet, an estimated 500 bicycle-related fatalities and 151,000 nonfatal head injuries would be prevented each year—one death per day and one injury every four minutes (Sacks, Kresnov, Houston, & Russell, 1996).

The most common complaints of children and adolescents are that helmets are not fashionable or "cool," their friends do not wear them, and they are uncomfortable (usually too hot). Riders also convey that they do not think about the importance of bike helmets, nor about the need to protect themselves from injury, particularly if they are not riding in traffic. Twenty-one states and the District of Columbia have enacted some form of bicycle helmet legislation. Most of these laws pertain to children and adolescents (Bicycle Helmet Safety Institute, 2010).

Injury Prevention Concepts

Prevention provides an opportunity to realize significant reductions in human morbidity (measurement of sickness or disease in a particular population) and mortality (measurement of death in a particular population) with a manageable investment. As a whole, the healthcare system is evolving from an emphasis on providing highly technological, curative care to improving health through prevention and wellness. The objective is to prevent people from ever requiring costly medical care (NHTSA, 1996). Engaging in prevention activities is the responsibility of every healthcare practitioner, including those involved with the provision of EMS (NHTSA, 1996).

Primary injury prevention, **secondary injury prevention**, and **tertiary injury prevention** represent three areas where EMS providers can have an impact on decreasing the morbidity and mortality from injuries. The goal of primary prevention is to prevent injury from occurring in the first place. Examples include wearing a seat belt or helmet and installing smoke detectors. Strategies that attempt to minimize further injury or death after the initial trauma or injury event has occurred are called secondary injury preventions. Medical treatments, such as securing the airway or C-spine immobilization, are included in tertiary injury prevention.

Injury prevention and control is the process of using knowledge about the injury event to design prevention programs and evaluate their success. Perhaps the most important principle of injury prevention and control is to understand that injury is a disease that can be prevented or modified by changing the transmission of energy (such as force) to an individual (host).

The components of the injury process (host, agent, vector) described earlier may be used to develop preventive measures for injuries. Before prevention measures to decrease morbidity and mortality are developed, it is helpful to identify the factors affecting the extent of the injury before, during, and after an injury. These components are examined as pre-event, event, and post-event. The Haddon Matrix can be used to identify factors affecting the extent of injury, from which prevention strategies or interventions may be designed.

Table 11-6 is a matrix taken from an injury prevention program targeted at reducing commercial fishing fatalities in Alaska, where the occupational fatality rate was more than 20 times the national average (NIOSH, 1997). Identifying factors affecting the extent of an injury during a specific phase event and developing a program targeted at changing or modifying these factors are crucial in creating a successful injury prevention program.

Interventions

Injury prevention interventions are generally classified into three groups: engineering, enforcement, and education, known as the **three E's**. These interventions are methods used to identify injury prevention and control methods. For example, a program to decrease head injuries from bicycling may incorporate the three E's by designing helmets that cover more of the head (engineering), lobbying for and enforcing helmet laws (enforcement), and teaching children about bicycle safety (education).

Surveillance

Lastly, **surveillance**, or the collection of information, may be used. Surveillance tells us how common the injury problem is, where it is, and who is affected. This information allows decision makers to allocate programs and resources where they are most needed. For example, prehospital care providers play

Table 11-6 Injury Prevention Program Matrix			
Phase	**Host/Human**	**Agent/Vehicle**	**Environment**
Preevent	Captain and crew fatigue Stress Prescription or illegal drugs or alcohol Inadequate training or exposure	Unstable vessel Unstable work platform Complex machinery and operations	High winds Large waves Icing Short daylight Limited fishing seasons Vessels far apart
Injury Event	Captain and crew reaction to emergency PFD not available or not working	Listing or capsized vessel Delayed abandonment Emergency circumstance not understood Man overboard (MOB)	High winds Large waves Darkness Poor radio communications Cold water
Postevent	Poor use of available emergency equipment Hypothermia Drowning Lost at sea	Vessel sinking Poor crew response to MOB	High winds Large waves Cold water

a crucial role in the documentation of the mechanism of injury in great detail. Surveillance data also tells us how well we are doing over time, where to shift resources, or to set a different direction. EMS information systems, including the National EMS Information System (NEMSIS), now make surveillance easier. Surveillance is discussed in more detail in chapter 13.

EMS and Injury Prevention

The 1966 report "Accidental Death and Disability: The Neglected Disease of Modern Society," released by the National Academy of Sciences/National Research Council, recognized injury as a disease that could be treated and prevented. This document, along with others, spurred the involvement of EMS in the prevention of injuries.

Over the past 45 years, American society has come to expect that EMS will be there when needed. EMS has progressed from the hearses of 60 years ago, which took acutely ill and injured individuals to the hospital between funeral runs, to today's high-tech EMS systems that employ the latest tools to save lives. As highly evolved as today's EMS systems may be, one crucial flaw in the paradigm of EMS delivery still exists: The primary function of an EMS system is reactive—responding after something has happened—rather than proactive—preventing the incident from happening at all. Many of today's EMS system leaders believe that the future of EMS will be as much proactive as it is reactive. The question that always comes to mind is: What injuries can be prevented? In this section we will examine the role that an EMS system can play in the injury prevention process.

EMS providers are the first members of the healthcare community to respond to most injuries and illnesses and are ideal individuals to lead injury prevention campaigns. Given the unique perspectives EMS providers possess on injuries, they are invaluable advocates, prevention program designers, and public educators capable of preventing injuries from occurring. In essence, their dedication to primary prevention positions EMS professionals as key leaders in community health, including to establish or improve relationships with other agencies and community organizations (EMSC, 1998).

To help reaffirm this commitment to primary prevention, in 1996 a group of EMS professionals and injury prevention experts developed the *Consensus Statement on the EMS Role in Primary Injury Prevention*. This document states:

> *Emergency medical services (EMS) organizations and individual providers must participate in primary injury prevention activities. This participation will benefit patients, communities, and the EMS system ... implementation of primary injury prevention activities is an effective way to reduce death, disabilities, and health care costs. EMS has an obligation to actively participate in primary injury prevention activities. (USDOT, 1996)*

Through developing this statement, the consensus committee identified key primary injury prevention activities for EMS system leaders, decision makers, and individual providers to carry out across the nation. The following recommendations can be used in developing injury prevention strategies.

Essential activities for EMS leaders and decision makers include:

- Protecting individual EMS providers from injury;
- Providing education to EMS providers in the fundamentals of primary injury prevention;
- Supporting and promoting the collection and utilization of injury data;
- Obtaining support and resources for primary injury prevention activities;
- Networking with other injury prevention organizations;
- Empowering individuals to conduct primary injury prevention activities in the local community;
- Interacting with the media to promote injury prevention; and
- Participating in injury prevention interventions in the community.

Essential injury prevention knowledge areas for individual EMS providers are:

- Principles of primary prevention;
- Personal injury prevention and role modeling;
- Safe emergency-vehicle operation;
- Injury risk identification;
- Documentation of injury data; and
- One-on-one safety education.

The *EMS Agenda for the Future* (NHTSA, 1996) identified 14 key areas in EMS that require further development, one of which is prevention. The agenda identifies prevention as a worthwhile investment that would provide significant reductions in mortality and morbidity. It recognizes that prevention activities are the responsibility of every member of the healthcare community. The agenda describes current status, goals, and direction on how to attain the goals.

The current status described is reflective of the shift in healthcare management paradigms. One of the key shifts that has taken place is the concept of improving health through prevention and wellness, thus reducing or even eliminating the occurrence of a medical condition. This is a significant change from the idea of waiting for an incident to occur, which would require high-tech, high-cost medical intervention. The ultimate goal is clear—"to prevent people from ever requiring costly medical care" (*EMS Agenda*, 1996, p. 39). Also identified in the current status is that injury is the third leading cause of death and disability in all age groups, accounting for more years of potential life lost than any other health problem.

Supporting evidence for highly effective public safety-driven prevention programs is also presented. Such evidence includes the fire service's efforts to affect the three E's related to fire safety, which has led to significant reductions in the numbers of fire-related injuries and deaths. An example of this is the "stop, drop, and roll" campaign for responding if one's clothing catches fire. Law enforcement agencies have also played a significant role in injury prevention. Through programs targeted at aggressive enforcement of impaired driving laws, significant reductions in traffic-related deaths and injuries secondary to impaired driving have been observed. EMS agencies themselves have proved their own ability to effectively reduce preventable injuries. Programs in New York to prevent falls from height, and drowning programs in Pinellas County, Florida, and Tucson, Arizona, have demonstrated that EMS can have an impact. Unified efforts are underway, although still early in development. An example of this is the Safe Communities concept, which involves a systematic approach to address all injuries and emphasizes the need for coordination among prevention, acute care, and rehabilitation efforts. EMS systems can provide crucial injury-related data pertinent to the study of injuries and to the design of risk-reduction strategies.

Ideally, the goals for injury prevention programs focus on EMS programs incorporating prevention into everyday practice. Ideally, EMS systems and providers should be continuously engaged in injury and illness prevention programs. Prevention programs should be developed based on system-specific needs, identifying injury and illness patterns prone to that service delivery area. Promotion of prevention-oriented environments throughout the EMS system (both internally within the system and externally in the community) is paramount. Continuing education will convey the prevention principles discussed in this chapter to all providers in the system, providing an understanding of how prevention activities as well as outreach activities relate to providers themselves.

Attaining these goals requires EMS systems to work with other community agencies as well as healthcare providers who possess expertise and interest in prevention activities (e.g., other public safety agencies, safety councils, public health departments). The purpose of a multiagency approach is to identify appropriate targets for prevention as well as to share the implementation of the programs. The agenda stresses the importance of EMS systems in identifying potential roles within partnerships to prevent injury and illness. Also included is EMS acting as an advocate for legislation geared toward injury and illness prevention. Prevention principles and their role in improving both individual and community health need to be incorporated into the core contents of EMS provider training programs. Lastly, EMS must continue to document the incidences of injury and illness along with specific circumstances, and convey this information to other entities and individuals.

Developing an Injury Prevention Program

As stated earlier, EMS can play a critical role in injury prevention. This does not mean, however, that EMS must develop and implement prevention programs; in fact, there are many existing agencies that can provide assistance in developing and implementing such programs. Several approaches to prevention programs already exist, such as injury prevention for children (EMSC, 1998). To create an injury prevention program in their community, EMS services can:

- Support an already developed activity;
- Provide leadership and advocacy for another agency's work; or
- Develop a new injury prevention program in collaboration with other agencies.

The most effective prevention strategies use a collaborative, systems-based approach that incorporates all allied health care disciplines and the appropriate agencies. See appendix C for a guide to developing or expanding an injury prevention effort.

Remember that every state has unique issues and resources, so carefully review all available information associated with injury and injury prevention in your state. This will be the most important action you will take.

WRAP UP

Summary

The exchange of information with the public is essential to the operation of any EMS system. Such exchange is not limited to the traditional form of newspaper articles on annual service events, but must encompass all means of communication. EMS systems use public education for both organizational and preventive aspects of EMS. Through a combination of public information, public education, and public relations (PIER), EMS systems extend their message and image to the community. Development of effective PIER programs involves planning, resources, and evaluation to reach the right people with the right message to bring about planned change.

How EMS systems conduct public education is changing with technology; to remain effective, they must adapt to this technology.

Traditionally, injury prevention has not been associated with EMS. However, as EMS expands its role and moves more in line with current focuses in health care, injury prevention becomes an important component for EMS. As a major source of trauma and death, injuries are in most cases preventable. By understanding the nature and cause of injury, EMS can use its unique position in the community to foster injury prevention, both for its constituents and for EMS providers.

Key Terms

agent

environment

epidemiological model

Haddon Matrix

host

injury

injury prevention and control

injury prevention interventions

intentional injuries

morbidity

mortality

primary injury prevention

public education

Public information, education,
   and relations (PIER)

public information

public information officer
   (PIO)

public relations

public service announcement
   (PSA)

secondary injury
   prevention

surveillance

tertiary injury prevention

Three E's of injury prevention

unintentional injuries

vector

violence

years of potential life lost
   (YPLL)

Review Questions

1. Define PIER.
2. List three examples of activities associated with each component of PIER.
3. List the general goals of any public education activity.
4. Discuss how a community CPR program can benefit an EMS system, the general public, and EMS providers.
5. Briefly describe a PSA related to EMS or public safety that you have seen in the media and local efforts.
6. Select a current communication technology and describe how it can be used to provide public education.

7. Cite examples of common causes of injury in the United States.
8. Diagram the relationship between the components of the injury event.
9. Cite at least five examples of intentional and unintentional injuries.
10. Discuss how the three E's of injury prevention can be used to reduce injuries.
11. Discuss the role of EMS in injury prevention.

Additional Resources

Bronstein, A. C., et al. (2009). 2008 Annual report of the American Association of Poison Control Center's national poison data system (NPDS): 26th annual report. *Clinical Toxicology. 47*, 911–1084.

Bicycle Helmet Safety Institute. (2010). http://www .helmets.org/mandator.htm. Accessed Jan. 6, 2010.

Campbell, J. E. (1998). *Basic trauma life support for paramedics and advanced EMS providers* (3rd ed.). Upper Saddle River, NJ: Prentice Hall.

Centers for Disease Control and Prevention, National Institute for Injury Prevention and Control. (2000). *Fact book 2000*. Washington, DC: U.S. Government Printing Office.

Centers for Disease Control and Prevention. (2008). http://www.cdc.gov/Homeand RecreationalSafety/Water-Safety/waterinjuries -factsheet.htm. Accessed Jan. 6, 2010.

Centers for Disease Control and Prevention. (2008). http://www.cdc.gov/NCIPC/factsheets /poisoning.htm. Accessed Jan. 6, 2010.

Centers for Disease Control and Prevention. (2009). http://www.cdc.gov/Homeand RecreationalSafety/falls/adultfalls.html. Accessed Jan. 6, 2010.

Corso, P., Finkelstein, E., Miller, T., Fiebelkorn, I., & Zaloshnja, E. (2006). Incidence and lifetime costs of injuries in the United States. *Injury Prevention*, 2006(12), 212–218.

Emergency Medical Services for Children Resource Center. (1998). *Preventing childhood emergencies: A guide to developing effective injury prevention initiatives* (2nd ed.). Washington, DC: Author.

Gibson, J. J. (1961). The contribution of experimental psychology to the formulation of the problem of safety: A brief for basic research. Reprinted from: *Behavioral approaches to accident research*. New York: New York Association for the Aid of Crippled Children.

Gordan, J. E. (1949). The epidemiology of accidents. *American Journal of Public Health*, 39, 504–515.

Haddon, W. (1963). A note concerning accident theory and research with special reference to motor vehicle accidents. *Annals of the New York Academy of Science*, 107, 635–646.

Judge, J. O., Lindsey, C., & Underwood, M. (1993). Balance improvements in older women: Effects of exercise training. *Physical Therapy*, 73, 254–265.

National Committee for Injury Prevention and Control. (1989). *Injury prevention: Meeting the challenge*. New York: Oxford University Press.

National Highway Traffic Safety Administration and Federal Emergency Management Agency. (1994). *EMS PIER manual: Public information, education and relations in emergency medical services (FA-151)*. Washington, DC: U. S. Government Printing Office.

National Highway Traffic Safety Administration. (1996). *EMS agenda for the future*. Washington, DC: Author.

National Highway Traffic Safety Administration. (2009). *Traffic safety facts 2008* (Early edition). Washington, DC: Author.

National Institute of Occupational Safety and Health. (1997). *Commercial fishing fatalities in Alaska: Risk factors and prevention strategies*. Washington, DC: U.S. Department of Health and Human Services.

National Research Council. (1985). *Injury in America: A continuing public health problem*. Washington, DC: National Academy Press.

Sacks, J. J., Kresnow, M., Houston, B., & Russell, J. (1996). Bicycle helmet use among American children, 1994. *Injury Prevention*, 2, 258–262.

Thompson, R. S., Rivara, F. R, & Thompson, D. C. (1989). A case-control study of the effectiveness of bicycle safety helmets. *New England Journal of Medicine*, 320, 1361–1367.

Tinetti, M. E., Speechley, M., & Ginter, S. F. (1988). *Risk factors for falls among elderly persons living in the community. New England Journal of Medicine*, 319, 1701–1707.

U.S. Department of Transportation. (1996). *Consensus statement on the EMS role in primary injury prevention*. Washington, DC: Author.

12

Emergency Medical Services and Disaster Response

Objectives

Upon completion of this chapter, the reader should be able to:

- State the importance of disaster planning for an EMS organization.

- Define disaster.

- Differentiate between types of disasters based on magnitude and cause.

- Identify disasters as either natural or technological.

- List four key phases of disaster management and define each.

- Describe a hazard analysis.

- State the role of EMS in disaster mitigation, disaster preparedness, disaster response, and disaster recovery.

- Define ICS and list the key components of ICS.

- Recognize the federal role in disasters.

Disasters

A **disaster** is any destructive, dangerous, or life-threatening situation that overwhelms the resources of a community. A disaster, sometimes in only a matter of minutes, places enormous strain on any emergency medical services (EMS) system. The September 11, 2011, terrorist attack on the Pentagon killed 125 people, and EMS transported more than 80 injured victims to Washington, D.C. metro hospitals. While there were some issues concerning coordination of the emergency response, victims received immediate medical evaluation, treatment, and emergency transport to hospitals. The more seriously wounded people remained in the building and awaited rescue. They were unable to help themselves because of the severity of their wounds or because they were trapped in the wreckage. The EMS system, in partnership with law enforcement and fire, had to respond quickly and efficiently or more lives could have been lost and injuries compounded. Procedures used in everyday, routine situations had to be drastically modified to aid the EMS system in accomplishing its primary mission.

Some EMS systems managers believe that their programs are too small in scope to accommodate disaster management. They take on the belief that "it will never happen here" and ignore the issue of preparing for a disaster or only give it cursory attention. They forget that some of the worst disasters in history occurred in small, isolated areas that had very limited resources. The Hinton railroad disaster occurred in a remote part of Alberta, Canada. Swiss Air flight 111 crashed in the Atlantic Ocean just off the coast from Peggy's Cove, a tiny community in Nova Scotia. Another tiny town called Barneveld, Wisconsin, was virtually wiped off the map when a tornado struck in 1984. The casualty count was 9 dead and 55 seriously wounded. Many others received minor wounds. Overall, the town sustained a 42% casualty rate! Natural disasters ranging from hurricanes to massive snow storms can hit anywhere and cause an EMS emergency in both small towns and large cities.

Every EMS system, regardless of its size, is vulnerable to a disaster. EMS systems that are equipped to respond to disaster situations, aided by well-developed disaster plans and well-trained staff who have practiced the procedures outlined in those plans, have been far more successful in responding to disasters than those systems that have not prepared. Understanding disasters, planning for them, and training and drilling in advance ultimately saves lives, limits disabilities, and hastens recovery of the victims of tragedies. Every community has the responsibility to actively participate in disaster planning and preparation. Every effort needs to be made to ensure that EMS plans are linked to those of fire, rescue, and law enforcement services. Disasters are everybody's business. This is especially so for EMS and other emergency services agencies.

The purpose of this chapter is to provide an introduction to disaster planning and disaster response for EMS students. This chapter does not provide comprehensive coverage of the disaster topic. Many other books have been written on disaster planning or response. Instead of attempting to be comprehensive, this chapter simply outlines the core concepts required for EMS systems' personnel to understand and appropriately respond to one of the greatest operational challenges an EMS system can face—the disaster.

What Is a Disaster?

Every day, EMS systems around the world handle many thousands of illnesses, accidents, and incidents that threaten life, cause destruction, and may even result in death. Yet, these are not considered "disasters." They are called "emergencies" and they require immediate attention to reduce the threat of life loss, to save property, or to maintain public health and ensure safety. They are not called disasters because it is within the capabilities of local resources to effectively manage these situations.

A disaster, on the other hand, overwhelms an organization's or a community's ability to manage the situation alone, with its own resources. A disaster is any situation that causes severe property damage, deaths, or multiple injuries and that is beyond the capabilities of local resources. From an emergency health services perspective, some of the local resources that may be overwhelmed or inadequate in size and scope are:

- Medical personnel and responders;
- Medical facilities;
- Emergency interoperable communications;
- Medical vehicles;
- Transportation resources;
- Medical supplies; and
- Fuel.

A large-scale disaster is one in which the local resources are overwhelmed and an effective response requires regional mutual aid and state-level resources, such as the National Guard or the state's environmental protection agency. A major disaster is any disaster, regardless of the cause, that, in the determination of the president of the United States, has caused damage of sufficient severity and magnitude to warrant major disaster assistance from the federal government to alleviate damage, loss, hardship, or suffering. A catastrophe is a disaster of extreme proportions and terribly overwhelming impact.

Some disasters produce no direct casualties. That is, there are no human deaths or wounded people as an immediate result of the disaster, though there may be horrific economic or environmental effects. Examples would be droughts that kill crops or oil spills that soil the environment and kill fish and other forms of wildlife. EMS systems would obviously have a limited or perhaps no role in such a disaster. The cleanup or restoration after such events, however, still requires state or federal resources that are beyond the capabilities of the local community and so such events are therefore still considered disasters.

Most EMS incidents involve a single patient. There are other incidents that produce various levels of human loss, and specific terms have been developed for those situations. An event with between 2 and 10 victims is called a **multiple patient incident**. A situation with between 11 and 100 direct victims is called a **multiple casualty incident**. Any disaster situation in which there are over 100 direct victims is called a **mass casualty incident**. Depending on the resources a community has, any of these levels can overwhelm local EMS resources and necessitate mutual aid assistance from other agencies. Additionally, an agency gets the opportunity to exercise its multiple patient and disaster plans at any level of incident. Plans should be scalable.

Natural Disasters

The word "disaster" comes from the ancient Latin language and meant "evil or sick star." The Romans and other ancient peoples believed that when someone saw a "falling" or "shooting" star in the sky, it was a sign that a horrible catastrophe was about to happen. Early astronomers were often soothsayers and prophets who predicted that the gods were sending catastrophes upon the Earth to express their displeasure with human beings or simply to show their power. The catastrophes were usually associated with some natural event, such as an earthquake, a volcanic eruption, or a terrible storm.

Today, we know that the movements of stars cannot accurately predict natural phenomena such as storms and earthquakes. The prediction of disasters is still quite inaccurate even with the most scientific equipment and procedures currently available. Emergency personnel, in particular, are mostly trained to react after an event has occurred. Knowledge of the natural phenomena that occur most commonly in one's area of operation, however, can help emergency personnel to meet the challenges presented by natural disasters.

A **natural disaster** is any disaster produced by the forces of nature—that is, those forces associated with earth, air, fire, and water. A list of natural disasters includes:

- Earthquakes;
- Thunderstorms;
- Lightning;
- Floods;
- Tornadoes;
- Hurricanes;
- Tsunamis;
- Freezes;
- Blizzards;
- Ice storms;
- Heat;
- Drought;
- Fire;
- Volcanoes;
- Windstorms;
- Dust storms;
- Avalanches; and
- Epidemics.

Technological Disasters

Technological disasters are the second major group of disaster situations. A technological disaster is any disaster produced by humans or by the things humans make or use. Examples of technological disasters include:

- Hazardous materials;
- Nuclear energy leaks;
- Utility failures;

- Pollution;
- Explosions;
- Transportation incidents;
- Fires;
- Civil disturbances and riots
- War;
- Acts of terrorism;
- Strikes and work slow downs;
- Massive demonstrations;
- Prison breaks and riots;
- Energy shortages;
- Material shortages;
- Embargoes;
- Nuclear attacks;
- Biological attacks;
- Chemical attacks; and
- Explosive device attacks.

There is an important reason for dividing types of disasters into natural and technological categories. Technological disasters, more often than natural disasters, have additional dangers associated with them, such as the presence of toxins or explosive conditions. Emergency personnel might be faced with violence, hostage situations, deliberately set secondary explosions, communicable diseases, or other dangerous conditions. When such potential dangers are present, the response of emergency personnel to a disaster must be modified and more carefully controlled to protect the emergency personnel. Rushing into volatile situations can be deadly to emergency operations personnel. At the very least, operations personnel can make a bad situation worse if they are not aware of the dangers. They need to be cautious when deployed to any disaster situation. Deployment to a technological disaster, however, requires a greater degree of caution because of the additional dangers to the operations personnel.

It is, of course, possible to have a combination of natural and technological disasters. An example would be an earthquake that causes a dam to burst. A flood may then result that, in turn, reaches a town and kills or injures the inhabitants. Or, that same earthquake might cause a chemical leak at a manufacturing plant. The chemical leak can then threaten lives in the plant and possibly even in the community. Hurricane Katrina in 2005 had an overwhelming combination of natural and technological disasters, including hurricane winds, flooding, levy ruptures, refinery fires, civil disturbances, animal infestations, and infectious diseases, just to name a few. It is important that responding personnel know the type of disaster they are responding to and its potential dangers. A full assessment of each disaster situation is essential before units are deployed and personnel are assigned to work within a disaster zone.

Disaster Management

A well-organized and efficient disaster management program is no accident. Communities and their EMS systems must sharpen their disaster management capabilities by planning and practice over a long period of time. It takes time, money, commitment, planning, education, coordination, practice, evaluation, and refinement to build an effective disaster management system.

The Federal Emergency Management Agency (FEMA) is the lead federal agency that is responsible for disaster management in the United States. Other federal agencies also play an important role, particularly in executing the emergency support functions (ESF). The U.S. Department of Health and Human Services (DHHS) has the lead role for ESF#8—Public Health and Medical Services, which includes EMS. **Table 12-1** outlines the entirety of federal responsibilities for the 15 ESFs.

FEMA has summarized the various aspects of disaster management into four key phases. When communities follow the federal guidelines for disaster management in those four phases, they can develop comprehensive and consistent programs that match up with other community disaster programs. Then, when one community has to call upon other communities for assistance, they are able to work together more efficiently because their plans and procedures are very similar. FEMA has identified four major phases for developing disaster programs:

1. **Mitigation**;
2. **Preparedness**;
3. **Response**; and
4. **Recovery**.

Mitigation

Mitigation refers to any efforts to identify, classify, and eliminate hazards and reduce their potential to produce a disaster. Mitigation also refers to efforts to reduce the damages encountered if a disaster cannot be prevented. Labeling hazardous materials and erecting fences and warning signs to keep people out of danger zones are just a few of the many methods to lessen the potential for a disaster to occur. A community is also mitigating the destructiveness of a potential danger when it prohibits people from building on earthquake fault lines or within flood plains.

EMS Role

EMS systems play significant roles in each of the four phases of disaster planning and management. EMS personnel need to be part of the mitigation phase because it would be more dangerous for them to be deployed into disaster situations when they do not know very much about the **hazards** they are likely to encounter. They should know the potential hazards in their areas. They should be able to see potentially dangerous environments marked on a community map. EMS personnel should join with fire service personnel to make building inspections or site visits. They need to know what is manufactured or stored, or what tasks are performed in specific areas and how dangerous the materials in a particular setting are.

Table 12-1 Emergency Support Functions

Emergency Support Function	Scope	Lead Agency
ESF#1—Transportation	Aviation Ground transportation	Department of Transportation
ESF#2—Communications	Coordination of telecom Restoration of infrastructure	Department of Homeland Security
ESF#3—Public Works and Engineering	Infrastructure protection Infrastructure restoration	Department of Defense
ESF#4—Firefighting	Coordination of federal firefighting activities (wild land)	Department of Agriculture
ESF#5—Emergency Management	Coordination of incident management and response	Department of Homeland Security FEMA
ESF#6—Mass Care, Emergency Assistance, Housing	Mass care, shelters, housing Human services	FEMA
ESF#7—Logistics and Resource Management	Logistics and resource support Contracting	Department of Homeland Security FEMA
EHS#8—Public Health and Medical Service	Public health Medical services and EMS	Department of Health and Human Services
EHS#9—Search and Rescue	Search and rescue Operations	FEMA
ESF#10—Oil and Hazardous Materials	HazMat response Environmental cleanup	Environmental Production Agency
ESF#11—Agriculture and Natural Resources	Nutritional assistance Food safety and security	Department of Agriculture
ESF#12—Energy	Energy infrastructure repair Energy industry coordination	Department of Energy
ESF#13—Public Safety and Security	Public safety and security support, security planning	Department of Justice
ESF#14—Long-Term Community Recovery	Long-term assistance to states and local governments	FEMA
ESF#15—External Affairs	Public information Media and community relations	Department of Homeland Security FEMA

Hazards

A hazard is a dangerous event or circumstance that can lead to an emergency or possibly even a disaster. Hazards are all around us in our daily lives. A driver's failure to stop at a red light is a hazard that endangers the driver as well as other people. Suppose a vehicle that failed to stop at a red light hits a truck carrying volatile chemicals. There is a massive explosion that flattens an entire city block and kills 62 people and injures over 100. Fires rage throughout the area and threaten other areas of town. Local emergency resources are inadequate to manage the situation without outside help. Other communities have to be called in to assist with the situation. That community would then be dealing with a mass casualty incident and a type of technological disaster.

Mitigation is the best method of dealing with hazards to prevent them from becoming emergencies or turning into disasters. It is important to identify hazards, locate them, and do whatever is possible to eliminate them entirely or to make them less dangerous.

If hazards cannot be eliminated or made less dangerous, then efforts need to be made to shield the community so that if the emergency or disaster occurs, it will do the least amount of damage. Mitigation is about lowering the risks associated with a hazard.

A **risk** is the degree of susceptibility of individuals or an entire community to the hazard becoming an emergency or a disaster that can lead to destruction, injury, or death. There are four important factors that create risk. They are:

1. Hazards;
2. Exposure;
3. Location; and
4. Vulnerability.

Hazards are the dangerous conditions that could generate an emergency or a disaster. Exposure refers to the lack of protection of a community from the hazard. Exposure refers to the hazard being unprotected from conditions such as weather that might cause the hazard to produce an emergency or a disaster. Location refers to the placement of a hazardous condition. The storage of explosives in a warehouse within a city is far more dangerous than the storage of the same materials in a remote area. Vulnerability is associated with the potential that a hazard could be attacked, stolen, impacted, or manipulated so as to become more dangerous and increase the chance that a disaster could occur. For example, not providing fences or other security devices around hazardous materials makes them more vulnerable to contact by people who do not know how to handle them or who might deliberately use those materials to harm others.

Hazard Analysis

Hazard analysis is the method by which hazards are identified, located, assessed for risks, and mapped on the community map. Maximum threat areas need to be identified and secondary hazards must also be identified. A hazard analysis has three segments. First, hazards are identified and listed. Second, information on the hazards is collected; this includes geographical as well as demographic information. Detailed information on the specific hazards must be carefully reviewed. This would include the types of hazards, the primary and secondary effects of each, the historical occurrences, the vulnerable populations, and the possible mitigation programs. Third, a report must be developed that clearly outlines the potential hazards, their exposures and locations, and their vulnerabilities to conditions that might cause a problem. Specific recommendations should advise community leaders and emergency personnel on how to limit the risks of having a disaster and what to do should a problem arise.

A well-executed hazard analysis can then be used to justify resource allocation. It can help to motivate the community to mitigate the hazards and prepare for a potential disaster. A hazard analysis sets the stage for the development of a disaster plan. A good hazard analysis can also serve as a platform for public education and information that might avert a tragedy.

EMS personnel should be on committees that evaluate hazards and threats to health and safety. There are **emergency planning committees** at the local and regional levels. Every possible effort should be made to rank the hazards from the most serious to the least serious. EMS expertise in emergency medical practices and procedures can be extremely helpful to the community disaster committee. Other emergency services groups, such as the fire department and law enforcement agencies, do not have the same level of expertise. EMS personnel should be active in making recommendations that mitigate the potential for an emergency or a disaster.

Preparedness

Preparedness has to do with resource identification and allocation as well as the training and drilling of disaster personnel. Planning, coordination, education, and practice are the mainstays of this particular area. FEMA runs intensive training courses for disaster management personnel, and has developed many planning documents since September 11 and Hurricane Katrina. The **National Response Framework (NRP)** and the **National Incident Management System (NIMS)** set out the goals of disaster preparedness and the organizational structure for disaster response, which details the different roles that federal, state, and local entities play and how they are coordinated. Part of NIMS is the **Incident Command System (ICS)**, which is the national guideline for emergency responder command and control at the incident level. Every emergency responder in the nation is expected to have taken the online introductory training that FEMA offers on the NRF, NIMS, and ICS. These documents help communities to develop disaster response plans. FEMA also pre-positions disaster response equipment. Every time a community runs a disaster drill, it is participating in a preparedness program.

EMS Role

The EMS role continues in disaster management by actively participating in the community's disaster planning process in the emergency planning committees. Additionally, EMS agencies must develop their agency-specific plans. Once the hazards in a community have been identified, evaluated, and labeled on a map, policies need to be established and plans need to be developed.

A policy is a statement from a government on a principle, an objective, or a procedure that is used to guide its activities to help to achieve its goals. For example, a city or county government might write a policy that states its emergency services organizations will work in a united and coordinated manner following the ICS guidelines to manage a disaster. This policy requires a unified command structure should a disaster occur in that community. Failure to work together without appropriate justification would violate the stated policy, and department or agency leaders could be reprimanded for their failure to cooperate with another agency during a disaster.

Some policies are set up in advance of a disaster to allow emergency personnel to immediately rescue and treat victims. Other policies must be established as the needs of particular situations arise. Usually, during a disaster, governmental leaders convene to monitor the situation. Once informed of changing circumstances in the field, they can review existing policies and make new ones if necessary to allow emergency personnel to do their work in and around the disaster site. For instance, routine policies may only allow 10 hours of overtime per week in a particular community. During a disaster, governmental officials might have to amend the routine policy and authorize additional overtime hours if such a waiver had never been written into the original policies.

Once policies have been written, then plans can be prepared. Emergency planning committees must plan for command and control functions, communications, utilization of special resources, and involvement of resources outside of the community-mutual aid. Plans should:

- Be based on the FRP, NIMS, and ICS;
- Prepare for evacuation of some or all of the population;
- Designate staff and supply for shelters;
- Coordinate with voluntary disaster intervention groups;
- Gain access to specialized emergency equipment;
- Modify procedures in the event of terrorism;
- Provide for the safety and security of response personnel;
- Establish perimeter control;
- Determine how to establish response priorities;
- Designate who will and how to provide the EMS functions of **triage**, **treatment in the field**, and **transportation**;
- Provide for public information needs and media relations;
- Arrange for debris removal;
- Activate prearranged **mutual aid** from neighboring, regional, and state resources;
- Manage the influx of volunteers; and
- Provide for security and other law enforcement issues.

Plans should be brief. It has been found that plans longer than seven pages are almost never read and are rarely used in an actual disaster. Plans are only guidelines; actual situations may demand alterations to the plan under field conditions. Plans, therefore, need to be flexible and scalable to the size of the incident. Plans that are not practiced before disasters occur often fail to work well when needed and thus prove to be useless.

Preparedness goes well beyond policy and plan development. Preparedness also includes education, training, and practice. The organizations that have been the most successful in managing disasters are those that have spent a great deal of time educating and training their personnel and drilling them in the steps to take in an actual disaster. It is also important to train field officers on how to be innovative and improvise when plans become unworkable under field conditions or when communications with upper-level command fails. This is why training in the ICS is so important for every responder.

Planning, education, training, preparation, practice, and refinement of procedures pay off in the long run. Lives are saved, injury rates are lessened, and damages are limited. EMS systems cannot afford to be excluded from the preparedness functions in disaster management. No one can be expected to perform well in a situation for which they have not prepared.

Response

The response phase of disaster activity addresses the immediate and short-term effects of a disaster. Any actions that are required to save lives, limit destruction, and meet basic human needs fall under the response phase. Mobilizing the American Red Cross, the state's militia, or the National Guard is an example of an activity in the response phase of a disaster. In some cases, emergency personnel, such as firefighters, paramedics, and police officers, need to be brought from other states to a disaster area to supplement the resources in the local community. The **Emergency Management Assistance Compact** is a federally enabled system that all states have signed on to that allows states to send mutual aid in the form of personnel and resources to disaster-stricken states. This is routinely utilized, especially for hurricanes, such as Katrina in 2005 and Gustav in 2008. Sometimes satellite communication systems must be set up because the communication system of a community has been destroyed. All of these activities and many more occur in the response phase of a disaster.

EMS Role

All the mitigation and preparedness activities should make the actual response to a disaster run more efficiently and effectively. Disaster research indicates the three important elements of disaster management that fail most frequently in an actual disaster—command, communications, and interagency cooperation. Proper planning and practice for disaster operations helps to avoid these three main failure points when the EMS system is called upon to respond to a disaster.

EMS units are usually among the first operations units on the scene of a major incident. In some instances, they are the only units on the scene for several minutes before other help arrives. Before getting directly involved in patient care, first-arriving units must take numerous steps to ensure that the situation is properly managed and to avoid any chaos and confusion that could quickly worsen the situation. EMS units that arrive on the scene first must:

- Access the situation;
- Assess the situation;
- Determine the magnitude of the incident;
- Determine if there are additional dangers to themselves or to other responding personnel;
- Assume temporary command;
- Establish communications;

- Declare that an incident is in progress;
- Call for assistance;
- Inform the communications center of the situation, its magnitude, and identifiable dangers;
- Request specific resources for deployment to the site;
- Establish a temporary command post;
- Establish a perimeter;
- Choose a staging area;
- Select a triage–treatment area;
- Prioritize rescue and life-saving functions;
- Communicate with incoming units;
- Assign incoming units to specific functions until higher-level command personnel arrive and assume command;
- Ensure that initial operations are as safe as possible; and
- After an initial report, transfer command functions to appropriate command personnel upon their arrival and then turn attention to access, triage, treatment, transportation, logistics, or other functions as required.

It is very hard for trained EMS people, who arrive first at a disaster site, to take the steps outlined earlier and not become directly involved in triage, treatment, and transport functions. Jumping into the triage and treatment aspects of a disaster may feel right at the time, but it is the wrong thing to do first. It will only add to the chaos and confusion of a disaster, because incoming units will have to assume the neglected functions. Ultimately, jumping right into action delays the organization of the disaster situation and the care for all the victims and also endangers responders to the site.

Incident Command System

The EMS response to a disaster needs to be organized in accordance with the guidelines of the ICS (**Figure 12-1**), which outlines an organized method of managing a large-scale incident such as a search for a missing child, a major wildfire, or a disaster. It was developed in California in 1972 after a series of large, uncontrolled fires destroyed vast areas of forest, homes, businesses, and other structures and killed numerous people and countless numbers of animals. At the time of those fires, thousands of firefighters worked independently of one another in separate departments in a totally uncoordinated manner. There was no unified command structure, no standardized procedures or equipment, no interagency communications, no common terminology, and no standardized training. The losses encountered in those fires motivated emergency organizations to formulate an integrated and coordinated system to manage large fires and other major incidents. The ICS has regularly been formulated, tested, refined, and retested since 1972. Today, it has become a standard operating procedure in most emergency services organizations and part of the NIMS. Communities throughout the world are using the system. Lives have been saved, injuries have been lessened, and destruction has been mitigated by

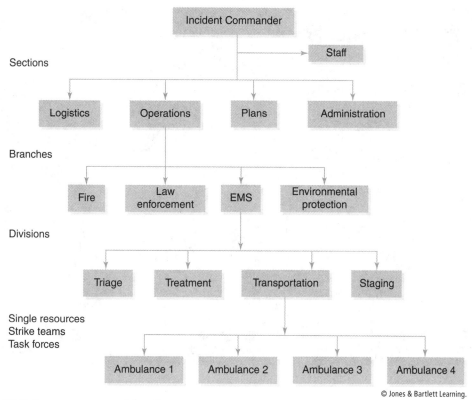

© Jones & Bartlett Learning.

Figure 12-1 Emergency support functions.

the coordinated and standardized procedures of the ICS. Without the ICS, disaster management today would be chaotic, inefficient, and ineffective (**Figure 12-2**).

The ICS was designed to address the eight primary components of a good emergency management system. They are:

1. Common terminology;
2. Modular organization;
3. Integrated communications;
4. A unified command structure;
5. Consolidated action plans;
6. Manageable span of control;
7. Designated incident facilities; and
8. Comprehensive resource management.

The ICS is a management tool characterized by a unified command structure in which the leaders of all of the agencies participating in a disaster come together under one key leader. They develop

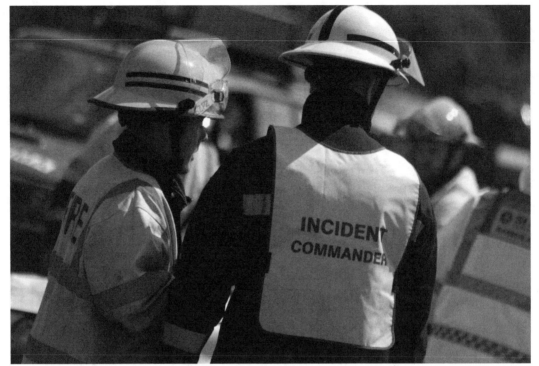

© Aled Llywelyn/Alamy.

Figure 12-2 Without the ICS, disaster management today would be chaotic, inefficient, and ineffective.

a strategic plan and then follow the primary leader, who orchestrates the overall response strategy. The word "strategy" means the big plan of the disaster. A strategy is directed toward a large goal. For example, a strategy in a typical disaster is to extinguish the fire, control the situation, and rescue the wounded without causing additional deaths or injuries. To carry out the strategy, a number of smaller tasks must be achieved by a series of steps or specific procedures. These steps or procedures are called tactics. In other words, tactics are the steps that need to be taken to increase the likelihood that the overall strategy can be accomplished.

The ICS uses commonly accepted and standardized terminology, procedures, training, communications, and equipment to perform the tactics and accomplish the strategy. One key characteristic of ICS is the use of sections (modular structure). A section (sometimes called a sector) is an area of responsibility. Examples of sections would be operations, logistics, command, administration, and plans. Section leaders have the responsibility to help develop the overall strategy and to manage the major areas of responsibility at the disaster.

The ICS utilizes a concept of manageable span of control. This means that a command officer has the responsibility for only between three and seven people. This helps to avoid overwhelming the commanders with too much input from too many people or with too much responsibility for too many people. The incident commander (IC), the person in charge of all the personnel working at a disaster, only receives information and feedback from five or six key commanders in charge of sections.

The personnel who are in charge of sections receive input from and have the responsibility for a limited number of commanders under their area of responsibility. The person in charge of all EMS-related activities, for instance, would be considered a "branch" officer. That person would report to the operations officer (a section officer). So would the individuals in charge of law enforcement activities, fire, and communications. Each of them would be a branch. All of them would report to the operations section officer.

The branch officer in charge of all EMS-related activities would then have five or six people who would provide input and feedback. These people would be called division officers. The division officers for triage, treatment, and transportation would report to the person in charge of the EMS branch. Similar arrangements exist for law enforcement and other main areas of responsibility. Division officers develop the actual tactics in a disaster. They usually direct single resources, task forces, or strike teams that carry out the specific tactics assigned to them.

In summary, the typical response of an EMS system in a disaster might follow the description in the following paragraphs. EMS units would be deployed to the scene. The first arriving unit would access the situation, assess it, communicate with its dispatch center, and advise them of the nature of the incident and request a multiagency disaster response. The first-arriving unit would assume temporary command until higher-ranking personnel arrived on the scene. Staging areas would then be chosen and a temporary command post would be established. Other responding units would be directed to assume certain tasks or to report to specific areas to begin their work. Early tasks would include the establishment of a perimeter and a patient collection and triage area. As soon as additional EMS personnel arrived, they would be assigned to triage, treatment, and transportation functions—but only if scene security and safety could be ensured. If not, personnel and equipment would be staged until specialized resources could secure the scene and ensure the safety of the response personnel.

Once higher-ranking personnel arrived, they would be briefed on the incident and command would be transferred to them. The ICS system would then be established and arriving EMS units would be assigned as required by the situation. The highest-ranking EMS officer (branch officer) would report to the operations chief and ensure cooperation and communication with the other branch officers. Division commanders in the EMS field would most likely include the personnel in charge of medical staging, supplies, triage, treatment, transportation, and communications with the hospitals. Each of those command personnel would have under their control individual resources, strike forces, or task forces to carry out the tactics. Individual resources mean one unit, such as one ambulance, one fire engine, or one police car. A strike force means a combination of same-type single resources, ideally five personnel assigned to a specific function under the leadership of a supervisor. For example, five advanced life support (ALS) ambulances might be assigned to serve one function of the overall operation. A task force is a combination of unlike resources that are assigned to deal with one problem in a disaster.

EMS field operations would continue in a disaster as long as the need for EMS resources remains. If a disaster is prolonged, the number of EMS units assigned to the scene may be downgraded once most of the wounded have been removed from the scene. In many cases of a prolonged search after a disaster, some EMS units are held at the scene in case another survivor is located. The EMS personnel are also held near the scene in case one of the other operations personnel is injured during the operation.

Figure 12-1 illustrates a typical incident command structure. It focuses on EMS aspects of incident command. Note carefully the primary segments of the ICS, with its sections, branches, divisions, and resource leaders.

Recovery

Recovery includes any activities designed to put the community back on its feet—a return to normalcy. During the recovery period, victims' needs are assessed, cost estimates are established, and resources are coordinated and deployed for the long-term care of victims. The recovery period is also a time when lessons from the disaster can be learned and a new and improved disaster plan can then be drawn up, practiced, and refined for the mitigation and preparedness phases. Debris removal, loans to small businesses, and the reconstruction of highways and bridges are all recovery activities. So are activities such as post-disaster counseling and temporary housing for people who have lost their homes.

EMS Role

Once the disaster has moved to the recovery phase, EMS systems may be requested to provide the community with medical education or information that might assist in the community's recovery. In situations in which the normal medical system has been badly disrupted, EMS systems may be asked to make field visits to assess medical needs or to provide limited medical care. These services are most needed by children and the elderly, especially those living in poverty. There may be the need to provide medical services to shelters and temporary housing as well. There have been a few instances in which EMS systems were requested to temporarily supplement nursing staff in hospitals after nurses were killed or injured during the disaster and insufficient staff members were available to keep the hospital running.

It is also common for other EMS systems to assist by providing direct EMS response services when the initial EMS system has encountered a severe loss, such as a line-of-duty death or such severe disaster effects that the personnel are directly affected. A flood situation would be one in which personnel may need to attend to personal family issues before they can return to normal work shifts. Relief from other EMS agencies is greatly needed during the recovery phase of a disaster. It is also during the recovery phase that EMS systems can review their procedures, write after-action reports, and decide what alterations to the disaster plan should be addressed in the mitigation and preparedness phases of disaster management.

It is important for EMS agencies to address the powerful psychological impact a disaster can have on their own personnel. A comprehensive, systematic, and multicomponent approach to psychological support for personnel should be in place for normal operations. This is even more necessary in the aftermath of a disaster. Support programs for emergency personnel are called **critical incident stress management** (CISM) programs. The research in the CISM field strongly indicates that people who are able to discuss their experiences in a disaster or other distressing events recover faster and return to normal work functions with less disruption than people who tend to hold distressing events within their minds without the benefit of talking to others. When properly organized, CISM programs provide education and planning services before a disaster strikes. They also provide on-scene support services while an incident is ongoing. After a disaster has concluded, a wide range of support services are provided to assist personnel in recovering from the emotional effects of the incident. Most personnel who receive the proper support are able to return to normal work. Support services should include, but are not limited to, the following:

- Stress education;
- On-scene support services;
- Demobilizations and group informational briefings;
- Defusing;
- Critical incident stress debriefings (CISD);
- Individual support services;
- Family support; and
- Follow-up services and referrals.

Mass Events

The EMS role in mass gatherings can be considered a special application of EMS disaster response. The four stages of disaster management apply, and ICS is the command and control methodology. These events range from events at large sports arenas, to festivals, to demonstrations or other gatherings. There is the preparation for and management of medical emergencies as they would occur in any population. There is also the mitigation, planning, and responding to events that are not part of the event but that could endanger the people at the event, such as a stage collapse, crowd stampede, or terrorist attack. Some events are planned for at a national level, such as the Super Bowl, presidential nominating conventions, and inaugurations, in which months of planning at the local, state, and federal levels culminates in a massive and coordinated operation that includes EMS assets.

Federal Role in Disasters

Most disaster management actions are the responsibility of local and state jurisdictions. The federal government's role is relatively small in situations that have not been declared disasters by the president. It does, however, provide disaster management strategic guidance and education and training to local and state disaster managers and emergency services personnel. It also provides additional assistance with hazard assessment and mitigation to most communities on a regular basis. In addition, the federal government provides other types of services in disaster mitigation, response, and recovery. The Army Corps of Engineers conducts an extensive flood control program in the United States. The Centers for

Disease Control and Prevention monitors and aggressively responds to communicable diseases that threaten the overall health of the nation.

Even without a **presidential declaration** of a major disaster, the federal government provides assistance to local communities for search and rescue operations. The National Park Service has assisted communities in large-scale search operations. The U.S. Air Force coordinates land-based aerial search and rescue support, and the U.S. Coast Guard takes responsibility for search and rescue operations on the seas, rivers, bays, and tributaries of U.S. waters. In major wildfires, the Bureau of Land Management and the U.S. Forest Service provide fire-suppression assistance.

There are many other ways in which the federal government provides direct and indirect support in local disasters that do not receive a presidential declaration. But, the magnitude and the sources of assistance are significantly increased once a presidential declaration is made.

Presidential Declaration of a Disaster

The federal government provides assistance in disasters in accordance with the Robert T. Stafford Disaster Relief and Emergency Assistance Act. Periodically, the act is amended by Congress to better meet the needs of disaster victims. Formal declarations of federal disasters are provided only in major disasters.

To begin the process of requesting a federally declared or presidential disaster, the local and state resources must be overwhelmed. Only a governor of a state or an acting governor can request a presidential declaration in a disaster situation. The governor contacts the regional office of FEMA. Local, state, and FEMA representatives survey the affected area. Disaster specialists determine the extent of the private and public damage and estimate the extent of federal disaster assistance that will be required. Further consultations with the FEMA regional office to determine eligibility for federal disaster assistance are conducted. FEMA officials are then notified that the governor intends to request federal aid.

The governor's staff prepare the formal request and indicate clearly in the document that an effective response is beyond the capabilities of the state, and that the state's resources have already been deployed and are overwhelmed. The governor's office must certify that the state will assume any costs not covered under the federal disaster assistance laws. Detailed estimates of the types and amount of federal assistance must be included in the document. The governor signs the request, which is then forwarded to the FEMA regional office. The regional office evaluates the request and makes recommendations to the administrator of FEMA. The administrator makes the final recommendations to the president. The president reviews the documents and decides whether a formal declaration will be signed. The governor's office is notified if the declaration is approved and then Congress and the participating federal agencies are notified. FEMA appoints a coordinating officer and develops and forwards to the governor's office lists of the types of assistance. Available resources are then matched with the types of assistance required. From that point on, the resources of the federal government are brought together to assist the community in managing and recovering from the disaster. Few disasters are predictable, but hurricanes are a most notable exception. In the case of hurricanes, governors expecting their states to be hit can request a presidential declaration in advance of landfall. If the declaration is implemented, personnel and materials can be pre-positioned and residents can be evacuated.

Federal Role and EMS

There are several federal departments that impact EMS agency disaster response. Besides the guidance that FEMA provides through the NRF, NIMS, and related training, the Department of Homeland Security (DHS), of which FEMA is a part, has other programs that affect EMS. There is the Office of Health Affairs (OHA) and the chief medical officer in DHS, who has a focus on medical first responder coordination and safety. The DHS has major initiatives in the area of developing nationwide interoperable emergency communications and administers grant monies to states and localities for that purpose. Finally, DHS administers grant programs for disaster preparedness, awarded to states to support equipping, training, and exercising first responders. Unfortunately, over the first five years of the program, only four percent of the dollars went to EMS agencies.

The Office of the Assistant Secretary of Preparedness and Response (ASPR), part of DHHS, would manage the ESF#8—Public Health and Medical Function in the event of a disaster. ASPR also has the responsibility for the National Disaster Medical System, which is a federal asset deployed to disasters that include Disaster Medical Assistance Teams (DMAT). Local EMS personnel are often part of the staff of these teams (**Figure 12-3**).

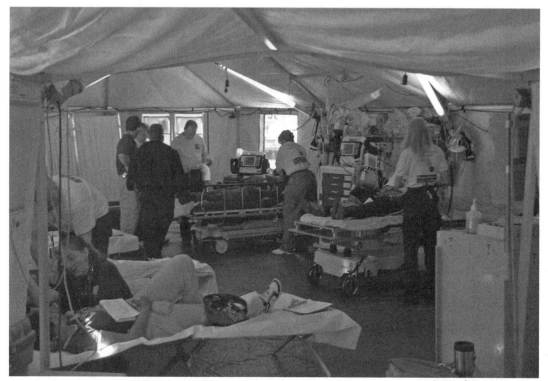

Courtesy of Marvin Nauman/FEMA.

Figure 12-3 Local EMS personnel are often a part of the staff of DMAT.

The National Highway Traffic Safety Administration (NHTSA) Office of EMS developed the Pandemic Influenza Guidelines for Statewide Adoption, released in 2007, and is engaged with states to assess the status of preparedness. The NHTSA EMS also conducts state EMS assessments, which includes disaster preparedness components. In 2009, the NHTSA, CDC, DHHS-ASPR, and DHS-OHA collaborated to issue guidance to EMS providers related to the H1N1 pandemic influenza.

WRAP UP

Summary

Disasters are the most significant operational challenge for EMS systems. Although somewhat rare in most communities, they are so demanding that EMS agencies and other emergency response organizations must spend a considerable amount of time preparing for them. A lack of preparation leaves a community vulnerable to a disorganized response that can be costly in terms of lives lost, injuries intensified, and destruction to the community. The energy and expense put forward now to prepare for a disaster will pay great dividends in an efficient and effective response once one is necessary.

A community does not have to wait for a big disaster, however, in order to reap some benefit from disaster preparations. Immediate benefits are available. They include better working relationships between the various emergency response organizations. They also include enhanced leadership and decision-making for more routine events. Practice for the major event enhances performance on the everyday emergencies. Up-to-date resource lists are frequently useful in unusual or complicated emergency responses that are clearly not disasters. If EMS organizations can see that disaster preparations make their communities safer and their emergency services more efficient, they will be more willing to expend the resources that are necessary to make a real difference once a disaster strikes in their jurisdiction.

All four phases are essential in disaster management and all four depend on one another to ensure a comprehensive, coordinated, and systematic approach to handling the extraordinary demands of a community-wide crisis event. Disaster management programs start off with mitigation and preparedness and then move on to response and recovery. After recovery, a community reviews its performance during the disaster and attempts to draw whatever lessons it can from the experience. The community can then utilize what it has learned to further mitigate the potential for future problems and to prepare for the next potential disaster. The mitigation–preparedness–response–recovery cycle continues indefinitely in a community. Improvements can always be made to a community's disaster program. Furthermore, to properly manage a disaster, local, state, federal, and private organizations must be willing to work together for the common good in each of the four phases. A great deal of effort must be put into gaining cooperation of the various segments of a community and into coordinating their efforts should a disaster occur. Continuous programs for the prevention of disasters or for community preparation for disaster management is a challenging and time-consuming process that demands interagency cooperation and leadership. EMS systems should not only be a cooperating entity in disaster programs, they should also play an active leadership role.

Key Terms

critical incident stress
  management (CISM)
disaster
Emergency Management
  Assistance Compact
emergency planning
  committees
hazards
hazard analysis
Incident Command System (ICS)

mass casualty incident
mitigation
multiple casualty incident
multiple patient incident
mutual aid
National Incident Management
  System (NIMS)
National Response
  Framework (NRF)
natural disaster

preparedness
presidential
  declaration
recovery
response
risk
technological disasters
transportation
treatment in the field
triage

Review Questions

1. Define disaster.
2. List three examples each of natural and technological disasters.
3. Discuss the relationship of the four key phases of disaster management.
4. Compare and contrast hazard assessment and hazard analysis.
5. Using a bulleted list, state the key points associated with EMS involvement in all phases of a disaster.

6. Diagram the ICS structure for a natural disaster involving a flood in your local area.
7. Describe the procedure to obtain federal assistance in a disaster.
8. Discuss the federal departments that have a role impacting EMS related to disasters.

Additional Resources

Auf der Heide, E. (1989). *Disaster response: Principles of preparation and coordination.* St. Louis, MO: C.V. Mosby Company.

Comfort, L. K. (1988). *Managing disaster: Strategies and policy perspectives.* Durham, NC: Duke University Press.

FEMA Staff, Emergency Management Institute. (1986). *Emergency management USA.* Washington, DC: U.S. Government Printing Office.

FEMA Staff, Emergency Management Institute. (1990). *Integrated emergency management course: Hazardous Materials.* Washington, DC: U.S. Government Printing Office.

FEMA Staff, Emergency Management Institute. (1994a). *Federal response plan for public law 93-288, as amended.* Washington, DC: U.S. Government Printing Office.

FEMA Staff, Emergency Management Institute (1994b). *Integrated emergency management course: All hazards.* Washington, DC: U.S. Government Printing Office.

FEMA Staff, Emergency Management Institute. (1995a). *ICS/EOC interface workshop: Participant handbook.* Washington, DC: U.S. Government Printing Office.

FEMA Staff, Emergency Management Institute. (1995b). *Consequences of terrorism: Integrated emergency management course: Student manual.* Washington, DC: U.S. Government Printing Office.

Grant, H. D., et al., & Rescue Training Associates, Ltd. (1985). *Action guide for emergency service personnel.* Bowie, MD: Brady Communications Company, Inc.

Hildebrand, M. S., & Noll, G. G. (1999). *Propane emergencies.* Washington, DC: Propane Education and Research Council.

Mitchell, J. T., & Everly, G. S. (1996). *Critical incident stress debriefing (CISD): An operations manual for the prevention of traumatic stress among emergency services and disaster workers.* Ellicott City, MD: Chevron Publishing.

Ursano, R. J., McCaughey, B. G., & Fullerton, C. S. (Eds.). (1994). *Individual and community responses to trauma and disaster: The structure of human chaos.* Cambridge, UK: Cambridge University Press.

Information Systems and Evaluation

Objectives

Upon completion of this chapter, the reader should be able to:

- State the importance of information in EMS.

- Recognize the role of a strategic information plan in EMS system management.

- List barriers to information system integration.

- Differentiate between data and information.

- List the three general types of data collected in EMS.

- Discuss the various EMS data collection tools.

- State the role of analysis in producing useful EMS system information.

- Relate quality, cost, and value to system performance.

- Define a high-performance EMS system using the series of equations presented in this chapter.

- Identify the role of planning in quality management.

- Defend the need for key performance indicators in process measurement.

- State the needs of a data system to support measurement of key performance indicators.

- Describe process assurance.

- Describe process improvement.

Information Systems

Contemporary emergency medical services (EMS) systems have access to large volumes of data from many different sources, such as 9-1-1 systems, patient care records (PCRs), computerized dispatch systems, global positioning systems (GPS), physiological monitoring devices, and billing systems. The challenge for senior managers of EMS systems is to take the raw **data**, append intelligence to it, and transform it into **information** that can be used to manage and improve the system. Data is just records of events in time. Alone, it is useless. But when data is placed in a framework or context, it acquires meaning and becomes information. Senior managers of EMS systems play a crucial role in transforming data into information and using information by:

- Creating and fostering an organizational culture that makes decisions based on facts instead of opinions;
- Analyzing information in light of population-based health initiatives, including hospital outcomes;
- Encouraging the sharing of information; and
- Establishing a clear information strategy.

This chapter covers some of the issues to consider when developing and maintaining an information system for a contemporary EMS organization.

Strategic Information Planning

Developing a sound information strategy begins with a clear mission and vision that states why the organization exists and what the organization wants to become. Overall strategic planning is used to decide how the organization is going to get there. A **strategic information plan** is a plan of the information needs of an organization so that it can meet its mission and vision by answering the following questions:

- How will it develop the needed information system capabilities to support the overall organizational strategy and goals? What types of hardware, software, and staff are needed to collect the data and transform it into information that will be useful to the organization? This is an important step and is more than just buying a computer and a commercial software package. It involves determining the information needs of the entire organization and then working backward to determine what hardware and software can provide this information. A common mistake made by organizations is to purchase hardware and software and then try to "fit" the organization's needs into the information provided by the system.
- How will it provide the people employed by the organization with the skills and tools they need to support the organization's information strategy? Data and information are only as good as the data captured by an information system. If the end users are not trained and motivated to properly collect data, the system will be inaccurate at best and most likely useless. It is important that organizations plan for training personnel to use the information system, as well as how to use the information the system provides. Training must include both initial competency and familiarization followed by ongoing quality assurance. By valuing the purpose of an information system, users are more inclined to input correct information and use the system in a positive way.

- How will the organization monitor its progress toward implementation of its information strategy? Planning alone does not equal success. Evaluation is an integral part of the implementation process. Therefore, it is necessary during the planning process to identify milestones or critical events that will provide an indication of implementation status. For example, a milestone might be completion of the initial phase of training for field personnel in data entry using a palm computer.

- How will the effectiveness of an organization's information strategy be measured? In the early days of computing, the saying "garbage in, garbage out" was commonly used to stress the importance of entering proper data into a computer. A computer is not capable of improving the data entered into it—it can only manipulate it in accordance with the user's wishes. Therefore, it is important for an organization to have a strategy for determining if the strategic information plan is working. This can be assessed by reviewing how information is used by the organization to increase efficiency and make better decisions. Whatever evaluation system is used, it must be shared at all levels to show the effectiveness of the system and the importance to the company, the provider, and patients.

- What regulations must the system meet? With the wide acceptance of information systems in EMS, organizations must now conform to local, state, and federal regulations. HIPAA regulations clearly require data encryption and safety measures that must be provided throughout the system (www. cms.hhs.gov/SecurityStandard/). Since the adoption of the **National EMS Information System (NEMSIS)**, many states (such as Connecticut) have required that all providers use **Electronic Patient Care Records (ePCRs)** on all calls.

- How will the system integrate within the overall healthcare system? With hospital systems now allowing data integration, organizations must consider more than their own needs and requirements. The information system should be able to both transmit and receive data from local hospitals to ensure continuity of care.

One of the most significant influences on EMS information strategy has been the explosion of Internet-based services and technologies. Wireless access is now built into most phones, and vehicles may have their own Wi-Fi systems. High-speed data connections, both hardwired and those through Wi-Fi or cellular networks, are making it economical to assemble and maintain the infrastructure components for a robust information system. EMS managers need to think through the implications and possibilities of having hospitals, suppliers, institutional customers, and the entire workforce equipped with Internet-connected devices.

Information System Integration

An EMS system is one component of a community's overall healthcare system. The various components of these healthcare systems are becoming increasingly reliant upon information systems to guide decisions and extract greater efficiencies and efficacy from healthcare processes. Most of these gains in efficiency and efficacy are found by looking at health care from a systems perspective rather than just looking at individual service components. Consequently, this is creating a growing demand for integration of information from all components of the healthcare system, including EMS, in order to reap those rewards (**Figure 13-1**).

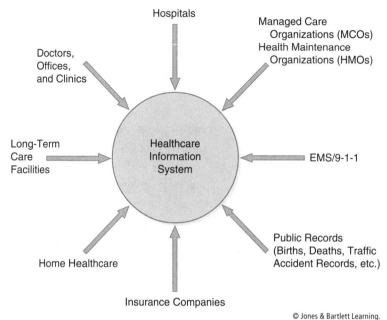

© Jones & Bartlett Learning.

Figure 13-1 Integration of EMS system data.

Contrary to these incentives for integration, EMS faces significant social, political, legal, and technical barriers. Of these, the social and political barriers can be the most formidable. There are often very strong competitive factors wedging themselves between entities in healthcare systems. Legal barriers to integration stem from issues of privacy and confidentiality. Technical barriers come from both software and hardware compatibility issues. In the long run, the incentives and quality improvement efforts are more than likely to prevail against the barriers, but it will be a struggle that EMS should be prepared for. The speed at which the integration occurs will likely be directly related to the magnitude of the mutual economic incentives to do so.

Information System Design Considerations

EMS systems must consider the wide variety of information needs in the organizations they interact with. These needs must be kept in mind when developing specifications or making actual selections of hardware and software components for information systems. EMS must work through the issues in facilitating data exchange with:

- *Other internal functions.* For example, if EMS is part of a larger organization, how would a central billing office integrate payment from a third-party payer if all other organizational functions are direct billed?
- *Institutional customers and other types of customers.* Institutions such as hospitals and nursing facilities may be able to link to an organization's electronic data records.

- *Billing systems.* Nearly all third-party payers have a mechanism to electronically receive billing information as well as to provide claim-processing data to the claimant.

- *Regulatory agencies.* Agencies such as the Centers for Medicare and Medicaid Services require regular reporting, which can be done electronically and can also be incorporated into report-generating software.

- *NEMSIS.* The National EMS Information System (NEMSIS) was developed to help track and identify nationwide trends, and data must comply with NEMSIS standards.

- *Other entities involved in patient care to maintain clinical continuity.* This is an especially important requirement and one that continues to plague healthcare information systems. In most cases, there is no universal identifier to link a prehospital patient care report with hospital medical records and rehabilitation facility records.

- *Quality management activities.* To ensure quality care, it is necessary to review reports and information for correctness and proper patient care. Software is available that can review data for accuracy and completeness and provide exception reports that identify questionable reports and inconsistent information.

- *Research activities.* These activities depend heavily on data. The ability to exchange raw field data with statistical software packages will greatly facilitate research.

- *Patients.* Some systems have now even allowed real-time access to both billing and medical records for patients. Providing patients access may cause a variety of issues in all areas of system design.

The information system will need hardware and software components for data input, transfer, encrypted storage, analysis, and output. The overall information system design should also consider costs for daily operation, maintenance, repair, and upgrades. Upgrade costs are a particularly important consideration in the face of rapidly changing information technologies.

Often overlooked in information system design are the challenges and costs associated with initial, advanced, and refresher training for the organization's staff. Ideally, some general concepts on the needs and benefits of information systems are covered in the EMS curricula used for training clinical staff. At some point in the evolution of information system utilization in an EMS organization, some level of computer literacy may be appropriate to consider as a requirement for employment. More specific training on the hardware and commonly used software applications might be included in the new-employee-orientation process. Continuing education might include in-depth software and data-entry training.

Changes in society have made computer use a commonplace event within some populations. The digital divide between "digital natives" (those who grew up with computers) and "digital immigrants" (those who learned computers later in life) still exists, but it is getting smaller. Generational changes, including wide acceptance of computers and smartphones, mean that incoming staff may be more aware of the use of information systems and thus may only need their skills retooled for an EMS information system. Before starting any initial information systems training, an EMS system may be better served by surveying the current level of competence and possibly creating different training programs to address providers' differing skills and abilities.

Data analysis and reporting is one of the last steps in most information system processes, but it should be one of the very first steps in designing an information system. The ability to do analyses and reports is the main reason that organizations have information systems in the first place. If the mission and vision for the organization are known, a strategy can be developed to achieve these goals. With a chosen strategy, the information needed to build, implement, and manage information can be identified. That information is typically in the form of reports that are used by managers and staff to manage, support, operate, maintain, and continuously improve their processes. Starting with the larger processes and working down to the smaller component processes, managers and staff can design the reports they need to accomplish their tasks and meet their goals. From those report designs, the data elements (specific items of data recorded) and calculations needed to generate those reports can be identified. All too often, the exact opposite approach is taken. Managers and staff make an itemized list of data they can collect, have collected in the past, or think might be helpful at some point in the future. Just because it is possible to collect a piece of data does not mean that you should. While adding an individual data element can seem a trivial matter matter in the design phase, consider the time it takes to collect it, enter it, quality check it, correct it (if needed), transfer it, and store it—multiplied by the number of times that data element is collected in a given time frame. If it is a data element on a PCR, a report completed by the EMS provider for each patient contact, in a busy system, the cost and hassle associated with superfluous data elements can be huge. Therefore, it is wise to limit data collection to items that are needed for a specific purpose for a specific internal or external customer.

Once it has been decided which data to collect (based on the design of reports to be used as the end products of a data system), managers can now confidently move forward in the design process to:

- Identify a source for each of the pieces of data needed;
- Determine the format in which the data are needed;
- Decide how to collect the data;
- Decide how to validate the data;
- Decide how to move the data from the point of collection to the point of storage;
- Decide how to securely encrypt and store the data;
- Decide how to move the data from the point of storage to the point of analysis;
- Decide how to move the information from the point of analysis to a point of storage; and
- Decide how to move the information from the points of storage to the internal and external customers who need the information.

Data Formats

Data formats precisely define each piece of information and in what form the information is obtained and stored. There are several data formatting standards related to EMS, but the most notable is the **National Standard EMS Data Set** developed by the EMS Office of the National Highway Traffic Safety Administration (NHTSA) and NEMSIS (www.nemsis.org) requirements. The standards list the information to be collected and the format in which the data is recorded for a typical prehospital EMS event. Another widely recognized set of healthcare data standards are the so-called Health Level Seven (HL7) standards. The HL7 is a standard for the collection, integration, and exchange of clinical patient care data among healthcare data systems (www.HL7.org). Both the National EMS Data Set and the HL7 attempt to provide a national standard that facilitates the movement and sharing of information among the various producers and users of healthcare information. The types of data collected by these standards are discussed later, under data collection. Regardless of the external standards an EMS organization might adopt, none of these standards are likely to include all the pieces of data an EMS organization needs to monitor, manage, and improve its key processes.

NEMSIS was designed to develop a national EMS database. All states in the United States have signed on to the memorandum of understanding, agreeing to conform to the NHTSA Uniform Prehospital dataset for upload to NEMSIS. NEMSIS has integrated the National EMS Data Set, HL7, and XML standards to provide for a uniform data source to report trends, improve quality, and nationally monitor the EMS system. These same data points not only can be used for local information but also will allow for comparison with other EMS agencies and communities.

Another strong factor in EMS data format standards is the variety of commercial EMS software packages available, such as EMScan/Keydata, EMS Charts, Fire Programs 2000TM, Firehouse Software, and SweetSoft. When an EMS system chooses to use a particular EMS data collection software package, the software usually comes with a very comprehensive data set and formatting standard. These software packages often include the National Standard EMS Data Set, NEMSIS reporting, and the ability for some customization to allow collection of unique data elements needed by a particular EMS system.

Data Collection Tools

There are many ways to collect data in the field during an EMS response, but the most preferable are those that allow crews to maintain their focus on their patients. Adoption of ePCR programs on tablet computers has made data collection easier, but every system has strengths and weaknesses.

Paper Forms

Paper forms are the most commonly used tool for field data collection, although their use is starting to diminish. Their main advantages are portability, ease of use, ability to generate multiple copies (with special papers), flexibility, legal acceptance, ease of filing, and moderate costs. The costs for printing forms on paper that can generate multiple copies can be quite substantial, but the value of having instantly available copies to provide to receiving facilities usually justifies the expense. The main disadvantages are potential legibility problems with handwritten entries, limited ability to provide real-time data validation, large forms or multiple forms being necessary to collect large data sets, and the expense of labor and cycle time delays when typing in data from the paper reports for billing and other reporting purposes. The design of paper forms is almost an art form. A good form is easy to read and understand, is easy to fill out, and uses space very efficiently. Trade-offs are made between clear, complete labels for each field on a form and using as little space as possible in an effort to collect the desired information on a single page.

Hybrid paper forms use electronic processes to reduce the need for manual keyboarding into a computer system. Optical mark recognition forms use one or more small circles filled in by pen or pencil to return a value for a particular data element, akin to the bubble sheets used in many multiple-choice question exams. These can work well when crews are careful to neatly darken the circles. These types of forms tend to take up a lot of space. Paper forms can also use optical character recognition (OCR) technology, making spaces for individual characters. These are read by a computer scanning device and converted to computer text, numbers, and symbols. These forms should be written legibly by the field crews. Another paper–computer hybrid is provided by optical imaging. The entire form is scanned with a scanner, fax, or similar device. A more robust type of handwriting recognition software that does not have the same strict spacing requirements as standard OCR methods is used. Some blocks of text that do not need to be electronically processed may be simply saved in an image and kept available in the database record for that particular patient care record. Other hybrid technologies may incorporate handheld barcode readers that allow crews to input certain types of information.

Paper strips with text and physiological waveforms (i.e., EGG, pulse oximetry, capnography) are often generated by medical devices. Paper patient care record designs often include spaces for attaching these strips of information with tape or adhesive strips added to the form in the printing process, which may then be scanned in. Alternatively, connections between cardiac monitors and computers are now completed via Wi-Fi or Bluetooth technology. These technologies allow the rhythms, and in some cases the entire patient summary, to be uploaded and stored electronically, where they can then be analyzed.

Stationary Computer Workstations

Another paper–computer hybrid strategy uses paper forms in the field. The information from the forms is typed by the crews into computer workstations at their crew quarters or in the receiving hospital. This option can work well for systems in which crews have sufficient time to enter their own data into the workstations between calls. The big advantage here is that the computers being used are housed in an environment that is less susceptible to the dirt, moisture, temperature changes, and mechanical forces that a field computer is subjected to.

Field Laptops

Light and durable laptops used directly in the field can offer many benefits. One of the most common reasons they are used is to streamline the billing and payment process by collecting information in a computerized format at the point of care. These efficiencies alone can often provide a sufficient return on investment to pay for the hardware and software. These systems can then be used for the many other administrative and quality management benefits that field computers have to offer. Other advantages of field laptops include the real-time quality and validation checks that can be performed on the data. This can lead to even further reductions in data collection costs. The disadvantages include high initial costs, loss of data in the event of system failures, susceptibility to damage or malfunction in the field environment, short service lives due to rapid technical obsolescence, and the bulk and weight of many of the hardware platforms. The good news is that laptops suitable for the field are getting smaller, faster, lighter, less expensive, and more durable. Laptops are now being marketed that have specifically been created to handle rough situations, such as the Panasonic Tough-book, but they are often heavy in comparison to standard laptops. Newer-generation field-capable lap-tops and medical devices are equipped with Wi-Fi or cellular capabilities and Bluetooth to allow the information that would previously have been transferred on paper strips to be moved electronically and added to the ePCR.

Data entry into field laptops typically requires a keyboard or touch screen–stylus technology. The technology for voice recognition, which allows a provider to speak and have the words be recognized by the software, is rapidly advancing and may soon be a practical and affordable way for crews to enter their data into their field computers. When combined with smaller hardware components configured into wearable devices, this technology will allow crews to enter data with both hands free to provide patient care.

Mobile Data Terminals

Mobile data terminals (MDTs) (**Figure 13-2**) have long been in use by police departments but have now gained popularity in EMS systems. Police departments have been using these systems for pulling records, creating reports, and communicating, and MDTs are now standard equipment on most police vehicles. In EMS, MDTs most recently have been adopted for communication with dispatch centers and for their GPS routing abilities. While MDTs are not yet standard equipment in all ambulances, the increased efficiency for large services means that adoption of data systems built into ambulances will most likely become a core of EMS operations in the same way as every ambulance has a radio. These devices provide critical information for system planning, such as response times, routing, closest unit availability, and accountability, but there has been a reluctance to use MDTs to collect patient data. Police officers regularly complete their "paperwork" in their vehicle while EMS professionals tend to complete their PCRs in the hospital or at their service, limiting the acceptance of using MDTs in the ambulance for PCRs.

Data Collection

There are three general types of data collected in EMS: clinical, operational, and support process data.

- **Clinical data** is data directly related to the assessment, treatment, and clinical outcomes of injuries and illnesses (e.g., cardiac care).
- **Operational data** is data related to the nonclinical activities taking place in direct support of field operations (e.g., fleet management and dispatch).

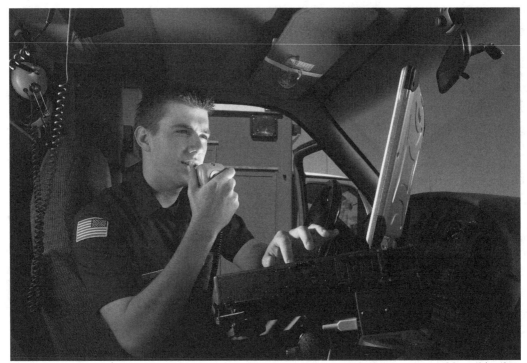

© Bounce/Cultura/Getty.

Figure 13-2 Mobile data terminals (MDTs) are now commonly used in EMS systems.

■ **Support data** is nonclinical and nonoperational data that comes from processes used to lead, manage, and support the overall organization (e.g., administration, payroll, human resources, training).

Data from operations and support activities is generally easier to obtain because the processes usually take place in fixed locations in controlled environments. Well-tested generic computerization and data collection systems are widely available for these processes from a wide range of business hardware and software providers. Data from the field EMS setting is far more challenging because of the highly variable and relatively uncontrolled settings in which field EMS crews perform their duties.

One of the biggest problems in EMS data systems has been making sure the data entered into a paper or electronic system is complete and correct. This is where strong leadership, management, and training must come together to make sure that:

■ The processes of field care are designed to include data collection. Protocols should integrate documentation into the process steps for assessment and care.

■ Training processes for field care include data collection. ACLS, BTLS, PHTLS, and other commonly used EMS scenario training programs all but ignore data collection in their processes. Therefore, it should not come as a surprise that EMS data collection suffers, because the designs of clinical processes and training fail to incorporate data collection. As a result, field crews are often inadequately trained to collect data during their care and assessment processes.

Data Validation

After all the time, effort, and expense to collect data, it is of no value if the data is not valid. Invalid data can actually have a negative value because it can lead staff and managers to costly mistakes. Fortunately, **data validation** can be addressed at several levels. Data collection tools can often be designed to increase the likelihood that data collected is valid. Paper forms can limit the range of inputs to valid choices with checkboxes and lists or a specific number of digits or characters. Reminders can be included on a data collection tool to help define valid entries.

Computer-based data collection tools can be designed to perform real-time checks on data for proper format and validity and advise how to correct the entry in many cases. For example, when 360 is entered for an adult pulse rate, the computer could give back an error message that states the range of values it will accept as valid. Care has to be taken in setting up error messages because the same system might consider a pulse of 0 to be invalid when it may actually be the patient's current condition.

Data Transfer, Secure Storage, and Analysis

Once the data related to a prehospital EMS event or out-of-hospital transport is collected in the field, it must be transferred to a central data storage point to be aggregated with other PCRs for analysis and centralized billing, accounting, and reporting activities. How the transfer occurs will depend on the type of data collection used. This could include paper reports, USB drives, wired or wireless Internet, and Wi-Fi and Bluetooth connections. The widespread availability of Internet technologies is making it possible to use cables and wireless Internet connections to move data from the field or crew station directly to the EMS organization's headquarters, without having to physically transfer a data source. Because these records contain sensitive and confidential information, any such data sent across the Internet must be adequately safeguarded with encryption, a firewall (a protective measure that limits direct access to a computer or program), and other appropriate security measures to protect patient privacy and ensure data integrity. Federal regulations have established certain standards that EMS systems must abide by when moving and storing patient information across the Internet. HIPAA regulations provide for substantial fines if personal data is not kept secure, and penalties may even include a jail term.

EMS leaders must also consider other types of threats to data security. For these reasons, organizations should make electronic backups of their data files and store those backups in another physical location that offers security against manmade threats and natural disasters, such as a safety deposit box in a bank or a data center.

Analysis is necessary to transform simple data into actionable information that can be used for different processes and to improve the overall system. Most of the types of analyses performed should be traceable from the mission to the vision, to the strategic plan, to performance and process measures associated with the strategy, to top-level reports, to the data sets and the individual data elements collected in the field and elsewhere in the system.

Data Usage

One of the most common problems with EMS data systems is that they collect vast quantities of data not used by managers for any specific purpose or benefit to the system. This may be due to a variety of reasons, including data reliability, usability, and the manager's lack of understanding. EMS managers need to make sure that there is a legitimate and valuable purpose for each piece of data being collected. When field personnel don't feel that this is the case, their efforts to ensure that all data is completely and correctly collected rapidly diminishes, and justifiably so.

In addition to using data to monitor performance and process measures, data and information are useful tools for all levels of an organization and all of their customers, both internal and external. For example:

- Management uses information to make better decisions. Any time a decision is made, there is some risk involved unless the manager knows for certain what the outcome of the decision will be. To reduce risk, the manager needs information that will help to decide the best alternative with the most acceptable amount of risk.

- **Internal customers** are customers within an organization. Internal customers have various other internal customers and function both as consumers and as producers of services. Information is important in both roles. For example, the supply manager for a large commercial ambulance service has the organization's fleet of vehicles and field crews as customers. In order to provide a constant and consistent supply of equipment and expendables to the units, the supply manager needs information. She or he needs to know, for example, the number of units on the road and the number and types of responses handled by the units. By linking the supply operation with data collected in the field, the supply manager can better anticipate the restocking needs of the fleet and prevent supply shortages without having to resort to having costly volumes of inventory sitting on warehouse shelves.

- **External customers** receive the services provided by the organization. As an example, a nursing care facility may have a contract with a commercial ambulance company to transport all of its residents to physician offices and other healthcare facilities. By linking the unit-availability status of the ambulance company to the scheduling database of the nursing facility, delays and reschedules can be reduced or avoided. And conversely, providing the ambulance company with the needs of the nursing facility allows the company to better schedule and utilize units for more efficient and reliable service.

Quality and Performance Evaluation

One of the most fundamental responsibilities of an EMS management team is to monitor and improve the quality and performance of its organization's services. Yet most EMS systems have relatively primitive quality and performance management systems. The most common reason is that the agencies that oversee or regulate EMS activities have similarly primitive systems for assessing quality and performance. NEMSIS was created in part to help raise the bar and provide a national database, but that database is still only a representation of the data collected and used at the local levels. Most people involved want to improve quality and performance but have difficulty making measurable progress. This discussion is intended to provide insights and exposure to some strategies and tools that can make real improvements in the quality and performance of EMS systems.

Quality, Cost, and Performance

To place the information in this chapter into proper context, the relationship between quality, cost, and performance should be clearly understood. Quality is a measure of how well a given process is working. It might be expressed in measures such as response-time intervals, survival rates, customer satisfaction ratings, or employee turnover rates. Cost is a purely financial expression, usually in terms of dollars (or other currencies), of how efficiently a process is working. It might be expressed in terms of cost per fleet mile, cost per advanced life support unit hour, average cost per resuscitation attempt, cost per bill, or cost per new-employee recruitment and orientation. Performance, in the context of this chapter discussion, is synonymous with value. It reflects the combined effects of quality and cost, as expressed in the equation below:

$$\text{value or performance} = \text{quality/cost}$$

Measuring Overall Performance

One of the first issues managers confront when trying to take an organized and logical approach to quality and performance management is determining their current level of quality and performance. One of the best ways to measure overall quality and performance is the **Baldrige Criteria for Performance Excellence**. These criteria were developed as part of the National Quality Improvement Act of 1987 (Public Law No. 100-107), which established the Malcolm Baldrige National Quality Award. Despite the award, the real focus is on the use of the Baldrige Criteria as a framework for organizations to improve overall performance. These criteria are widely recognized for their validity and utility. The criteria and a host of related information and resources are available online at no cost from the National Institute of Standards and Technology (NIST) website at www.quality.nist.gov.

The EMS Office of the National Highway Traffic Safety Administration (NHTSA) undertook a project in the mid-1990s to develop a model for EMS system quality improvement. The result was not a new program, but a discovery and strong endorsement of the Baldrige Criteria as the best available model. A special information package on the Baldrige Criteria and EMS quality management, called the Leadership

Guide to Quality Improvement of EMS Systems, is available at no charge from the NHTSA EMS Office website at www.nhtsa.gov/people/injury/ems/leaderguide/. The Leadership Guide provides EMS managers with an excellent primer to quality management concepts and tools. It also has an excellent bibliography on EMS-specific quality management literature. As the NEMSIS data becomes available, some findings may change, but the Baldrige Criteria still work no matter what the format of the data is.

Examining organizational performance with the Baldrige Criteria is not a pass–fail process. It is more like measuring an organization's performance with a very long tape measure. These same criteria can be used over and over again to measure EMS system progress from year to year. The overall results are expressed on a scale of 0 to 1000. The Baldrige Criteria results are divided into seven broad areas:

1. Leadership system;
2. Strategic planning;
3. Information and analysis;
4. Customer systems;
5. Human resources;
6. Process management; and
7. Results.

The feedback report from a properly performed organizational assessment using the Baldrige Criteria provides an objective and detailed analysis of the organization's overall performance. The feedback is not prescriptive but gives insights on how well things are going in terms of an organization's approach to performance improvement, how well those efforts are deployed throughout the organization, and how effective those efforts have been in yielding meaningful results.

Conducting a complete Baldrige assessment is a significant task in itself. Many organizations begin the assessment portion of their quality and performance management journey by using one of several less elaborate assessment tools that are based on the criteria. The survey-style tool developed by Mark Graham-Brown (Graham-Brown, 1994) based on the 1995 Baldrige Criteria is one very useful example of this type of tool. Many states have their own versions of the Baldrige Criteria and corresponding sets of abbreviated assessment tools, such as the State of Florida's Sterling Challenge. (NIST now provides a self-assessment tool for the Baldridge Criteria that can help identify areas of improvement and serve as a framework for quality improvement in the healthcare fields.) With the Centers for Medicare and Medicaid Services looking at ways to improve quality, it is likely that they will use existing programs such as the Baldridge Criteria to evaluate organizations in addition to patient-level reporting.

Regardless of which version or which type of Baldrige assessment an EMS organization uses, the feedback provides an excellent starting point for the strategic planning process. In many successful organizations, the Baldrige assessment process is conducted annually and the feedback is used to start a new annual cycle of strategic planning, budgeting, implementation, and reassessment.

High Performance EMS Systems

Jack Stout is well known in the field of EMS systems for the concept of designing high-performance EMS systems (Stout, 1983, 1996). He effectively makes the case that it is relatively easy to have high costs and high quality, but these factors do not make for a high-performance system. For example, a system can easily lower response times and thereby improve survival from cardiac arrest by putting many more ambulances or rescue units with defibrillators on the street. Plugging numbers into the value equation shows that spending more money might get a higher level of quality, but the corresponding level of performance may not change because the numerator and the denominator are both increasing in that scenario. Similarly, it is not difficult to build a system with a few units and low survival from cardiac arrest for low costs and low quality. Lower costs and lower quality also do not make a change in performance in this equation.

The challenge is to build a high-performance EMS system in which costs are held constant or lowered while simultaneously increasing quality. In the example, this translates into making improvements in survival without increasing costs. Preferably, survival (quality) increases while costs simultaneously decrease. The goal is to make smarter financial decisions, by spending money on the processes that really matter. A good starting point for improving quality in an organization is with an examination of its mission. The mission states why the organization exists. For many EMS organizations, the mission may be to simply provide out-of-hospital care and medical transportation services to a specified community. The vision of an organization describes what it aspires to be while fulfilling its mission. Lofty words, such as the best, finest, and excellence, are often used in statements of an organization's vision. If an EMS organization has a vision to provide the highest level of quality in out-of-hospital care and medical transportation services, the strategy of the organization needs to identify how the organization plans to achieve that vision.

Most organizations with successful long-term efforts have discovered that quality is far more than a program or function. It is something that cannot be delegated to the "quality manager." It is a philosophy of management that gets woven into the very culture of the organization. It is something that every person in the organization should participate in. This philosophy is based on several fundamental premises, including the following:

- Every organization (or system) is composed of interrelated processes that must collectively fulfill its mission and serve the needs of its customers.
- The performance (or value) of a process is the result of the combined effects of quality and cost. The goal is to be a high-performance organization, one that provides a high level of quality at a low level of cost (a point that deserves frequent repetition).
- People cannot effectively manage what they cannot effectively measure.
- The performance of almost every process can be directly or indirectly measured.
- The performance of almost every process can be improved (by improving its quality, reducing its cost, or both).

- Every process in an organization should contribute toward fulfilling its mission.
- The people who best understand how a process really works and how it can be improved are those who work inside that process and those who directly use the products or services that come from the process.

Leadership System

The role of the senior leader and the senior management team is essential to the success of a quality and performance management system. The leaders must focus the organization on the mission; create and communicate a vision; and take clear steps in their policies, procedures, and processes to steer the organization toward achieving their vision. Too commonly, leaders talk about lofty quality themes and values while their actions are inconsistent with their words. This is one of the quickest ways for leaders to undermine such efforts and diminish their own credibility within their organization. High-performance leaders in high-performance organizations not only "talk the talk," they "walk the walk" of continuously improving quality, performance, and value.

Improving quality and performance in an organization must also be recognized as a never-ending process. Many liken it to a never-ending journey in which the organization reaches many exciting milestones along the way, but there are always higher levels of quality and performance to aspire to. In a business like EMS, with the lives and well-being of the community at stake, there should never be a point at which an EMS organization is content and no longer seeks to make further improvements in decreasing the morbidity, mortality, and suffering of the citizens it serves.

Strategic Quality Planning

Most organizations use strict financial performance measures and budgetary planning as a routine part of their business activities. The senior managers of the organization are held accountable for meeting specific budgetary targets related to expenses, revenues, and other financial measures of performance. This same type of planning, measurement, and accountability can be applied to meeting quality-related performance targets.

The overall strategy of the organization identifies how it plans to achieve its vision. The strategic planning process should provide sufficient detail to enable plans to be made on how to attain goals that reflect attainment of that vision. Many of those goals will relate to issues of quality, cost, and returns on investment (in both public and private sector EMS organizations).

Strategic quality planning starts by articulating all of the quality-related goals that stem from the organization's vision. From those goals, the next step is to break them down into specific quality objectives. Each of those objectives can be broken down even further into specific milestones with associated timelines, budgets, and measures that will indicate how well the goals and objectives are met. Some of these goals might be attainable sooner than others. Because the overall strategic planning and budgeting process in most organizations works on an annual cycle, the strategic quality plan should also be organized into one-year increments.

For example, one component of an EMS system's vision is to have the highest rate of survival from cardiac arrest. That might be articulated in even more specific terms—the highest rates of survival from cardiac arrest per the Utstein Guidelines on reporting survival from cardiac arrest (Cummins et al., 1991). The **Utstein Guidelines** are an international set of standards and templates for the recording of prehospital cardiac arrest resuscitation outcomes. Assuming that the organization is early in its quality journey, the main objectives for the first year might be to establish a reliable data collection and analysis process that will enable the system to measure its current rate of survival as a baseline. For most EMS systems, this is no small task. Working through all of the initial process design problems and then refining the process to a high level of reliability could easily take a year or more. Meeting this objective will require planning, budgeting, and establishing managerial accountabilities, just as those organizations have for financial planning and performance. Assuming this objective is met in year one, the goal for the next year might be to improve survival to a higher level, based on lessons learned in the first year. Experience gained in those first two years will be extraordinarily helpful in identifying opportunities for further improvement and setting realistic goals for the following years. This same approach can be taken to all functions of the organization, from fleet management to human resources, billing and collections, supply and dispatch, and administration.

Information and Analysis

The performance measures for **key processes** in an EMS organization, whether clinical, operational, or administrative, are referred to in quality management terminology as key performance indicators. These key processes may be broken down into smaller and smaller levels of component processes and corresponding performance indicators. Regardless of whether they are "key" performance indicators or components thereof, ideally they should all be developed to include both the quality and cost aspects of performance. When developing a **quality indicator**, it is helpful to ask, "What changes would I expect to see if this process were working very well or very poorly?" Measuring these changes may be the basis for a quality indicator. Try to choose indicators that are influenced only by the process under examination, or as close to this ideal as possible. Vehicle emissions from an EMS fleet might reflect on the performance of engines and exhaust system, but using the citywide pollution index is not specific enough to these EMS vehicles to be a useful indicator. A direct measurement of emissions from the tailpipes of the EMS vehicles would be a more specific, and therefore a more useful, performance indicator.

Careful judgment is necessary in choosing indicators, because in some cases, the less direct indicators may be more useful. For example, the time spent on scene could be used as a quality indicator for the EMS processes used in the care of acute coronary syndrome (ACS) patients. But with deeper consideration, a better process might have slightly longer EMS scene time to obtain a prehospital 12-lead ECG and administer appropriate medications, but have a lower total time from the onset of symptoms until a decision is made for providing thrombolytic therapy or other definitive treatment. The time interval from the onset of symptoms to the time a decision is made regarding definitive treatment may be a better indicator, although it is not as specific as we might like it to be. Overall survival rate for ACS patients may look like a better measure, but it would not be appropriate because it represents the entire treatment of the patient including in-hospital treatment, not only the actions of the EMS organization.

When developing a **cost indicator**, it is helpful to ask, "What costs do I have from this process?" Some of those costs may be direct and others may be indirect. As with the quality indicators, careful consideration is necessary to choose good cost indicators. Using the acute coronary care example again, the cost of all equipment and supplies used in the field on a suspected acute myocardial infarction might be a good direct cost indicator for that clinical process. A lower cost process might suggest a better performing process. On deeper consideration, a better process in some systems with longer transport times might include prehospital administration of thrombolytic or antiplatelet drugs or both. This early timing of drug administration might increase the EMS costs both in time and the cost of the drug, but decrease the total costs of care.

A quality indicator can be combined with a cost indicator to derive a **value indicator**, as referred to in Equation 1. For example, an EMS fleet might use the number of breakdowns per 100,000 fleet miles in each month as a quality indicator. A cost indicator might be the monthly average cost per fleet mile. If the fleet runs 334,562 miles in a particular month and had 17 breakdowns, that would equate to 17 ÷ 334562 or approximately 5.1 breakdowns per 100,000 fleet miles. That same fleet had an average cost per fleet mile of $34.18.

To use the value equation mentioned earlier, the quality numbers in the numerator must be expressed in such a way that better results have higher values and worse results have lower numbers. A lower number of breakdowns is better than a higher number of breakdowns. To flip the direction of the breakdown numbers to be usable in the value equation, use the reciprocal (1 ÷ number of breakdowns per 100,000 fleet miles). In the cost values for the denominator, the opposite must be true. A higher number needs to reflect a higher cost. The use of dollars in the denominator is also acceptable. The resulting fleet value indicator is shown in the following equation:

$$\frac{1 \div 5.1 \text{ breakdowns per } 100,000 \text{ fleet miles}}{\$34.18 \text{ average cost per fleet mile}}$$

$$0.196 \div 34.18 = 0.00573$$

If the fleet was able to reduce the frequency of breakdowns over the next month to 4.5 per 100,000 while keeping its average cost per fleet mile steady at $34.18, the fleet value indicator would go up to 0.00650, as shown in the next equation:

$$\frac{1 \div 4.5 \text{ breakdowns per } 100,000 \text{ fleet miles}}{\$34.18 \text{ average cost per fleet mile}}$$

$$0.222 \div 34.18 = 0.00650$$

If the breakdowns stayed at 5.1 per 100,000 fleet miles but the average cost per fleet mile went down to $30.50, the fleet value indicator would go up to 0.00643, as in this equation:

$$\frac{1 \div 5.1 \text{ breakdowns per 100,000 fleet miles}}{\$30.50 \text{ average cost per fleet mile}}$$

$$0.196 \div 30.50 = 0.00643$$

There might be a smaller improvement in the number of breakdowns per 100,000 fleet miles to 4.7 and a smaller decrease in the average cost per fleet mile to $32.25. But the value equation would reflect their combined effects, as shown in this equation:

$$\frac{1 \div 4.7 \text{ breakdowns per 100,000 fleet miles}}{\$32.25 \text{ average cost per fleet mile}}$$

$$0.212 \div 32.25 = 0.00660$$

It is interesting to consider other commonly used EMS quality indicators, such as survival rates from cardiac arrest or response times, in combination with appropriate cost indicators to derive value indicators. These types of value indicators can be far more useful to EMS system managers than quality or cost indicators alone. In order to calculate any of these quality or cost indicators, it is necessary to carefully design, implement, and manage data processes that address all of the data system creation components highlighted earlier in this chapter:

- What specific pieces of data are needed?
- Where does each piece of data come from?
- How will each piece of data be collected?
- How will each piece of data be moved from where it is collected to where it needs to be stored and used in calculations?
- How will the accuracy for each piece of data be ensured?
- How can it be ensured that all pertinent data has been collected?

Putting the infrastructure in place for a data management system that addresses these issues is another significant challenge. (See chapter 14.) It is an absolutely vital step for building a robust quality and performance management system.

Process Assurance and Improvement

Having data collection and analysis processes is a great step forward, but the journey to high performance is just beginning. The next step is to make sure that the processes under evaluation are followed consistently. Consider a situation in which an EMS system is studying the performance of its clinical process (protocol) for the management of chest pain of suspected cardiac origin. On the quality side, the providers are looking at changes in the patient's level of pain on a scale of 0 to 10. The protocol (or clinical process) calls for the administration of a 0.4 mg sublingual nitroglycerin spray every five minutes for as long as the patient reports continuing pain or discomfort and the patient's systolic blood pressure remains above 100 mmHg. The data from the first month of study might show that for patients starting with a pain level of 7 and having transport time intervals of 10–12 minutes, the pain level only goes down to an average of 6 by the time they arrive at the hospital emergency department (ED) doors. For those patients whose systolic BP remains above 100, there should be at least 3 doses of nitroglycerin in that time frame (at minutes 0, 5, and 10). Closer study of the data reveals that these patients are receiving an average of only 1.4 doses. Discussion of the process by the cross-functional team (to be described later in this section), which includes field crews, suggests that some of the problems may be related to difficulties in keeping track of the elapsed time between nitroglycerin doses. With many tasks to accomplish, it can be difficult for crews to keep track of the five-minute intervals. The team comes up with the idea of putting timers in the drug kits that could be set to beep every five minutes once they are activated. Crews are asked to turn the timers on when they give the first dose of nitroglycerin. The month after the timers are installed, the cases starting at a level of 7 go down to a level of 3 on average. The average number of doses is now 2.86 out of 3 available doses.

This example illustrates **process assurance**. Initially, the protocol was not being followed consistently. Over the next couple of months, these and other problems in process assurance were discovered and corrected to the point that the results from month to month were consistent and the cross-functional team felt that it now had a good idea of what their clinical process was capable of accomplishing in terms of pain relief. Until the process was being followed as written by all crews, the results did not reflect how well the process was capable of performing. In an unknown number of cases, the results were clouded by noncompliance to the stated nitroglycerin dosage protocols. The challenge then becomes maintaining these levels over the long term and sustaining improvements.

Once an organization has completed the first big steps of putting processes in place to collect and analyze data that reliably measure its levels of performance, it will be ready to begin the next phase: process improvement. In this phase, processes are examined to find ways to make them perform with higher quality and ways to make them perform at lower cost. The goal is to bring the processes to a higher level of overall performance.

Many organizations use **cross-functional teams** to oversee and improve processes. Cross-functional teams are typically composed of people who supply a process (suppliers), those who work inside a process (processors), and those who use the outputs of a process (customers). The cross-functional teams are often charged with developing the performance indicators, designing the processes for data collection and analysis, evaluating the results, and coming up with ideas for improvements to the processes.

For example, a cross-functional cardiac team might take stewardship of the protocols for acute coronary syndromes, cardiopulmonary resuscitation, stroke, and congestive heart failure. The team members might consist of a field emergency medical technician (EMT), field paramedic, field supervisor, ED physician, critical care nurse, cardiologist, and a representative from a cardiac patient support group. To come up with ideas for protocol changes, the group might use brainstorming, literature reviews, surveys, polls, or ideas from other EMS systems that have had good results in their cardiac processes (benchmarking).

Care should be taken to involve all concerned parties in cross-functional teams. Not only do you need to involve those with direct patient care, but you may want to include a representative from your medical oversight office and union. Involving a union representative early on may help keep your organization out of trouble later. What may seem like only a clinical issue may involve the union if additional training hours or expanded duties are required.

Referring back to the chest pain example, a cross-functional cardiac care team might have come to recognize that the current protocol for pain relief in suspected acute coronary syndrome cases, with near 100% compliance, was not capable of providing complete relief of pain in cases in which the pain level started at a 7 or higher. In those cases, a quality improvement project might try to "test" a change in the protocol to see if a better level of performance can be obtained. The "test" should be conducted using the scientific method. (See chapter 14.)

A change in a process (protocol) represents a hypothesis that the new process will perform better than the current one. Therefore, quality improvement teams should develop strong skills in the design and analysis of experimental data.

The cardiac team members, after reviewing the literature and their own data, came to the conclusion that if the patient's chest discomfort was not completely relieved by three EMS nitroglycerin sprays, it was unlikely to make additional improvements. Therefore, the protocol (process) was modified to add 2 mg doses of morphine sulfate at three-minute intervals if three EMS doses of nitroglycerin failed to completely relieve the chest pain. The results of the new protocol can be compared to the prior protocol to determine if there was a statistically significant improvement under the new protocol. If the data from the new protocol (process), while being reliable and consistent, showed better performance, then the new protocol (process) change could be permanent. If it failed to show better results, another idea for improvement could be developed and tested. This continuous cycle of planning a change, implementing it, checking the results, and acting on results is referred to by several names in the literature: the Plan-Do-Check-Act (PDCA) Cycle, the Shewhart Cycle, or the Deming Cycle.

Scope of Performance Improvement Efforts

There are many administrative, operational, and clinical key processes in an EMS system. It is impossible for a designated quality improvement officer and the medical director to study, collect data, measure performance, analyze trends, maintain consistency, and generate improvement ideas, and then implement and test them all by themselves. Despite this fact, that is the way in which many EMS quality programs are currently designed. As a result, most EMS quality programs only look at a small number of performance indicators, most likely reflective of the personal concerns of those involved rather than sound data. Most of the available hours for quality efforts are spent on quality assurance activities and externally mandated data collection and reporting requirements. This leaves little to no time available for quality improvement efforts.

The organizations that have been most successful in their performance improvement efforts have overcome this issue (in EMS, healthcare, and non-healthcare industries) with a very broad scope of participation from a large portion of the workforce. The activities associated with performance improvement are designed into employee selection criteria, job descriptions, orientation, training, education, schedules, and budgets for all departments, divisions, workgroups, and work processes within the organization. For example, those working in fleet management participate on teams that address fleet processes and participate on cross-functional teams for other processes. The managers serve as coaches and remove roadblocks and hassles for the teams they work with. The performance-improvement-staff team trains the staff in the use of performance improvement strategies and in the use of analytical tools. They may also serve as facilitators and internal consultants for specific problems with which the teams might need additional assistance. Performance improvement staff might also consolidate reports between multiple teams and conduct global performance audits, such as an annual self-assessment with the Baldrige Criteria.

WRAP UP

Summary

EMS systems collect data related to patient care, operations, and support processes. In order for this data to be useful, it must be collected in the proper format, validated, and analyzed. Only then will the data become useful information. Information is an important tool for EMS system managers that helps them make informed decisions. For system information to be truly useful, it must be integrated into the total healthcare information network. Technological advances have the prospect of making integration easier as well as improving the capture and validation of EMS system data.

It is up to the senior leaders of an EMS system to make sure that performance (quality and cost) improvement components are deeply integrated into all job descriptions, budgets, managerial accountability goals, reward and recognition programs, and policies and procedures and are at the very core of what each person is expected to do within the organization. It has to be more than talk—it must be measured and held to the same level of accountability, and get as much (or more) time as the budget or other primary responsibilities of the management team.

Key Terms

analysis

Baldrige Criteria for
  Performance Excellence

clinical data

cost indicator

cross-functional teams

data

data formats

data validation

Electronic Patient Care
  Records (ePCR)

external customers

hybrid paper forms

information

internal customers

key processes

mobile data terminals (MDTs)

National EMS Information
  System (NEMSIS)

National Standard EMS
  Data Set

operational data

paper forms

process assurance

quality indicator

strategic information
  plan

strategic quality
  planning

support data

Utstein Guidelines

value indicator

Review Questions

1. What is the difference between data and information?

2. Support the need for a strategic information plan in an EMS system.

3. Identify current factors that inhibit integration of healthcare system information.

4. List at least five entities that EMS systems need to share information with.

5. What are data elements and how are they standardized nationally?

6. List the three types of data used by EMS systems.

7. Compare and contrast the various methods of collecting EMS data elements in the field.

8. Describe the role of analysis in the utilization of EMS data.

9. Define a high-performance system in terms of this equation:
   performance = quality ÷ cost.

10. What is the difference between an organizational mission and vision?

11. Describe the role of quality within an organization.

12. Discuss the Baldrige Criteria for Performance Excellence.

13. Defend the need for strategic quality planning.

14. Identify and describe key performance indicators within an EMS organization.

15. List members to include on a cross-functional team to study transport of fall patients from nursing facilities.

Additional Resources

Cummins, R. O., Chamberlain, D. A., Abramson, N. S., Allen, M., Baskett, P. J., Becker, L., … Eisenberg, M. S. (1991). Recommended

guidelines for uniform reporting of data from out-of-hospital cardiac arrest: The Utstein style. A statement for health professionals from a task force of the American Heart Association, the European Resuscitation Council, the Heart and Stroke Foundation of Canada, and the Australian Resuscitation Council. *Circulation*, 84(2), 960–975.

Graham-Brown, M. (1994, December). Measuring up against the 1995 Baldrige Criteria. *Journal for Quality and Participation*. 66–72.

Stout, J. (1983). Measuring your system. *Journal of Emergency Medical Services*, 8(1), 84–91.

Stout, J. (1996, June). High performance mobile healthcare services. Sponsored by the 4th Party and the University of Maryland, Baltimore County. St. Petersburg Beach, FL.

14

Research

Objectives

Upon completion of this chapter, the reader should be able to:

- Define research.

- List reasons why research is necessary in EMS.

- List the steps involved in the scientific method.

- Define various research designs.

- Identify the components of a research study.

- Differentiate between a null and an alternate hypothesis.

- Define reliability, validity, and bias.

- List reasons why research should be published.

What Is Research?

One way to define **research** is "organized curiosity." It is a way to ask questions and develop answers. It is a way to examine the world. Perhaps most importantly, it is a systematic method for understanding the world. Researchers use this understanding to predict a patient's response to medication, the effect of a procedure used for trauma patients, and the changes that can be expected from new policies or procedures.

Why Research?

Emergency medical services (EMS) personnel have been extraordinarily good at coming up with innovative solutions to problems, but not as good at sharing accomplishments. Perhaps this is because problem solving means that a problem exists, and some managers refuse to admit that their agency has a problem. Perhaps it is because there are few role models or mentors to help EMS personnel work their way through the research process. Whatever the reasons, it is now recognized that research is a crucial component of future EMS development. Other reasons to do research include to:

- Improve patient care;
- Improve the system;
- Understand the system;
- Reduce hazards;
- Provide legal protection; and
- Improve the profession.

Improve Patient Care

One of the most crucial reasons for healthcare professionals to conduct research is to improve patient care. An organized research project allows researchers to consider a number of interventions for a particular type of patient complaint or condition. As an example, consider the use of MAST (Military Anti-Shock Trousers). For many years, the MAST suit was considered the prehospital intervention of choice for hypotensive trauma patients. During those years, much anecdotal evidence was accumulated that seemed to demonstrate the efficacy of the trousers. Then Dr. Paul Pepe and a team of researchers conducted a number of scientific research studies (Bickell et al., 1985, 1987; Mattox et al., 1986, 1989; Pepe, Bass, & Mattox, 1986). As a result of those studies, they found that MAST did not improve patient outcomes, and in some cases may have even increased mortality. As a result of this research, MAST protocols have changed dramatically. Adoption of these changes often takes many years, yet it is the research that leads the way.

This process of using research to improve patient care has become known as evidence-based medicine (EBM). Evidence-based medicine has now become a standard of care within health care as a whole and will form the basis of EMS patient care in the near future.

Improve the System

Research can also be used to make improvements within an existing EMS system. In one study (Joyce, Dutkowski, & Hynes, 1997), a quality improvement (QI) program was evaluated for its impact on the EMS system. Using criteria such as appropriate treatment, adequate documentation, call time intervals, and protocol compliance, the authors found that the new QI program resulted in significant improvement in 13 of the 19 parameters evaluated.

Understand the System

Sometimes knowing whether an intervention works is not enough to improve the system. In order to improve the system, research may be needed. For example, a researcher may want to understand exactly how a sample of paramedics learn from their experiences in order to help others learn effectively. Research on understanding the system may also help to find areas that can be further researched to improve the system.

Reduce Hazards

Many hazards that are involved in EMS can be identified and reduced using research. In another study (Maguire & Porco, 1997a), the authors reported on a research experiment aimed at reducing ambulance collisions. In this case, the study was prompted by a number of dramatic ambulance collisions. Using a pre- and post-intervention evaluation model, the collision rate was calculated before and after the implementation of two interventions. The combined use of a mandatory driver training program and a change in the departmental driving policies was associated with a 50% reduction in collisions following the interventions.

Provide Legal Protection

Research projects can both identify the legal risks associated with EMS (Goldberg et al., 1990; Soler et al., 1985) and help protect practitioners who follow guidelines based on scientifically verified procedures. For example, researchers in Brooklyn, New York, conducted an eight-year retrospective review of all legal cases related to one hospital-based EMS agency (Maguire & Porco, 1997b). They found that 100% of the litigation was associated with motor vehicle collisions. They also discovered that the lack of seat belt use was a recurring factor in much of the litigation.

Improve the Profession

For the medical and healthcare communities, research is the language of professionals. It is the way professionals communicate with one another and it helps to separate the professions from the trades, thereby elevating EMS practice. It is the method that professionals use to improve their professions. Evidence-based medicine is quickly becoming the standard in both hospital-based and prehospital medicine. Having research evidence helps professionals to make informed decisions rather than to work based on experience and conjecture alone. Research now includes real-time patient data from the healthcare system and in the future may include real-time changes.

Introduction to the Scientific Method

As described earlier in the MAST example, the lack of an organized objective examination of the facts can lead to erroneous assumptions and beliefs. Therefore, researchers have developed a systematic inquiry approach called the **scientific method** that includes:

- Formulating a testable **hypothesis** from which verifiable predictions can be confirmed or deduced as true or false based on brute facts (facts not subject to controversy, interpretation, or dispute);
- Using neutral and repeatable **experimental procedures** to test a hypothesis to screen out biases and preconceptions about the validity of the hypothesis being tested;
- Submitting findings to the review of peers; and
- Organizing knowledge into a system of general laws that reveal causal connections existing in the world.

The scientific method has allowed the natural sciences to have the following characteristics:

- Self-correcting methods that provide an increasingly accurate picture of nature; and

- Consensus generation; that is, practitioners come to agreement on which hypotheses are to be accepted and rejected (this differs from philosophy and religion, areas in which disagreements do not necessarily diminish over time).

Statistics

Although a formal review of statistical methods is beyond the scope of this text, it is now essential for EMS professionals to be familiar with at least the basic tenets of statistics. One of the most important statistical concepts is that of population distribution. A **population** is the entire group of individuals that may be affected by an issue. Since it is impossible to study everyone, researchers work with **representative samples** to determine trends within the population. Population distributions are measured by calculating average scores and **standard deviations** in a sample. For example, if we measure the height of a randomly selected group of men from the population, we will find an average height and a distribution of heights that will be mostly near the average. So, if the average height is 5'8", most men will be approximately 5'8", fewer will be 6', and even fewer will be 6'5". If we graph the results using height as the *x* axis (the base), starting at under 4' on the left and going to over 7' all the way to the right, and if we put the number of subjects as the *y* axis, we will generate a picture that looks like **Figure 14-1**. This is known as the **standard distribution curve**.

The standard deviation is a calculation that allows predicting, for example, how many men will be within certain ranges. In a normally distributed population, 68% of the subjects fall within one standard deviation of the mean. If, for example, the standard deviation for the subjects we tested was 3", we would expect that 68% of the group are between 5'5" and 5'11". Two standard deviations encompass 95 percent of the population. So, we would expect that 95% of these men are between 5'2" and 6'2". Ninety-nine percent of the population will be within three standard deviations of the mean. In this example, this means that 99% of the subjects will be between 4'11" and 6'5".

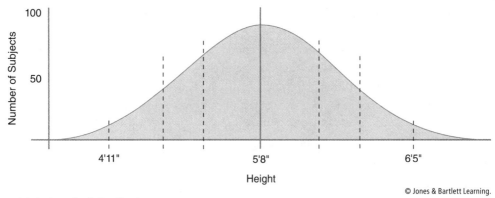

© Jones & Bartlett Learning.

Figure 14-1 Standard distribution curve.

Consider the measurement of IQ. The IQ test is written to generate an average score of 100 and a standard deviation of 15. This means that 68% of the population have an IQ between 85 and 115, 95% between 70 and 130, and 99% between 55 and 145. Because the population is normally distributed, we can also calculate the percentage of people who have, for example, an IQ over 130. We know that 95% of the population have an IQ between 70 and 130. That leaves 5% of the population. We also know that there is the same number of subjects above and below the average. Therefore, we can calculate that 2.5% of the population have an IQ above 130.

Once we know the average and the standard deviation, we can use those figures to determine if an intervention changes the average and standard deviation in our test population to a significant degree. Various statistical tests are used to measure that question under different circumstances.

Research Design
Quantitative and Qualitative Methods

Research can be broadly broken into subsections of quantitative and qualitative research. **Quantitative research** involves facts and figures to determine relationships between variables being studied or the occurrence of something within a sample. Most medical research is quantitative in nature and studies the impact of changes within a sample that is representative of the population as a whole. This method is convenient as it allows for statistical analysis and comparisons that show whether trends have changed or if an intervention had a statistically significant effect. Quantitative studies are convenient because the results are generalizable to similar samples and can be applied across a population if the significance is high enough.

Qualitative research is useful for understanding how a sample thinks, feels, or reacts within a certain situation. Qualitative research is a broad concept that covers several forms of inquiry and is useful for understanding and explaining the meaning of social phenomena. It is designed to gain an understanding from the participants' perspectives. Qualitative research relies on interviews, questionnaires, observations, sampling, and other data collection methods that help describe a phenomenon. The data are then analyzed for themes and are presented to "paint a picture" of the findings. Qualitative research is useful when it is important to get a greater depth of understanding about a topic, such as to determine why a sample from a quantitative study reacted in a certain way, or it may be used to provide examples for further research or practice. These studies have large sample sizes to increase generalization, control variables, and randomize subjects. Qualitative research pursues questions that are not easily answered by experimental methods. It is an inductive process that seeks to gain a deeper understanding of a patient's experience.

Some studies use mixed methods that employ both quantitative and qualitative methodologies to develop a complete understanding of a problem. While true mixed-method studies are rare, researchers often follow up a quantitative study with qualitative research or vice versa. For example, if a quantitative study found that 30% of patients surveyed rated their local EMS service as "poor" or "very poor," the data may help the service to do a qualitative study to understand why the patients had this perception.

In this case, the researcher might interview a sample of patients and ask them about their perceptions and feelings about components of the system to identify potential areas of improvement.

Qualitative research is all too often overlooked as a method, for various reasons. Medicine has relied heavily on quantitative research, as the statistics are relatively easy to understand, and the data is readily generalizable to a wide population as long as the sample is large enough and probability of error is low enough for the results to be statistically significant. Qualitative research, by its nature, is not generalizable to wider populations because it only represents the specific sample in the study. Qualitative research requires just as rigorous a design as quantitative research, but does not have as large a sample as quantitative studies—it would be nearly impossible to interview 100+ individuals and analyze the data in a realistic time frame.

Quantitative research projects can be divided into two broad categories: observational and interventional.

Observational Studies

In an **observational study**, events are monitored and analyzed without an attempt to manipulate or alter the outcome. The causation results are inferred based on the observed outcomes. The problem with observational studies is that they do not account for other variables. There is no way to control for the effects of outside influences. In fact, there is no way to know if you are even observing the proper variables. Observational studies are often done as a prelude to an interventional research project. They may define the problem or offer a baseline look at the prevalence of a condition or the incident rate of a factor to be studied.

Interventional Studies

In an **interventional study**, the researcher influences the process and then analyzes the effects. The Maguire and Porco (1997b) collision study is an example of an interventional project. In this case, the collision rate was calculated, an intervention was performed, and the collision rate was recalculated. It was found that there was a 50% reduction in collisions following the intervention.

Double-Blind, Randomized Control Studies

The gold standard in research is the **double-blind, randomized control study (DBRCS) experimental design**. This is a prospective (ongoing, not retrospective) research method. In this approach, the subjects are randomly assigned to the experimental and control groups (each subject has the same chance of being in the experimental group). When the experimenters and the subjects are both blind to the intervention being used on each subject, it is called double blinding. Let's use a hypothetical example.

A drug company has just released a new drug for experimentation. The hypothesis is that this drug will cause an increase in heart rate for all persons receiving the drug. If you are the experimenter, you might list the potential difficulties of performing such an experiment. For example, if you simply pick the next 10 people who come into the emergency department (ED) and administer the drug to them, you might have some confounding effects. Maybe the 10 people are all frightened of needles. Maybe they are all becoming hypotensive, or they are all becoming increasingly irate at being in the ED. Perhaps some (or all) of them consumed coffee (or another stimulant) right before coming to the ED. If you tell them that the drug will increase their heart rate, perhaps any noted increase was influenced by your suggestion.

In order to control for these types of variables, we begin by randomly selecting a group of subjects from the population. There are rigorous standards for subject selection, which will be covered later in the chapter. After selecting an adequate group size, we randomly assign each of the subjects to either the experimental (receives the intervention) or control (receives a **placebo** or no intervention) group. Next we prepare the drug. Syringes, which look identical except for an identification number, are prepared for each of the subjects. The subjects in the experimental group receive an injection of the drug; the subjects in the control group receive an injection of sterile water.

In order for the study to meet the criteria of "double blind," the person administering the medication must not know the contents of the syringe. Therefore, we select research assistants (perhaps medical students) to administer the drug. The research assistants are not told what the drug is supposed to do and they do not know the contents of the syringes. To control for bias, it is important for all participants and researchers involved to think they are getting the "active" materials rather than the placebo. Double-blind studies are set up this way because knowing which group received the active ingredient may alter the data, akin to when a patient changes respiratory rate while it is being counted or the way providers change their behavior while their supervisor is watching.

Prior to the day of the experiment, the subjects are all given the same instructions as to diet, physical activity, and travel to the site of the experiment. They are also asked to complete a questionnaire that asks them about any factors that might affect the outcome of the experiment (although the questionnaire may not have indicated the nature of the experiment to prevent bias). Participants are informed of the risks and rewards of the study and sign an informed consent form developed by the facility's **Institutional Review Board (IRB)**. On the day of the experiment, the subjects' vital signs are recorded, the drug or placebo is administered, and the subjects' vital signs are retaken at the appropriate time(s).

Using this step-by-step approach, we can be confident that if there is a significant increase in heart rate in the experimental group, and if there is a significant difference in heart rates between the experimental and control groups (i.e., their distribution curves are significantly different), then the effects can be attributed to the drug. The benefit of a double-blind, randomized control study is that the data are "pure" and reliable, but as shown in the previous example, these studies require considerable planning, procedures, and time, which may not be available in the field.

Quasi-Experiment

One of the problems with the gold standard is that some types of problems or environments do not lend themselves to randomization. If we were to do a study to test the effect of epinephrine on cardiac arrest in the field, we could not randomly assign subjects to the condition of cardiac arrest. Nor would many paramedics, or medical directors, feel comfortable with ambulances carrying syringes that might contain either epinephrine or water. In the MAST study, researchers could not randomly assign subjects to be hypotensive (or traumatized), and the rescuers could certainly not be blind to whether they were using the MAST. Under such circumstances, researchers use what is called the **quasi-experimental model**.

In the MAST study, patients who met the research criteria were assigned, on alternate days, to the MAST or no-MAST groups. After the study period, the two groups were compared on the basis of age, sex, race, injury etiology, injury severity score, and trauma score. In a total population of 784 patients, the two groups were statistically identical for those indices. Therefore, the researchers felt comfortable with their findings that the overall mortality of 31% in the MAST group compared to 25% in the no-MAST group was statistically significant ($p = 0.05$) (Bickell et al., 1987). The $p = 0.05$ equation means that there was a 5% or less probability that the outcome could have occurred.

The Research Study

The components of a research study include a series of steps to formulate the research question or hypothesis, test the hypothesis, analyze the results, and make the findings known. The steps of a research study are the following:

- Identify the problem or question.
- Review the literature.
- Formulate a hypothesis.
- Define the team.
- Design the study.
- Perform the study.
- Analyze the data.
- Use the information.
- Share the findings.

Identify the Problem or Question

Problem identification occurs the moment someone says that something is wrong and must be fixed, or that something can be done better. In some studies, researchers have made statements such as: "There are too many ambulance collisions;" "There are too many pediatric drownings;" and "Do MAST really work?" These types of statements promote thinking and help researchers realize the opportunities for improvement. They may also inspire others (e.g., funding agencies) to support the research project. The problem then has to be translated into a bounded question that can be researched. For example, "there are too many pediatric drownings" might be the perceived problem, but the research question might be "what effect does an outreach effort to encourage homeowners to install fences have on the number of pediatric drownings per year?"—a quantitative approach. Qualitative research on the same subject may consist of interviews and visits to a sample of the drowning sites to identify ways in which the sites and trends in the attitudes toward water safety can be improved.

Review the Literature

The next step, the literature review, is to see if anyone has already answered the question or if anyone has done research that will assist in answering the question. There is a wealth of available sources for this research that can be divided into a few different categories. The first is information available in scientific peer-reviewed journals. Peer-reviewed, referred journal articles are always the best sources of information, but there are a variety of sources available to researchers. In the medical profession, these papers are cataloged in databases such as Medline or PubMed. Other professions also have peer-reviewed papers cataloged in a variety of databases. EMS, nursing, and other health-care professions have peer-reviewed and non–peer-reviewed papers cataloged in a database called CINAHL.

A second common resource for information and data is the Internet, including online databases. Search engines can direct us to governmental databases, newspaper articles, and a variety of organizational and private webpages. Researchers must be cautious when using these sources. Peer-reviewed journal articles have been thoroughly critiqued by knowledgeable experts to ensure that the findings are valid and reliable. Information found on the Internet may not have had such rigorous evaluation. While there are good sources of information found on the web, such as Google's Scholar search engine (scholar.google.com), other sources such as Wikipedia (www.wikipedia.org) should be used sparingly, as anyone can change Wikipedia and it is neither peer reviewed nor referenced in most cases. Wikipedia should only be used for background information, not as a reference itself.

Finally, textbooks can also be a rich source of information. Libraries and commercial book retailers have searchable databases for textbooks. Textbooks tend to become dated quickly, but may provide a resource for foundational information of a study.

Formulate a Hypothesis

The hypothesis is the declaration to be proved or the outcome expected by the researcher; for example, "Drug x will cause an increase in heart rate" or "The prehospital use of MAST improves survival rates for trauma patients."

Researchers and statisticians use two terms when describing the hypothesis. The null hypothesis states that no significant difference will exist between the control (placebo) and experimental (intervention) groups; for example, "There is no difference in survival rates between prehospital trauma patients treated without MAST and those who were treated with MAST."

The alternate hypothesis states that a significant difference will be seen between the two groups; for example, "Subjects in the experimental group will experience an increase in heart rate," or "Prehospital trauma patients treated with MAST will have improved survival rates."

Statisticians operate under the assumption that the alternate hypothesis can never be proved. That is, they are never 100% confident that drug x, for example, really does increase heart rate. Therefore, the statistical tests are designed to either prove the null hypothesis or disprove the alternate hypothesis.

Define The Team

Determine who else is affected by the issue, who may benefit from the findings, and what expertise is required for the project (e.g., a statistician or epidemiologist). Are there specific skills that team members will need? Who has those skills? What other perspectives may be useful to answer the research question?

In the Pinnellas County example, paramedics teamed up with physicians, nurses, firefighters, public health officials, and local elected officials. All provided valuable perspectives and resources to the process. Having such a team may also be valuable when attempting to implement changes based on the research findings. For example, if an EMS agency experiments with a new type of intervention but does not include the medical community in the process, the agency may be blocked from implementing changes regardless of the research findings.

If human subjects are used in an experiment, it is important to get approval from the appropriate IRB before the experiment is conducted. The IRB, among other things, ensures that the following ethical guidelines are adhered to (Davis & Maio, 1993):

- Subjects give **voluntary consent**.
- All potential hazards are explained to the subjects.
- The research results may offer benefits to society.
- The research is based (when applicable) on animal models.
- Each subject can stop participating at any time in the experiment.

For some research, these guidelines may be untenable. Therefore, the U.S. Department of Health and Human Services (DHHS) has approved waiver regulations. To qualify for the waiver, four conditions must be met:

1. The research could not be practically carried out without a waiver.
2. Whenever appropriate, the subject will be provided with additional pertinent information after participation.
3. The research involves no more than minimal risk to the subjects.
4. The waiver will not adversely affect the rights and welfare of the subjects.

The agency medical director will likely be the liaison with the IRB. It is important to meet with the IRB early in the research-design phase and recognize that the IRB will be an integral part of the research team. The IRB may be part of the hospital the researcher is working with, the research organization itself, or a university. Requirements vary by board, and many IRBs have tightened their requirements, especially for waivers. Conducting prehospital research on subjects who cannot give informed consent, such as in research on cardiac arrest patients, may require public education efforts before the study and time for public comment before any research can be completed.

All types of research require IRB approval, even if the researcher is only looking back at old data or patient care reports. IRBs are designed to protect the welfare of the public and to ensure that the data is used responsibly. When in doubt, contact your representative IRB and ask what requirements it may have. Any data the researcher desires to have published should receive IRB approval before a publisher even looks at it.

Design the Study

Experiments can be quantitative or qualitative; observational or interventional; retrospective or prospective; open, blinded, or double-blinded; quasi-experimental or experimental. Observational and interventional models were discussed previously. **Retrospective** and **prospective** refer to the time the observations are made. For example, a typical retrospective analysis is a chart review of all patients who were seen in the past three years. The observational data is based in the past. A typical prospective study is the drug x example. A study is designed, a subject is selected, an intervention is made, and the results are recorded. The observational data is made in the present.

Open, blinded, and double-blinded refer to the knowledge of the participants and researchers. For example, in the drug x example, an open model, the subject and the physician both know the contents of the syringe. In a blinded model, the subject would not know the contents of the syringe, but the physician would. In a double-blinded model, neither the subject nor the physician knows the contents of the syringe. The quasi-experimental and experimental models were discussed previously.

Consider the data sources, what will be measured, and how the measurement will be performed. When creating data collection instruments (e.g., data from questionnaires, observations, response to stimuli), begin by assessing the reliability and validity of the instrument.

Reliability means that repeated observations by different people at different times are in agreement. A straightforward example is the pulse check in the hypothetical drug test discussed earlier. Different people taking the same patient's pulse at the same time should record the same rate. Furthermore, the results should be consistent every day of the experiment. There may be statistically insignificant variances in sampling procedure, but larger variances will decrease the statistical significance of the data.

Validity means that the instrument is measuring what it is meant to measure. For example, using MAST on healthy subjects may not be a valid means of determining the effect they will have on traumatized, hypotensive patients.

Controlling for Bias

A **bias** is an influence that distorts the results of a test. The best defense against inadvertent bias is to be aware of its common causes. They include:

- *History.* This may include personnel changes. For example, if the hypotension study was begun using senior physicians to take the blood pressure, and nursing students performed that role later, it may be possible that a change in blood pressure over time was in some way due to the change in the person performing the test.

- *Maturation.* Will subjects themselves change over time (e.g., will their blood pressure improve even without treatment)?

- *Repeated measure.* This is the change in the subjects' responses after being tested the same way repeated times.

- *Regression toward the mean.* This problem is most noticeable when subjects are chosen from the extremes of the distribution curve. In the hypotension study example, if only subjects with extremely high blood pressure were chosen in the beginning, subsequent measures will tend to be closer to the average, even without an intervention.

- *Instrument decay.* Change in the performance or operation of equipment from the beginning to the end of the experiment.

- *Subject selection.* Research will often be designed to predict the effects of an intervention on the general population. Therefore, subjects should be randomly selected from the general population and not from one particular group.

- *Loss of subjects.* Do the subjects lost to attrition differ in any way from the rest of the subjects?

- *Investigator bias.* The researcher, too, can unintentionally influence the outcome of an experiment. This is particularly true of qualitative studies in which the investigator may also be the investigation tool, as in conducting the interview. There is an old story of a horse that could count. People were amazed and came from miles away to see the horse. A person would shout out a number and the horse would tap his foot exactly the right number of times. A skeptical scientist put a sheet in front of the horse to block his view of the people. The horse suddenly lost his amazing ability. It turned out that the horse was simply reacting to the body language of the people in the room; he would tap his foot until they started smiling.

The same effect can be seen in medicine. A doctor believes a drug will work a certain way, the patient is told this is how it will work, and, after administration, the patient begins to behave as if the drug worked in the described manner.

Sample Size

The question of adequate sample size has perplexed many researchers. The competing objectives are:

1. To have enough subjects to ensure that any changes noted are the result of the intervention and not the result of chance. When researchers indicate "$p < 0.05$," it points to the results of a statistical test proving that there was less than a 5% probability that the results occurred by chance. In order to arrive at this conclusion, the study must have an adequate number of subjects.

2. To avoid having too many subjects. An overabundance of subjects may make the research unwieldy, very costly, or both.

The best way to determine sample size is to employ a statistician to calculate the minimum number of subjects needed for the experiment.

Perform the Study

This is the moment to administer the drug, turn on the machine, teach the class, and so on. Extensive planning in the design phase will ensure that this component of the study is implemented appropriately. This is also when data is collected. The 2000 presidential election's "hanging chad" problem is an excellent example of the problems researchers may face during data collection. Because it was not specified in advance, there was a great deal of debate about whether ballots that were not punched through entirely should be counted. Anticipating these problems in advance may save a researcher (or an election worker) many hours of recounting.

Analyze the Data

The first issue to evaluate is whether the research answers the question. Also consider the demographic characteristics of the subjects: How do they relate to the population in terms of age, gender, race, and experience? What correlation exists between the interventions and the outcomes? What else was learned?

Use the Information

The information can be used in a variety of ways. The findings can help solve problems, reduce risks, and improve health. The findings are also used to constantly improve the process and outcomes. In many fields, there is usually no one "right" answer or "right" way to do something. Instead, managers, clinicians, and researchers use the "best" way based on currently available information. Ongoing research reevaluates this best way and seeks to find better ways.

Share the Findings

EMS professionals are typically very creative. Over the years, a plethora of innovative practices have been implemented. Unfortunately, many of the experiences have not been shared. This has meant that EMS agencies must repeatedly "reinvent the wheel." As a profession, we all pay the cost when limited resources are used on basic problems instead of on creating new opportunities.

An early example of one paper that had a great influence on the profession is the research article published by Pantridge and Geddes (1966). Their description of prehospital advanced life support inspired the world. There are other reasons to publish:

- It is what scientists (and professionals) do.
- It is a hallmark of the profession.
- It helps create a strong professional community.
- It is good for patient care.
- There may be some personal benefit in terms of professional, academic, or monetary recognition.
- It provides academic credibility for the profession.

Another way that EMS providers share their findings is through presentations at professional conferences.

Such conferences are an ideal means of not only sharing research findings but also of meeting people who are interested in either the findings or the research itself. Good research practices are outlined in **Table 14-1**.

Table 14-1 Good Research Practices

- Be open-minded.
- Use common sense.
- Think of yourself as the user as well as the supplier of information.
- Be creative.
- Be confident.
- Be consistent and care about the details.
- Develop your ability to communicate.
- Be honest.
- Have fun.
- Finally, a quote from one of the most important philosophers of the late 20th century, Gene Roddenberry: "In every revolution, there is one man with a vision." Be a visionary.

Future Challenges

The scientific method works especially well with precise experiments conducted in controlled laboratories. In the drug example used earlier, to test the efficacy of a new drug designed to increase heart rate, an experimenter would bring a group of subjects to the lab, take their pulse, administer the drug, wait x minutes, and retake the pulse.

When we combine this simple approach with an adequate sample size, random selection of subjects, placebos, and the double-blind method, we can be confident that our results will be both reliable and valid. We will be confident, based on the results, that the drug either does or does not increase heart rate.

If, on the other hand, the question is, "Does CPR work?" then the challenges include the following: we do not have controlled laboratories, we cannot randomly assign citizens (e.g., to the condition "cardiac arrest patient"), and we cannot randomly assign patients to the treatment (CPR) and placebo (no CPR) groups. In addition, many of the factors affecting outcome occur before patients arrive in the "laboratory" (the ambulance) and after they leave (i.e., their time in the hospital).

Furthermore, many EMS interventions cannot (or should not) be measured in isolation. That is, many EMS practices work, or do not work, largely because of influences from the entire system. For example, measuring cardiac arrest outcomes based on the quality of the field providers' CPR skills would obviously not account for the myriad influences on cardiac arrest outcomes. These influences include the entire chain of survival from pre-event system design through public education, 9-1-1 operations, EMS training, vehicles, equipment and hospital designation, resources, and staffing.

Using Research in EMS

As more research becomes available, the next challenge is how to integrate findings into everyday practice. The issue of how to use research or EBM in practice is not only a problem for EMS, but for medicine overall. The fact that providers are still utilizing MAST 25 years after this application has been shown to have accounted for higher mortality in patients (Bickell et al., 1987) helps illustrate that the system does not currently embrace research or have a method to change practice.

Methods are available to use data to change your system, but EMS needs to adopt EBM as a way of everyday practice. (See chapter 13 for discussion of use of data.) Protocols that are out of date, not based in sound research, or based on personal opinions need to be changed. Practitioners then must be educated on the research, put the changes into practice, and conduct further research to determine whether the changes were effective. This is a monumental task.

WRAP UP

Summary

To meet the challenges of EMS-related research, EMS professionals must be resourceful, knowledgeable, and creative. There must be support for research projects and all EMS personnel must be familiarized with the importance of ongoing research into all aspects of EMS operations. EMS professionals must keep up to date on changes in the literature and be able to read and analyze research to find ways to improve the EMS system as a whole.

Key Terms

alternate hypothesis
bias
double-blind, randomized
   control study experimental
   design (DBRCS)
experimental procedures
hypothesis
institutional review board (IRB)
interventional study

literature review
null hypothesis
observational study
placebo
population
prospective analysis
qualitative research
quantitative research
quasi-experimental model

reliability
representative samples
research
retrospective analysis
scientific method
standard deviations
standard distribution curve
validity
voluntary consent

Review Questions

1. Using an EMS-related magazine or journal, identify a study that supports the null hypothesis.
2. Discuss the difference between reliability and validity.
3. Discuss the reasons for using a team approach when doing EMS research.
4. Write an example of a null hypothesis.
5. Give examples of where both quantitative and qualitative research would be useful in your EMS system.

Additional Resources

Bickell, W. H., Pepe, R. E., Wyatt, C. H., Dedo, W. R., Applebaum, D. J., Black, C. T., & Mattox, K. L. (1985, March). Effect of antishock trousers on the trauma score: A prospective analysis in the urban setting. *Annals of Emergency Medicine, 14*(3), 218–222.

Bickell, W. H., Pepe, R. E., Bailey, M. L.,Wyatt, C. H., & Mattox, K. L. (1987, June). Randomized trial of pneumatic antishock garments in the prehospital management of penetrating abdominal injuries. *Annals of Emergency Medicine, 16*(6), 653–658.

Davis, E. A., & Maio, R. F. (1993, January-March). Ethical issues in prehospital research. *Prehospital and Disaster Medicine, 8*(1), Supplement S11–S14.

Goldberg, R. J., Zautcke, J. L., Koenigsberg, M. D., Lee, R. W., Nagorka, F. W., & Kling, M. W. (1990, May). A review of prehospital care litigation in a large metropolitan EMS system. *Annals of Emergency Medicine, 19*(5), 557–561.

Harrawood, D., Gunderson, M. R., Fravel, S., Cartwright, K., & Ryan, J. L. (1994, June). Drowning prevention: A case study in EMS epidemiology. *Journal of Emergency Medical Services, 1–9*(6), 34–38, 40–41.

Joyce, S. M., Dutkowski, K. L., & Hynes, T. (1997, July–September). Efficacy of an EMS quality improvement program in improving documentation and performance. *Prehospital Emergency Care, 1*(3), 140–144.

Maguire, B. J., & Porco, F. V. (1997a, June). An eight year review of legal cases related to an urban 911 paramedic service. *Prehospital and Disaster Medicine, 12*(2), 83–86.

Maguire, B. J., & Porco, F. V. (1997b, November). Vehicle safety issues related to the provision of emergency medical services. *Emergency Medical Services, 26*(11), 39–78.

Mattox, K. L., Bickell, W. H., Pepe, P. E., & Mangelsdorff, A. D. (1986, September). Prospective randomized evaluation of antishock MAST in post-traumatic hypotension. *Journal of Trauma-Injury Infection & Critical Care, 26*(9), 779–786.

Mattox, K. L., Bickell, W., Pepe, P. E., Burch, J., & Feliciano, D. (1989, August). Prospective MAST study in 911 patients. *Journal of Trauma-Injury Infection & Critical Care, 29*(8), 1104–1111; discussion 1111–1112.

Pantridge, J. F., & Geddes, J. S. (1966). Cardiac arrest after myocardial infarction. *Lancet, 1:* 808–808.

Pepe, P. E., Bass, R. R., & Mattox, K. L. (1986, December). Clinical trials of the pneumatic antishock garment in the urban prehospital setting. *Annals of Emergency Medicine, 15*(12), 1407–1410.

Soler, J. M., Montes, M. F., Egol, A. B., Nateman, H. R., Donaldson, E. A., & Greene, H. H. (1985, October). The ten-year malpractice experience of a large urban EMS system. *Annals of Emergency Medicine, 14*(10), 982–985.

Fire and Emergency Services Higher Education (FESHE) Course Correlation Grid

FOUNDATIONS OF EMS SYSTEMS

Course Description:	An overview of the design and operation of EMS systems, delivery of services, and the echelons of care. The history of EMS, the interface of public and private organizations, and review of the various personnel who comprise these systems will be examined in relation to their impact on the health care delivery system.	***Foundations of EMS Systems, Third Edition*** Chapter Reference
Prerequisite:	None.	
Outcomes:	1. Define EMS System.	1
	2. List the 15 components of EMS Systems and the 14 attributes.	1
	3. Recall important milestones in the evolution of EMS.	2
	4. Describe the federal role in EMS.	2, 10
	5. Describe the role of state government in EMS.	2, 10
	6. Identify laws and legislation associated with EMS.	10
	7. Describe the levels of prehospital care providers.	3
	8. Describe medical oversight.	6, 8
	9. Identify various configurations of EMS delivery systems.	5
	10. Summarize the recommendations and findings in *"EMS Education Agenda for the Future."*	4
	11. State the role of public education and prevention in EMS.	11
	12. Describe the role of EMS in disasters.	12
	13. State role of communications and communications technology in EMS.	7
	14. Identify the fundamentals of emergency medical dispatching.	7
	15. Describe the sources of EMS funding.	9
	16. Describe the role of information systems and evaluation in EMS.	13
	17. Summarize the role of research in EMS.	14

14 attributes Essential components of an EMS system listed in the EMS Agenda for the Future.

2002 Guidelines for Educating EMS Instructors Guidelines prepared by the National Association of EMS Educators (NAEMSE) for the EMS Office of NHTSA to provide the basis for most instructor training courses.

A

Academy The focal point of training in the fire service.

Accident rooms Foreign terminology for an Emergency Room.

Accountable care organization A form of healthcare organization where the healthcare system (hospital) is financially responsible for patient outcomes.

Accreditation Approval that a program meets the minimum requirements of the national guidelines.

Administrative law Laws related to the rules and regulations passed by a governmental agency.

Advanced EMT (AEMT) A provider level standard for prehospital providers who provide advanced care above the EMT level.

Advanced life support (ALS) Emergency medical care for sustaining life, including defibrillation, airway management, and drugs and medications.

Agent Energy.

Air medical transport The transportation of critical patients by aircraft, usually a helicopter.

Air medical units Helicopter or fixed-wing aircraft used to transport critical patients.

Algorithm A flowchart that outlines patient care for specific emergencies from patient assessment to management.

Allied healthcare A group of medically prescribed health care services, such as occupational therapy, speech pathology, and physical therapy, provided by licensed professionals.

Allied health professionals Professionals who provide allied health care services.

Alms houses Facilities that developed to care for individuals, such as the poor, orphans, and the insane, who did not have families to provide care.

ALS intercept A nontransport vehicle staffed with advanced life support providers who respond to upgrade basic life support teams.

Alternate hypothesis A statement that a significant difference will be seen in the two groups involved in an experiment.

Ambulance diversion Ambulances taking patients to other hospitals as a result of overcrowded emergency departments or system deficiencies.

Ambulance Service Manager An individual who oversees daily operation of an EMS service.

American Red Cross Standard and Advanced First Aid The de facto training standard for ambulance personnel until the early 1970s.

Analysis The assessment of data collected and the transformation of the data into actionable information that can be used to improve the overall system.

Antiseptic techniques The process of providing for a clean process.

Assessment The detailed process of determining the physical and mental status of a patient.

Asynchronous learning Availability of resources for learning that can occur in any place and at any time.

Automatic tracking and status notification System used to continuously update a computer-aided dispatch system via radio.

Automobile extrication The process of removing a vehicle from an entrapped patient to gain access.

B

Bad debt Fee-for-service charges that go unpaid for some reason.

Baldrige Criteria for Performance Excellence Criteria established to use as a tool by organizations to evaluate their overall performance and effectiveness.

Basic and Advanced Red Cross First Aid First aid courses developed by the American Red Cross. Standard training for EMS personnel prior to EMT.

Bias An influence that distorts the results of the test.

Biotelemetry Electronic transmission of patient physiological parameters such as an ECG.

Black box The transformation process wherein the input is processed or changed in some way by the system or is affected by it with the resulting product being the output.

Block grants A lump sum of money to be used in broad targeted areas, giving the states more leeway in how to spend it.

Boarding The process of leaving patients in either the ED or on an EMS stretcher due to lack of facilities to admit a patient to a floor of a hospital.

Burnout Result of working and stress in an understaffed, high-demand system.

C

Cadavers Dead bodies, especially intended for dissection or skills practice.

Call takers Persons who answer 9-1-1 line.

Cardiopulmonary resuscitation (CPR) The uses of mouth to mouth ventilations and chest compressions to revive an individual suffering from heart attacks and sudden death.

Career provider An individual whose primary job is in the emergency services.

Categorical funding Funding given by the government to support specific programs or initiatives.

Categorization A process whereby emergency departments in a particular region designate the services they are capable of providing.

Centers for Medicare and Medicaid Services Federal agency responsible for managing payments for federally and state-funded healthcare programs in the United States.

Central transmission system System capable of delivering a signal over the entire service area.

Certification Testing of an individual to ensure that they meet the minimum competency level.

Certifying examination The process whereby an EMS provider proves competency by both written and practice examinations.

Chase vehicle A motor vehicle that is used to transport personnel (nurses, physicians, paramedics) with advanced training to the scene of an incident to aid the basic level personnel.

Chief Medical Officer (CMO) (1) Person who heads the Office of Health Affairs at DHS. (2) The senior operational officer of an EMS service.

City dispensary A facility developed to provide medical care to the poor.

Clinical behaviors and judgments Appropriate actions completed to treat and assess a patient in the field.

Clinical Time in the field (hospital or pre-hospital) that provides on the job training experience.

Clinical data Data directly related to the assessment, treatment, and clinical outcomes of injuries and illnesses.

COBRA See Consolidated Omnibus Budget Reconciliation Act.

Code of Federal Regulations (CFR) Federal regulations derived by federal agencies.

Combination departments Departments where volunteers and career staff work together for fire and/or EMS services.

Commercial insurance Health insurance provided by a commercial company.

Commission on Accreditation of Allied Health Education Programs (CAAHEP) An organization formed to review and recommend accreditation of allied health programs.

Committee on Accreditation of Emergency Medical Services Professions (CoAEMSP) A body of the CAAHEP that serves to review and recommend programs for accreditation of all levels of EMS provider.

Common law Rules and regulations derived from English common law based upon judicial precedent.

Community paramedic A new model of care which utilizes EMS providers in non-emergency roles including long term and preventative care.

Competency Condition of being sufficiently qualified to perform a particular action. To achieve this condition, one must possess the proper knowledge, skills, training, and professionalism.

Component processes Measures of the processes within the key performance indicators.

Computer-aided dispatch (CAD) The use of computer software to track unit status and dispatch appropriate equipment to an incident.

Congressional caucuses They serve to organize members of Congress that have a particular interest in supporting a specific cause.

Consensus standards Rules and regulations developed by professional associations and trade groups related to a particular occupation or service.

Consolidated Omnibus Budget Reconciliation Act (COBRA) Requires hospitals that receive Medicare funding to provide initial assessment and stabilization for any individual presenting to an ED or for a woman in active labor. It also presents a guideline for patient transfers; also known as EMTALA.

Constitutional law Rules and regulations derived from the U.S. Constitution; examples are civil rights and due process.

Contact hours A measurement of the field or clinical experience of an EMS provider.

Continuing education Helps field providers to remain updated with current developments as well as provides a means for reviewing areas identified through quality assurance assessments as needing attention.

Continuing Education Coordinating Board for EMS (CECBEMS) A board established to approve continuing education programs and assign CEU to particular programs.

Continuing education unit (CEU) For courses taken to maintain minimum levels of certification a designated unit is assigned per number of hours of course work.

Continuous quality improvement (CQI) Monitoring the quality of care provided and ensuring that quality is maintained and continually improved based upon outcome evaluation.

Core content It represents the breadth of EMS clinical practice, outlines the content at risk for examination in EMS, serves as a guide in the development of provider and continuing medical education programs for those involved in the delivery of EMS care.

Cost indicator A measurement of the costs related to implementation of a process.

cost shift Process of covering costs of unreimbursed care by increasing the cost of reimbursed care.

Crash Injury Management for Law Enforcement Officers (CIMFLEO) The original 40-hour course that evolved into Fire Responder training program and now EMR training.

Critical care intensivists Nonsurgical physicians dealing with the continued care of critical patients.

Critical care transport The moving of a critical patient (one needing life support measures) from one facility to another.

Critical incident stress management (CISM) A systematic approach to prevent and mitigate traumatic stress in emergency personnel.

Critical patient areas Patient populations that require some specific specialized care.

Cross-functional team A group composed of suppliers, processors, and customers in a system.

D

Data A record of an event in time.

Data formats Pieces of information that are precisely defined in regard to the form in which the data is obtained and stored.

Data validation A method of ensuring the accuracy of the data obtained and entered into a system.

Defibrillate The use of electrical shocks to stimulate the heart to pump.

Definitive care Refers to care provided to patients which fixes or solves their current medical issues.

Department of Homeland Security (DHS) Department formed by combining numerous federal law enforcement and emergency management agencies into one entity post-9/11 to provide oversight for national safety and response.

Designation The process whereby a hospital is legally approved to provide a specialized service.

Destination protocols Protocols created while regionalizing EMS services to properly direct the patients to the right hospitals that will provide the best possible care for their particular emergency.

Didactic Classroom instruction. EMS professionals require to complete this course to obtain certification.

Direct medical oversight Real-time physician involvement in a patient encounter with EMS providers; also known as online medical oversight.

Disaster Any destructive, dangerous, or life-threatening situation that overwhelms the resources of a community.

Disease process The lifecycle of a condition for a patient over time.

Dispatch center A central location for receiving and dispatching 9-1-1 calls and coordinating system communications. May be the PSAP or part of the PSAP.

Dispatch life support (DLS) Describes emergency medical dispatching, priority dispatching, and prearrival instructions.

Distance learning, distance education, distributed learning, technology-enhanced learning See asynchronous learning.

Double blind, randomized control study experimental design Each subject has the same chance of being in the control group as the experimental group and neither the researcher nor the subject is aware of the interventions being used.

E

National EMS educational standards National set of expectations for the training of EMS professionals.

Educators Teachers of EMS and other programs.

Electronic Patient Care Records (ePCR) A computerized method of documentation of patient care.

Emergency department A department within a hospital that provides stabilizing care for urgent and emergent conditions. Formally known as the Emergency Room.

Emergency Management Assistance Compact A federally enabled system that most states have signed on that allows states to send mutual aid in the form of personnel and resources to disaster-stricken states.

Emergency medical dispatch (EMD) The process of sending the right units to the right location with the right resources.

Emergency medical responder (EMR) The lowest level of EMS provider.

Emergency Medical Services at the Crossroads An IOM report which detailed the current status of the EMS system in the United States and made a series of recommendations for improvement.

Emergency medical services attributes The 14 attributes that are used to assist local planners and administrators in establishing EMS systems and as benchmarks for evaluating existing programs.

Emergency Medical Services for Children (EMS-C) A program established to focus on the special needs of children in the EMS system.

Emergency medical services (EMS) system System that provides for the arrangement of personnel, facilities, and equipment for the effective and coordinated delivery in an appropriate geographical area of health care services under emergency conditions.

Emergency Medical Services Systems Act of 1973 Governmental legislation that established the 15 components of an EMS system and provided federal funds for systems meeting these requirements.

Emergency Medical Technician (EMT) The basic provider level standard for ambulance attendants.

Emergency Medical Technician-Ambulance (EMT-A) standards Standards established in the 1960s that the ambulance attendants had to be trained to meet.

Emergency Medical Technician—Basic An individual trained to assess and manage patients at the BLS level. The minimum level of training for ambulance personnel.

Emergency Medical Technician—Intermediate An individual who provides minimal advanced life support for medical and trauma patients.

Emergency Medical Technician—Paramedic An individual who can provide advanced life support using a diagnostic approach. The highest level of prehospital providers.

Emergency Medical Treatment and Active Labor Law (EMTALA) Requires hospitals that receive Medicare funding to provide initial assessment and stabilization for any individual presenting to an ED or for a woman in active labor. It also presents guidelines for patient transfers; also known as COBRA.

Emergency planning committees Committees established at the local and regional levels to evaluate hazards and threats to health and safety.

EMS Agenda for the Future A consensus document that outlines a future approach for EMS.

EMS coordinator Person designated by an agency to be the official liaison between the agency and local EMS services.

EMS Education Agenda for the Future: A Systems Approach An extension of the EMS Agenda for the Future, the education agenda provides guidelines for implementation of curriculum, testing, and accreditation.

EMS national standard training curriculum Curriculum for which the federal DOT's EMS Division within NHTSA used to guide education of EMS providers throughout the United States.

Engine company personnel Personnel from a fire engine company who were historically not trained to provide even rudimentary first aid.

Enhanced 9-1-1 System Provides the PSAP with the caller's phone number and the street address.

Environment The surroundings in which an injury occurs.

Epidemiological model A projection and explanation of the expected progression of a disease outbreak such as pandemic flu.

Essentials Minimum standards to meet for accreditation.

Evacuation The process of ridding the body of fluids that disrupted balance and tone.

Event-driven resource deployment A type of delivery system that matches resources to predicted demand based upon data and historical patterns.

Evidence-based best practices Best practices developed implementing methods of diagnosis and treatment on the basis of the best available current research.

Evidence-based medicine The use of scientific data to confirm that proposed diagnostic or therapeutic procedures are appropriate in light of their high probability of producing the best and most favorable outcome.

Experimental procedures Neutral and repeatable procedures used to test a hypothesis to screen out biases and preconceptions about the validity of the hypothesis being tested.

External customers Customers receiving the services provided by the organization such as the public.

F

Federal Interagency Committee on EMS (FICEMS) A joint agency headed by NHTSA to organize multiple federal agencies that oversee EMS.

Fee-for-service A transaction in which the patient pays directly for the services that are rendered.

Fee schedule A form of prospective payment.

Field instruction Instruction that takes place within an operational EMS system.

Fire and Emergency Services Higher Education project (FESHE) EMS management curriculum model developed by the National Fire Academy to provide an educational pathway for EMS Professionals within college environments.

Firefighter First Responder (FFFR) A course developed to train firefighters in first aid.

First aid clubs Historically clubs formed in mining and industrial towns to teach first aid to workers.

First responder An individual trained to provide initial lifesaving assessment and intervention using minimal equipment.

Fixed-post staffing A type of delivery system in which all response teams operate from a fixed station and the same number of units are available at all times.

Flight nurse A registered nurse who is trained to provide emergency care while in flight.

Flight paramedic A paramedic trained to provide care while in flight.

G

General anesthetics Anesthetics used to induce general anesthesia, that is, the induction of a state of unconsciousness with the absence of pain sensation over the entire body.

General fund Fund maintained by the government for various EMS activities and services, where excess funds available are returned to.

General hospitals Hospitals designed to provide a wide range of medical services within a community setting.

Geographic information systems Systems that present different layers of information about local response areas and infrastructure from many different perspectives; facilitate mapping and comparing incident demand and type with local demographics.

Global positioning system (GPS) A worldwide system utilizing satellites to provide precise geographic location information.

Guidelines for Air Medical Crew Education Published by the association of air medical services, provides guidelines for additional skills beyond the Paramedic, RN and RRT levels, specifically for air based medicine.

H

Haddon's matrix A concept used to determine factors affecting the extent of injury from which prevention strategies or interventions may be designed.

Handheld radios Small, portable radios that allow personnel to remain in contact with the dispatcher when away from their vehicle over a limited distance.

Hazard A dangerous event or circumstance that may or may not lead to an emergency or disaster.

Hazard analysis The methods used to identify, locate, assess risks, and map risks on a community map.

Heroic medicine The aggressive treatment of disorders through the use of techniques such as evacuation and restorative therapies.

High-fidelity human simulation A simulation model developed to impart an educational experience as real and intense as actual patient encounters. Simulators breathe, speak, have a pulse and otherwise mimic actual patients.

High-volume systems Systems in which the number of emergencies handled are high.

Host An injured person.

Humoral theory Theory that explained illness in terms of imbalances in the four humors: blood, phlegm, black bile, and yellow bile.

Hybrid paper forms Forms that utilize paper and electronic processes to reduce the need for manually entering data into a computer system.

Hypothesis A tentative explanation for an observation, phenomenon, or scientific problem that can be tested by further investigation.

I

Incident command system (ICS) An organized method of managing a large-scale incident.

Indirect medical oversight Physician input that is administrative, involving all facets of emergency medical service, but remote from patient care; also known as off -line medical oversight and system medical oversight.

Information Data placed within a framework or context to give it meaning.

Injury Any unintentional or intentional damage to the body resulting from acute exposure to energy.

Injury prevention and control The process of using knowledge about the injury event to design prevention programs and evaluate their success.

Injury prevention interventions Methods used to identify injury prevention and control methods. Classified into three groups: engineering, enforcement, and education.

Input Input is what enters a system.

Institutional review board (IRB) A group of individuals whose purpose is to ensure that an experiment is being done following ethical guidelines.

Instructional guidelines Guidelines that provide additional information to assist the instructor in the transition to the National EMS Educational Standards from the traditional national standard curriculums.

Intentional injuries Damage caused by the desire to induce harm upon one's self.

Inter-facility transports Transporting a patient from one healthcare facility to another.

Internal customers Customers within an organization.

Interventional study Events are influenced by the researcher and then analyzed for the effects.

Issue caucuses A group of congressmen who support the issue and agree to work together to support legislation supportive of that issue.

K

Key processes Processes whether clinical, operational, and administrative that form the basis for quality management in an EMS organization.

KKK-A-1822 General Services Administration specifications of ambulances.

L

Lead agency The governmental agency at the federal or state level responsible for EMS-related issues and regulation.

Learning management systems Usually an electronic system that provides educational content and tracking (such as eLearning).

Legislation Bills or proposed laws that can affect the way practice is carried out and how EMS systems are controlled by the government.

Licensure Authorizes an individual to provide care based upon proof that the individual has met the minimum competency level.

Literature review Analyzing and researching documentation and publications to synthesize the state-of-the-art knowledge base about a specific subject.

M

Make ready Primary function of vehicle service technicians hired by providers where the technicians wash and stock ambulances and make them ready for the crew to start the service.

Mass casualty incident A disaster with over 100 victims.

Medevac Use of aircraft to transport critical patients.

Medicaid A program in which state and federal funds are used to compensate health care providers for services to program enrollees who otherwise are not able to pay for the services.

Medical command/medical direction Physician involvement in emergency medical service.

Medical communications All communication involved in online medical control and notification of receiving facilities.

Medical control Control provided by a physician who oversees the practice of EMS professionals. See also Medical Director.

Medical director A physician who oversees the practice of EMTs and paramedics.

Medical interrogation A process in the comprehensive pathway management system included in nonemergency triage, which involves interrogating to determine patients whose condition does not require an EMS response.

Medical oversight Physical involvement in emergency medical services to ensure quality of care and support.

Medical specialty The process of specializing in one area of medicine to develop an in-depth understanding of a small segment of patients.

Medicare Federally funded health care program for the elderly.

Medium duty ambulance A Type I ambulance mounted on a medium duty truck chassis.

Mitigation Any efforts to identify, classify, and eliminate hazards and reduce the potential that they might produce a disaster.

Mobile Army Surgical Hospitals (MASH) Hospitals introduced during the Korean conflict in the 1950s for rapid evacuation and treatment of wounded.

Mobile data terminal A mounted computer system, often in an ambulance or other response vehicle that provides 2-way digital communication and information.

Mobile health care The ability to take services to the patient instead of the patient coming to the hospital or facility.

Mobile Integrated Healthcare Practice (MIHP) The concept of building a health system that integrates all areas of care in treatment and prevention (including EMS).

Mobile intensive care unit Terminology used to describe an ALS ambulance.

Mobile unit A radio unit that is inside a vehicle.

Morbidity Measurement of sickness or disease in a particular population.

Mortality Measurement of deaths in a particular population.

Mortality rates The ratio of total deaths to total population in a specified community or area over a specified period of time for a specific disease process or event.

Mouth-to-mouth ventilation A technique used to resuscitate a person who has stopped breathing, in which the rescuer presses his or her mouth against the mouth of the victim and, allowing for passive exhalation, forces air into the lungs at intervals of several seconds.

Multiple casualty incident A disaster involving between 11 and 100 victims.

Multiple patient incident A disaster involving between two and ten victims.

Mutual aid Aid pre-arranged from neighboring, regional, and state resources.

N

National certification A proposal to have a certification system that serves the entire United States.

National EMS Advisory Council (NEMSAC) A federal advisory committee to the Secretary of Transportation of EMS providers and concerned citizens.

National EMS Core Content Presents a broad definition of what an EMS provider must know and be able to do.

National Emergency Medical Services Education and Practice Blueprint A historical guide for curriculum development and certification that identifies the four levels of providers and the core elements pertinent to all providers.

National EMS Education Standards Defines the terminal objectives for each provider level.

National EMS Information System System that helps track and identify trends nationwide; data must comply with NEMSIS standards.

National EMS Radio System A series of frequencies designated by the FCC to be used only for EMS transmissions.

National EMS Scope of Practice Defines the levels and skills needed for each provider.

National Highway Traffic Safety Administration (NHTSA) A division of the Department of Transportation; this organization was developed to oversee the development of initiatives to make road travel safer.

National Incident Management System (NIMS) One of the systems that set out the goals of disaster preparedness and the organizational structure for disaster response detailing the different roles federal, state, and local entities play and how they are coordinated.

National Registry of Emergency Medical Technicians A private organization that provides testing and national registration for EMS providers.

National Response Framework One of the systems that set out the goals of disaster preparedness and the organizational structure for disaster response detailing the different roles federal, state, and local entities play and how they are coordinated.

National response system Response system to both natural and man-made emergencies in which with very little prior support or formal arrangements, hundreds of providers in hundreds of ambulances converge on the area to support thousands in need.

National Standard Curriculum Standards and guidelines complete with objectives and lesson plans to guide the teaching of Emergency Medical Services that allows commonality across all areas of the United States.

National Standard EMS Data Set A uniform list of information that is to be collected and the format in which the data is recorded for prehospital event, developed by the National Highway and Traffic Safety Administration.

Natural disaster Any disaster produced by the forces of nature: fire, air, earth, and water.

NFPA 1917 Standard for automotive ambulance design and performance.

Noncredit program A program that offers training that does not lead to a degree.

Nonemergency access number A number for people to call for general information not related to an emergency.

Not-for-profit company A business that is organized under special provisions within the federal tax code; money comes from donations or loans.

Null hypothesis A statement that no significant difference will result in the two groups involved in an experiment.

O

Observational study Events that are monitored and analyzed without attempting to manipulate or alter the outcome.

Off -line medical oversight Physician input that is administrative, involving all facets of emergency medical service, but remote from patient care; also known as indirect medical oversight and system medical oversight.

Online medical oversight Real-time physician involvement in a patient encounter with EMS providers; also known as direct medical oversight.

Operational data Data related to the nonclinical activities in support of field operations.

Outpatient departments Facilities similar to alms houses that administered to the poor, but unlike alms houses they focused on medical care which later developed into outpatient departments.

Output The input is processed or changed in some way by the system or is affected by it with the resulting product being the output.

Overcrowded emergency departments A complex issue caused in part by the increase in number of patients seeking emergency care that can result in delays or patient boarding.

P

Paper forms Forms used in the field for data collection.

EMT-Paramedic A health professional certified to perform advanced life support procedures under a physician's direction, the highest level of EMS provider.

Paramedic engine company A fire service vehicle that staffs a paramedic and responds to ALS calls as an upgrade response vehicle.

Pathophysiology The functional changes associated with or resulting from disease or injury.

Pathway management A process by which an agency controls how a person enters into the health care system.

Patient dumping The transfer of patients to an alternate facility for economic rather than medical reasons.

Patient parking Delayed patient offload times at the ED, up to one to two hours or longer.

Peak hour The period of time in which the most ambulances are scheduled to be on duty at one time.

Peak load staffing Making additional personnel and resources available during times of suspected high use rates.

Performance clause The combined effects of quality and cost.

Performance measures The actions taken and the ability to evaluate those actions to bring about change.

Performance-based contracts Contracts that require the nongovernmental ambulance provider to meet specified performance standards.

Performance clause Specifies the required response time and response coverage.

Physician assistant One who has been trained in an accredited program and certified by an appropriate board to perform certain of a physician's duties, including history taking, physical examination, diagnostic tests, treatment, and certain minor surgical procedures, all under the responsible supervision of a licensed physician.

Placebo A substance containing no medication and prescribed or given to reinforce a patient's expectation to get well.

Population The entire group of individuals that may be affected by an issue.

Posting plans Plan for Staging a response vehicle in a location where it is anticipated that demand will be high.

Practical examination Examination of the practical skills of EMS providers by having them perform key skills or assessments.

Practice analysis A process of surveying EMS professionals who are currently employed to determine what skills and knowledge are used on a daily basis and the impact on patients.

Prearrival instructions Information provided by dispatchers to the 9-1-1 caller on.

Prehospital Intervention provided to patients before they reach hospitals.

Preparedness Resource identification and allocation and the training and drilling of disaster response personnel.

Preplanning Planning an emergency response, education, and keeping sound statistics in advance.

Presidential declaration A decree signed by the president of the United States to provide guidance and resources in emergency situations.

Primary care physician A doctor who provides general practice care to a patient.

Primary injury prevention Strategies to prevent an injury from occurring.

Priority dispatching The process of using a scripted series of questions to interrogate the caller and determine the proper level of EMS system response.

Process A collective means of fulfilling the mission of and organization and serving customers.

Process assurance Ensuring that all teams are performing the same procedures outlined by their system.

Program director An individual who is responsible and accountable for a program.

Prospective analysis The process of analyzing or studying something while it is occurring. The observations data are made in the present.

Protocol A preauthorized set of instructions that guide patient care.

Provider levels Levels granted to EMS service providers depending on the skills and expertise. For example, emergency medical technician, paramedic, and so on.

Public access The ability of an EMS system to respond appropriately to a caller's needs.

Public education The process of teaching the public about an issue of importance to EMS.

Public health The overall condition of the public at large.

Public information Any news that an EMS organization wants to tell the public in the community about.

Public information, education, and relations (PIER) An acronym to describe activities for disseminating public information developed by the National Highway Traffic Safety Administration.

Public information officer (PIO) An individual designated by an EMS agency to disseminate public information (news).

Public relations The process of shaping public opinion to support EMS initiatives.

Public safety agency A governmental agency that provides all public safety functions such as fire, police, and EMS.

Public safety answering point (PSAP) A center where call takers receive all 9-1-1 calls.

Public service announcement (PSA) Free advertising on broadcast media or in print media provided to public safety organizations to educate the public.

Public utility model A method of providing ambulance service through an established EMS authority that contracts with a commercial provider; the authority owns the equipment and establishes performance standards.

Q

Qualitative research Research that is useful for understanding how a sample thinks, feels, or reacts within a certain situation.

Quality improvement (QI) A process of reviewing practice to find ways that patient safety or treatment can be improved.

Quality indicator A measurement of the changes expected based on implementation of a specific process.

Quantitative research Research that involves facts and figures to determine relationships between variables being studied or the occurrence of something within a sample.

Quasi-experimental model A method of research that does not meet the standards of a doubleblind experimental design but attempts to measure data for research in a reliable method.

R

Recertification A continuous process of proving competency at regular intervals.

Reciprocity Acceptance of training and certification by another jurisdiction.

Recovery Any activities designed to move the community back to normalcy.

Refresher training A formal, structured educational activity often mandated for recertification or relicensure.

Regulation Addresses specific areas too detailed or dynamic to be codified in a public law.

Regulators Federal, state, and local officials who have the responsibility to regulate EMS operations.

Reliability Repeated observations by different people at different times are in agreement.

Relicensure Process of 'renewing' a licensure at the state level. Requirements vary by state.

Representative samples Part of a research process that ensures that the group being measured provides an accurate picture of the overall population.

Research A rigorous process of testing a hypothesis (can be either qualitative or quantitative).

Respiratory arrest When a patient has stopped breathing.

Response Actions required to save lives, limit destruction, and meet basic human needs in the immediate and short-term effects of a disaster.

Response coverage The process of ensuring that a certain percentage of emergency calls are covered for EMS response.

response package A set of resources to meet the needs of a particular emergency (such as an ambulance and a fire engine for a car accident).

Response time A measure of the amount of time it takes to get an EMS provider to the patient's side after a 9-1-1 call is placed.

Restorative The process of building a body back up to its normal stamina after an illness.

Resuscitation Act of restoring a person's consciousness, pulse, and/or breathing.

Resuscitation squads Squads formed to revive firefighters overcome by smoke and the products of combustion. They were equipped with oxygen-powered resuscitators.

Retrospective Refers to the process of review and examination of outcomes after occurrence.

Retrospective analysis The process of analyzing or studying something after it has occurred, such as reviewing completed incident reports.

Risk The degree of susceptibility of individuals or an entire community to the hazard becoming an emergency or disaster and causing death, injury, or destruction.

Rulemaking Process of developing rules and regulations.

S

Scientific method A systematic inquiry approach to allow organized, objective examination of the facts.

Scope of practice A national consensus document that outlines the knowledge and skills required for each provider level.

Secondary injury prevention Strategies that attempt to minimize further injury or death after the initial trauma or injury event has occurred.

Self-study One of the stages in the educational program accreditation process during which the program compares itself to a national standard.

Simulation Creating a learning environment that mirrors real life or a patient.

Site visit A program director and medical director visit the institution providing the program to verify compliance with the CoAEMSP guidelines.

Skills Psychomotor actions to treat or diagnose a patient.

Specialty EDs Emergency departments dealing with specialty emergency cases. For example, Trauma ED, pediatric ED, and so on.

Specialty referral centers Referral centers equipped to handle emergencies of a particular category. For example, spinal cord, burns, and so on.

Standards and/or guidelines Guidelines for education and training in areas of allied health education developed by an accrediting body.

Standard deviations A calculation that allows predictions based upon averages.

Standard distribution curve A continuous probability density function roughly characterizing a random variable that is the sum of a large number of independent random events; usually represented by a smooth bell-shaped curve symmetric about the mean.

Standing order Specific direction given by a physician to support already existing protocols.

Star-of-life ambulance Ambulances designed to meet the General Services Administration specifications.

Star-of-life emblem Federally registered emblem created for ambulances.

Statutory law Rules and regulations derived from a legislative body resulting in federal laws, state codes, and local ordinances.

Strategic information plan Defining the needs of an organization that will enable the organization to achieve its vision and mission.

Strategic quality planning Articulation of all the quality-related goals that stem from the organization's vision.

Student outcomes The results obtained by students, after being trained, that have to be evaluated to ensure quality and compliance of the educational program.

Subsidy A grant.

Subsystems Components of complex systems.

Support data Data that comes from processes used to lead, manage, and support the overall organization.

Surveillance Collection of information.

System A collection of three components—input, process, output.

System medical oversight The oversight of an entire EMS system provided by the system medical director.

System status management The process of preparing the system to produce the best possible response to the next EMS call.

Systems communications All communication involved in operating and coordinating an EMS system such as alerting EMS units, dispatching EMS units, and coordination of EMS units.

T

Technical training centers Training centers that impart technical training to EMS providers.

Technological disasters Any disaster produced by mankind or the things that human beings make or use.

Telecommunicator Another term for dispatcher; the individual who receives and directs EMS-related calls.

Telemedicine The ability of a physician to treat a patient in the field without even touching or seeing the patient through the use of technology.

Terminal objectives Measurements of learning at the end of an educational process.

Tertiary injury prevention Medical treatment for injuries upon occurrence.

The golden hour The time a seriously injured patient has to receive definitive care in order to survive his injuries.

Third-party insurance Liability cover purchased by an insured (the fi rst party) from an insurer (the second party) for protection against the claims of another (the third) party.

Third-party payers An insurance company or medical program pays for a portion of or all of the billed charges.

Third service A separate public safety service devoted to the delivery of EMS.

Three EEEs Engineering, Enforcement, and Education (components of injury prevention programs).

Three E's of injury prevention Interventions used in injury prevention: engineering, enforcement, and education.

Transportation Transporting injured people to the nearest hospital or medical facility.

Trauma care system A subsystem of an EMS system designed to provide rapid surgical intervention for moderate to severe trauma victims.

Trauma centers Facilities designated to treat patients seriously injured by trauma.

Trauma registry A uniform means of collecting data on trauma systems and trauma patients.

Traumatologist A physician who specializes in resuscitation of the trauma victim.

Treatment in the field EMS function of treating injured people at the place where the catastrophe occurred.

Trepanning Removal of a portion of the skull to relieve pressure on the brain.

Triaged A process for sorting injured people into groups based on their need for or likely benefit from immediate medical treatment.

Type I ambulance A type of ambulance that has a design similar to that of a pickup truck with the ambulance module in place of the truck bed.

Type II ambulance A type of ambulance that has a design similar to that of a van.

Type III ambulance A type of ambulance that has a design that combines both the modular style of a type I ambulance with the van style of type II; it is the most common configuration in use today.

U

Unintentional injuries Damage caused with no intent to do harm.

Universal access number A generic phone number used nationwide to request an EMS response; in the United States it is 9-1-1.

Utstein Guidelines An international set of standards and templates for recording of prehospital cardiac arrest and resuscitation.

V

Validity The instrument is measuring what it is meant to measure.

Value indicator A measurement of the outcomes of specific processes.

Vector Mechanism by which energy is transferred.

Ventricular fibrillation An often fatal form of arrhythmia characterized by rapid, irregular fibrillar twitching of the ventricles of the heart in place of normal contractions, resulting in a loss of pulse.

Violence The use of physical force with the intent to inflict injury or death upon oneself or another.

Voluntary consent Consent obtained from the subjects without any force.

Volunteer An individual who gives time and knowledge without compensation.

W

Wedworth-Townsend Paramedic Act The first legal recognition of paramedics; served as model legislation for other states.

White Paper A publication of the National Academy of Sciences that detailed the problems of trauma-related injuries in terms of deaths, disability, and cost; also known as Accidental Death and Disability: The Neglected Disease of Modern Society.

Wilderness medical training Specialized training for EMTs to meet the needs of those injured in extreme environments.

Y

Years of potential life lost (YPLL) A measurement of the impact injury and illness have on society.

Index

Page numbers followed by f and t refers to figures and tables, respectively.